Autism and Child Psychopathology Series

Series editor
Johnny L. Matson
Department of Psychology
Louisiana State University
Baton Rouge, LA, USA

More information about this series at http://www.springer.com/series/8665

Johnny L. Matson
Editor

Clinical Guide to Toilet Training Children

Springer

Editor
Johnny L. Matson
Department of Psychology
Louisiana State University
Baton Rouge, LA, USA

ISSN 2192-922X ISSN 2192-9238 (electronic)
Autism and Child Psychopathology Series
ISBN 978-3-319-62724-3 ISBN 978-3-319-62725-0 (eBook)
DOI 10.1007/978-3-319-62725-0

Library of Congress Control Number: 2017951390

Printed on acid-free paper

This Springer imprint is published by Springer Nature
The registered company is Springer International Publishing AG
The registered company address is: Gewerbestrasse 11, 6330 Cham, Switzerland

Contents

About the Editor

Johnny L. Matson, PhD is a professor and distinguished research master in the Department of Psychology at Louisiana State University, Baton Rouge, LA, USA. He has also previously held a professorship in psychiatry and clinical psychology at the University of Pittsburgh. He is the author of more than 800 publications including 41 books. He also served as founding editor-in-chief of three journals: *Research in Developmental Disabilities* (Elsevier), *Research in Autism Spectrum Disorders* (Elsevier), and *Review Journal of Autism and Developmental Disorders* (Springer).

Contributors

Neville Blampied University of Canterbury, College of Science, Psychology Department, Christchurch, New Zealand

Kayzandra Bond Department of Psychology, 985450 Nebraska Medical Center, Omaha, NE, USA

Claire O. Burns Louisiana State University, Department of Psychology, Baton Rouge, LA, USA

Amarie Carnett Department of Educational Psychology, University of North Texas, Denton, TX, USA

Michael A. Cocchiola Jr. Capitol Region Education Council-River Street Autism Program, Windsor, CT, USA

Delilah Mendes de Gouveia The Emerge Center, Baton Rouge, LA, USA

Terry S. Falcomata Department of Special Education, University of Texas at Austin, Austin, TX, USA

Raechal Ferguson University of Texas at Austin, Austin, TX, USA

Lauren B. Fishbein Department of Psychiatry, Indiana University School of Medicine, Indianapolis, IN, USA

Jill C. Fodstad Department of Psychiatry, Indiana University School of Medicine, Indianapolis, IN, USA

Rachel L. Goldin Department of Psychiatry, Indiana University School of Medicine, Indianapolis, IN, USA

Ansley C. Hodges Florida Institute of Technology, Melbourne, FL, USA

Xinrui Jiang Department of Psychology, Louisiana State University, Baton Rouge, LA, USA

Cassie D. Karlsson Department of Psychiatry, Indiana University School of Medicine, Indianapolis, IN, USA

Abigail E. Kennedy Department of Psychology, 985450 Nebraska Medical Center, Omaha, NE, USA

K.A. Kroeger Kelly O'Leary Center for Autism Spectrum Disorders, Division of Developmental and Behavioral Pediatrics, Cincinnati Children's Hospital Medical Center, University of Cincinnati College of Medicine, ML, Cincinnati, OH, USA

Giulio Lancioni University of Bari, Bari, Italy

Russell Lang Department of Special Education, Clinic for Autism Research Evaluation and Support, Texas State University, San Marcos, TX, USA

Katherine Ledbetter-cho Department of Special Education, Clinic for Autism Research Evaluation and Support, Texas State University, San Marcos, TX, USA

The University of Texas at Austin, Austin, TX, USA

Johnny L. Matson Department of Psychology, Louisiana State University, Baton Rouge, LA, USA

Laurie McLay University of Canterbury, College of Education, Health, and Human Development, Christchurch, New Zealand

Noha F. Minshawi Department of Psychiatry, Indiana University School of Medicine, Indianapolis, IN, USA

GenaLynne C. Mooneyham Department of Psychiatry and Department of Pediatrics, Duke University School of Medicine, Durham, NC, USA

Jessica Xiaoxi Ouyang Indiana University School of Medicine, Indianapolis, IN, USA

Caroline C. Redpath Capitol Region Education Council-River Street Autism Program, Windsor, CT, USA

Maura L. Rouse Department of Psychiatry, Indiana University School of Medicine, Indianapolis, IN, USA

Jennifer Smith Kelly O'Leary Center for Autism Spectrum Disorders, Division of Developmental and Behavioral Pediatrics, Cincinnati Children's Hospital Medical Center, University of Cincinnati College of Medicine, ML, Cincinnati, OH, USA

Xiaoning Sun Department of Special Education, Clinic for Autism Research Evaluation and Support, Texas State University, San Marcos, TX, USA

William J. Warzak Department of Psychology, 985450 Nebraska Medical Center, Omaha, NE, USA

Munroe-Meyer Institute, University of Nebraska Medical Center, Omaha, NE, USA

Stephanie Weber Kelly O'Leary Center for Autism Spectrum Disorders, Division of Developmental and Behavioral Pediatrics, Cincinnati Children's Hospital Medical Center, University of Cincinnati College of Medicine, ML, Cincinnati, OH, USA

David A. Wilder Florida Institute of Technology, School of Behavior Analysis, Melbourne, FL, USA

Hollie V. Wingate University of Texas at Austin, Austin, TX, USA

Historical Development of Toilet Training

Maura L. Rouse, Lauren B. Fishbein, Noha F. Minshawi, and Jill C. Fodstad

Introduction

The completion of toilet training is considered to be an early childhood developmental milestone. Wagoner (1933) defined the completion of toilet training as the "the development of voluntary control over the sphincters…" that "…involves both maturation and learning" (p. 224). Brazelton (1962), a fixture in the toilet training literature for his work in introducing child-oriented toilet training, wrote about successful toilet training as a step toward maturing into adulthood and identifying with adult society. The ultimate goal of completing toilet training in early childhood has remained relatively constant. However, the specific age at which this occurs, and the age at which initiation of training occurs, has not. History has seen differences in recommended ages of beginning toilet training from a few months to a few years old.

This chapter emphasizes the history of toilet training practices in the United States. Although there are similarities (e.g., physiology, general step-wise progression), toilet training practices vary widely across different cultures. Other researchers (e.g., Ainsworth, 1967; Varkevisser, 1973) have written extensively about the diversity of training practices in different nations and groups. Members of many cultures advocate beginning toilet training their children at early ages. For example, children born in some African, Chinese, and Indian cultures begin toilet training by the time they are a few weeks to a few months old (deVries & deVries, 1977;

M.L. Rouse • L.B. Fishbein • N.F. Minshawi • J.C. Fodstad, PhD, HSPP, BCBA-D (✉)
Department of Psychiatry, Indiana University School of Medicine, 705 Riley Hospital Dr., Suite 4300, Indianapolis, IN 46202, USA
e-mail: jfodstad@iupui.edu

J.L. Matson (ed.), *Clinical Guide to Toilet Training Children*, Autism and Child Psychopathology Series, DOI 10.1007/978-3-319-62725-0_1

Paradox, 2016). The majority of children in the United States, however, do not begin toilet training until 21–36 months (Joinson, Heron, Von Gontard, Butler, Emond, & Golding, 2009). It is noted that within the United States, many cultural variations exist. Authors have documented some of the many differences in toilet training practices among people of the United States from a variety of ethnic, socioeconomic, and religious backgrounds (e.g., Davis & Havighurst, 1946; Ojha & Pramanick, 1992; Schulze, Harwood, Schoelmerich, & Leyendecker, 2002). Cultural variations will not be discussed within this chapter to allow in-depth focus on the historical development of the trends of major toilet training practices within the United States.

Over several centuries, the teachings and methods used to toilet train children in the United States have drastically changed. This chapter provides a review of these changes, focusing primarily on the nineteenth and twentieth centuries till today. The authors present factors that have influenced toilet training practices. Several major practices are discussed, including Brazelton's (1962) child-oriented toilet training method and Azrin and Foxx's (1971) rapid toilet training (RTT). Additionally, future directions of toilet training are discussed.

Factors Influencing Toilet Training Practices

Prerequisite Skills

The process of toileting is a complex chain of events (Radford & Anderson, 2003). Appropriate toileting requires that an individual recognizes the need to void, communicate this need, mobilize him/herself to get to the bathroom, waits before elimination, voids into the toilet, engage in appropriate hygiene behaviors, and removes and replaces clothing (Keen, Brannigan, & Cuskelly, 2007). There are several prerequisite skills to consider prior to implementing behavioral toilet training: (1) Physiology: children should be able to recognize and interpret the sensation of a full bladder. Children must be able to physically control their bladder and bowel muscles to withhold urine or stool until they get to the toilet (Kiddoo, 2012). (2) Regular voiding: voiding on a regular schedule allows the interventionist to maximize opportunities for success and reinforcement. (3) Compliance and remaining seated on the toilet for several minutes: this helps with the ease of implementing the intervention. Compliance may need to be taught prior to formal toilet training if this skill is not present. (4) Gross and fine motor skills: children should be able to mobilize themselves to get to the toilet and to manage clothing removal and replacement. (5) Communication skills: children need to have the ability to communicate the need to use the bathroom as they learn to self-initiate going to the bathroom. (6) Social knowledge and awareness: children must learn where and when it is appropriate to go to the bathroom. (7) Absence of medical conditions that may interfere with or be exacerbated by toilet training procedures: physicians should be consulted prior to implementing toilet training procedures. It is important to rule out the presence of medical conditions that may interfere with or be exacerbated by toilet training procedures such as increasing fluid intake (Lowenthal, 1996).

Technology

The materials used in toileting have greatly influenced the course and timing of toilet training. As materials requiring less financial and time-intensive attention to toilet training became more available, the initiation of toilet training took place at later ages (Harrison, 2013). The materials used to cover infants' genitalia have changed over time. For example, many centuries ago in European countries with warm climates, mothers covered their babies with leaves, animal skins, moss, and grass, or would leave them bare. In cooler climates, infants were covered in swaddling bands made of linen and wool strips (Harrison, 2013).

The end of the 1800s and early 1900s marked the beginning of the use of cloth diapers in infants and toddlers. Diapers that were wet (i.e., with urine) were usually not washed, but instead they were hung to dry then reused. At the turn of the century, scientists and mothers became more aware of the possibility of illness from bacteria from unwashed diapers, which changed this practice. With the increasing threat of illness from dirty diapers, parents become more motivated to eliminate the use of reusable diapers. The first disposable diapers were invented in the 1940s and surpassed the popularity of the cloth diaper by the 1980s (Harrison, 2013). The wide availability of disposable diapers, even for older children (i.e., 5 year olds), likely impacted the trend toward a later age of toilet training initiation and completion in the latter half of the twentieth century (Engelhart, 2014). Because of the new relative ease of disposable diapers, many parents took advantage of the opportunity to initiate toilet training at later ages that disposable diapers offered.

Brief Overview of Approaches to Toilet Training

Toilet training is a complex process that is affected by physiological, anatomical, and behavioral factors. Norms for toilet training, such as when and how to train, are more culturally based than empirically -based. Families often seek advice from their pediatricians when they first initiate toilet training (Kiddoo, 2012). In 1990, Berk and Friman conducted a review of literature of the past 40 years of research on toilet training. In this review, the authors concluded that the majority of children are toilet trained between 24 and 36 months of age and almost all typically developing children are trained by 48 months of age. They also found that toilet training techniques that emphasized independent, voluntary control resulted in later development than training approaches focused on biobehavioral factors and caregiver attention to children's readiness for toilet training. Recently, toilet training has had a trend toward delayed approaches (i.e., approaches that do not begin until the child is between 2 and 3 years old). However, the importance of completing toilet training has increased due to a number of factors including the institutionalization of child care centers (e.g., daycare) and the risk for infectious diarrhea and hepatitis, as the incidence of these problems have increased in children in day care settings who are not yet toilet trained. Given these considerations, it is possible that approaches to toilet training will shift from delayed to earlier approaches (Berk & Friman, 1990).

The methods and approaches to toilet training have fluctuated over the last 100 years between more passive, child-readiness approaches to more structured, behaviorally based approaches. Since the 1950s, more child-oriented approaches to toilet training have been adopted by western societies. This has resulted in delayed toilet training approaches characterized by waiting to begin toilet training until the child is between 2 and 3 years of age (Joinson et al., 2009; Polaha, Warzak, & Dittmer-McMahon, 2002). Brazelton (1962) initiated the child-centered approach to toilet training, which provided the first toilet training recommendations supported by the American Academy of Pediatrics (AAP; Stadtler, Gorski, & Brazelton, 1999). Spock (1968) quickly followed Brazelton's lead when he published the third edition of his widely popular book *The Common Sense Book of Baby and Child Care* that promoted a child-oriented, unstructured approach to toilet training. Spock's emphasis on maturation served to popularize the gradual, passive approach to toilet training (Kiddoo, 2012; Luxem & Christopherson, 1994).

Toilet Training in Early Civilizations

Little data is available in peer-reviewed journals about the toilet training practices of individuals before the late 1800s and early 1900s. However, it is obvious that children were toilet trained before this time. The earliest civilizations documented in history used systems to eliminate their waste. For instance, the Roman Empire adopted the use of public bathhouses, flushing toilets, and sewer systems, as well as legislation related to waste management (Beck, 2016). As toilet usage was seemingly integrated in the lives of the Roman people, it then follows that parents would want their children to learn to effectively use toilets. The Romans are credited with developing the first example of a child's toilet; however, little is known about the methods they used in toilet training. In general, children's education emphasized obedience to authority and self-reliance, which provides some insight into the societal values during this time (Andrews, 2016).

Parent-Centered Toilet Training

During the late nineteenth and early twentieth centuries, the general practice of toilet training began when the child was approximately 3 months old. According to a review of popular women's magazines dating from 1890 to 1949, the emphasis on general child development was on physical development (e.g., nutrition), as opposed to the moral development of children (Stendler, 1950). The magazines purported that very young children needed to build strength to grow, and that holding them when they cry could deprive them of opportunities to build this strength. With this emphasis, mothers practiced rigidity in all schedules, including feeding, eating, sleeping, and toileting (Stendler, 1950). Pediatricians suggested that mothers allow their babies to continue to cry if they cried before the scheduled mealtime. This behavioral strictness is likely an effect of the rising influence of the teachings of Watson (1919) and behaviorism in general. Watson's teachings greatly influenced the behavioral strategies that were later used in behavioral methods of toilet training (e.g., Azrin and Foxx's Rapid Toilet Training; Azrin & Foxx, 1971).

Extending from the behavioral movement, classical conditioning was used to develop the daytime wetting alarm to toilet train children. This device was attached to a child's underwear and an alarm sounded when the child began to void. When the alarm sounded, parents placed children on the toilet (Kiddoo, 2012). In 1938, Mower and Mower published a paper, *Enuresis: A Method for its Study and Treatment*. This article helped popularize the bed wetting alarm for nocturnal urinary incontinence. This approach is thought to help children identify physiological sensations that cue them to void in the toilet (Kiddoo, 2012). The bed wetting alarm (i.e., Bell and Pad method) is still popular today as a treatment for nocturnal incontinence (Antony & Roemer, 2011).

Not all researchers adhered to this strict behavioral training model of infants and very young children. Woolley (1931) suggested that learning should be positive and that children should be praised for their efforts. Although he suggested praise for positive behaviors, he wrote that children should not receive special prizes; mothers' praise for positive effort (e.g., attempt to urinate in the toilet) should be sufficient to further encourage this behavior. He stated, "only failures deserve special notice" (p. 55).

As society entered into the 1930s, the focus of childrearing continued to be on the physical development of children, but with a leniency not witnessed in the past decades such that the rhythm and natural maturational processes of children's bodies were considered (deVries & deVries, 1977). Still, parents decided when children would begin toilet training. The emphasis of beginning toilet training and achieving successful toilet training remained quite young; researchers and parents wished to capitalize on the believed trainability of very young children (deVries & deVries, 1977). In the United States in the 1930s, children were expected to achieve dryness by the time they were 18 months old, with toilet training occurring between 12 months and 18 months (Woolley, 1931). If children were not toilet trained by the time they turned 2 years old, mothers were told to seek a special physical and mental health evaluation (Woolley, 1931), indicating that their 2-year-old children were in need of medical and/or psychological treatment.

The more lenient approach to toilet training in the 1930s was made clear when many authors of articles in popular magazines at this time wrote that there were some limitations to expectations of achieving toilet training so early in a child's life. For instance, these authors wrote that although children typically established a regular elimination schedule by the first 6 months of life, this schedule did not indicate that elimination patterns were under the child's control. Instead, mothers read popular articles stating that their children's bowel and bladder functioning was not under conscious control until their fourth year of life (Stendler, 1950). This was due to the time it took for nerve fibers in the muscles of the bladder and sphincter to properly mature such that children could recognize when to relax and contract these muscles (i.e., recognize full and empty sensations). Additionally, as children grow older, their elimination patterns become more regular and spread out. Although infants urinate two to three times per hour, 2 year olds are able to urinate and have bowel movements on a more regular schedule, such that maintaining dryness during the night was possible (Stendler, 1950).

Mothers in the first half of the century encountered problems when attempting to toilet train their infants and toddlers (i.e., achieve dryness by 18 months old). One of these difficulties was that mothers (because mothers did most of the childrearing at this time) were told to devote their time exclusively to their children's toilet training schedule. If they did this, the final steps of toilet training (i.e., maintaining dryness) should last only a few weeks; this was true if mothers provide their children with constant attention (Woolley, 1931). Idealistically, uninterrupted contact between mother and child seemed to be a wonderful goal; however, logistically, mothers experienced great difficulties in the day-to-day details of toilet training their 12–18 month olds, which may have led to feelings of guilt and failure in mothers.

Mothers were told to anticipate the elimination patterns of their children. With this advice, mothers placed their children on the toilet at the "right time." However, when children refused to urinate at that specific time, and mothers took them off the seat, children often urinated without warning. Fulton (1926) described this as a situation involving a problem of release and inhibition. He wrote that when children were learning to stay dry, they must learn the times to release their bladder and sphincter muscles and when to inhibit. Children that did not eliminate on the toilet seat inhibited for too long and did not learn to voluntarily release. When mothers and children entered into a pattern such that children inhibited and released at incorrect times, particularly if children had already established, at least to some degree, a regular toileting schedule, retraining could be very difficult. As Woolley (1931) noted, retraining after these backslides (often due to illness, changes in environment) was often more difficult than initial training because mothers were less patient the second time around. This sentiment points to the parent-centered approach and mindset that researchers, clinicians, and parents held in the beginning of the 1900s.

Child-Centered Toilet Training

Problems faced by parents and caregivers to toilet train children in the early twentieth century gave rise to a different approach and philosophy in the 1940s and 1950s. Although the beginning of the 1900s saw a parent-focused approach to toilet training (e.g., mothers decided when children were ready to begin toilet training), children who were toilet trained in the middle of the century experienced a child-centered approach. A child-oriented method to toilet training began to emerge as researchers (e.g., Huschka, 1942; Montgomery, 1947; Trainham & Montgomery, 1946) recognized the advantages of a more flexible training schedule with the child's natural rhythm of elimination taken into consideration. Instead of the standard of beginning toilet training at 6 months of age, physicians began to consider the physiological readiness of children before they encouraged regulation of their elimination schedules, such that providers did not suggest that mothers begin to train their children before 18 months old (Stendler, 1950).

The 1960s brought a significant change in the conceptualization and overall teachings of toilet training as the AAP outlined elements of child readiness for toilet training (Stadtler et al., 1999). The AAP based these assumptions and general principles of toilet training on Dr. Barry Brazelton's seminal paper written that outlines a child-oriented approach to elimination training (1962). In this paper, Brazelton described basic assumptions of early childhood training, which he based off of a program he developed using observations he made over approximately 10 years of 1170 children approximately 2 years old.

Assumptions

Brazelton's (1962) toilet training procedure was based on several theories, which described physical and developmental maturation when children are approximately 2 years old. Physically, although Brazelton wrote that children as young as 9 months old can be conditioned (i.e., when children are put on a toilet, they urinate), and noted that voluntary cooperation with parents can begin at 12–15 months old (i.e., children agree to use the toilet when suggested), he argued limitations in beginning toilet training at such a young age. Physiologically, Brazelton wrote that the "myelinization of pyriamidal tracts to these areas [bladder and bowel] are not completed until the 12th to 18th month" (p. 121). He also wrote that an "inner resistance to outside pressure" (p. 121) may be responsible for the difference in timing between reflexive conditioning or compliance and a developmental accomplishment of toilet training. Further, Brazelton wrote of the motor tasks children should be able to achieve before beginning a toilet training program. These requirements include sitting and walking independently. He noted that after 15–18 months old, children are able to perform these tasks with much more ease than when they were younger. As these physiological skills become easier and they require less effort to perform successfully, children are able to direct their cognitive focus toward sphincter control, a newer skill.

Brazelton (1962) also noted markers of developmental maturity that could signal children's readiness for toilet training. Again, his consideration of children's developmental stage illuminates the new child-centered approach to toilet training. Along with physiological readiness to begin toilet training, he also wrote about a psychological readiness to begin training. He highlighted the growing ability of young children, those approximately 18–30 months of age, to control their impulses (i.e., urinate and defecate). Brazelton wrote that children's realization that they are able and wish to control these impulses is influenced by several factors, including the parent–child relationship, children's wish to identify with and imitate parents, and children's wish to develop mastery and autonomy of selves and impulses. According to Brazelton, along with impulse control, other developmental factors that affect the early stages of toilet training are 2-year-old children's tendency to prefer personal cleanliness, organization, and setting things in their places. He also noted the trend toward negativism at this age, indicating a need for parents to be flexible in their responses to their children.

Consistent with a child-centered approach, Brazelton (1962) believed it was important to explore parental attitudes toward toilet training, as they were influential in the way in which parents' toilet trained their children. He discovered that parental attitudes and thoughts about sexuality (i.e., allowing children to watch as they toileted) significantly influenced how they carried out toilet training procedures. As Sears, Maccoby, and Levin (1957) wrote, the subjects of toilet training and sexuality are closely linked for parents. When interviewing parents about their toilet training practices, parents reported that by adhering to the American culture of modesty (i.e., covering genitals, especially in public) required a different method of teaching toileting behaviors than most other behaviors children learned (i.e., imitation). Essentially, parents' attitudes about sexuality influenced whether or not parents allowed their children to observe them using the toilet and imitating their toileting behaviors.

Brazelton (1962) also wrote about pressures from older generations on parents about methods and timing (i.e., when to begin) of toilet training. However, some parents may have also felt pressure to begin toilet training later with the new emphasis on the child-oriented approach, although they may have wished to begin at a younger age. Finally, while Brazelton highlighted the tendency toward cleanliness of children, he also noted that the cleanliness practices of parents influenced their methods of training their children.

Brazelton (1962) introduced a new conceptualization of toilet training. Theoretically, he highlighted physiological and psychological maturation that needs to take place within children before they are ready to begin a toilet training procedure. Without these markers of readiness, Brazelton noted that successful training is less likely, will take longer (although he noted questions about increased tension around training with a later onset of training, partially due to the negativism of 2 year olds), and children will have greater conditioning as opposed to reflexive compliance if parents begin later (i.e., 2 years old) than was previously practiced (i.e., within the first 6 months of life).

Procedure

As noted above, Brazelton (1962) observed the toilet training practices of 1170 children who were approximately 2 years old between 1951 and 1961, paying particular attention to the beginning stages of toilet training, age of successful training, and parenting practices. Brazelton's procedure served as the model for recommendations for toilet training practices for the AAP in the 1960s.

To begin toilet training, Brazelton (1962) told parents to introduce a potty chair on the floor to children as their own chair. Eventually, parents explicitly associate the potty chair and the toilet. At the same time each day (one time per day), mothers were instructed to take their children to sit on the chair with their clothes (including diapers) on to increase comfort with the chair. During this time, children and mother read and received a treat for complying. Children were able to leave the seat during this time. After 1 week of this procedure, children performed the same behaviors, but sat on the chair with their diapers off.

Once children demonstrated interest in "catching" their stool or urine, parents were instructed to take their children to the chair a second time during the day. Importantly, as children were still wearing diapers at this point, Brazelton (1962) suggested that waste from diapers be emptied into the potty chair and tell children that they will eventually make this action happen. With a combination of children's understanding of toileting and a desire to comply with toileting procedures, their general compliance to the first sit in a day increased. Therefore, Brazelton encouraged parents to watch for other times throughout the day when they could be taken to the chair. With increasing interest from children, Brazelton suggested that parents remove diapers or training pants for short periods of time. He also recommended that parents make the potty chair easily accessible to children by placing it in a bedroom or play areas. Although children might require reminders to use the toilet, parents were told to highlight their children's ability to toilet independently. At this point, parents were told that children could use training pants if needed, but children should remove them independently. This protocol aimed to gradually increase children's independence in toilet training.

In following this protocol, Brazelton (1962) noted that the majority (i.e., 80.7%) were successfully trained during the day by the time their children were between the ages of 2 years and 2.5 years (average age was 28.5 months) under situations of typical stress (i.e., no illness or major environmental changes). He wrote that when parents used coercive methods to train their children, children often developed constipation. No significant differences were noted between male and female children. Brazelton (1962) reported that most children began toilet training at 24 months of age, with the earliest being 12 months and the latest being 36 months. Interestingly, 150 of the 1170 children were not toilet trained by 42 months, 48 of which began training before 18 months. Clearly, this relationship is not causal, as there were children in this study who were successfully trained that began training at 12 months old, but it is worth noting nonetheless.

This study also presented a protocol for and examined the success of nocturnal toilet training. Brazelton (1962) suggested that parents begin nighttime toilet training with their children 1–2 years after successful daytime toileting had been accomplished; however, he noted that daytime and nighttime training often occurred simultaneously. He reported that out of the nearly 1200 children he observed, 80.3% were trained at night by 36 months old (average age of 33.3 months), only slightly later than daytime training was achieved. Contrary to daytime training, female children were trained an average 2.46 months before males.

Consistent with his theoretical assumptions, Brazelton (1962) emphasized the vital importance of parental involvement during training. Throughout the 10 years he observed this protocol in use, he noted factors that contributed to the success and delay of toileting. Specifically, he noted factors common to parents and family composition that influenced children's achievement of this developmental milestone. Children with older siblings were more likely to achieve toilet training earlier than first or only children; Brazelton wrote that this is probably because children use their siblings as models, which facilitates training. Results of this study indicated that children without siblings to serve as models were slower to achieve successful nighttime training by 1–7 months. Parent characteristics also impacted children's success. While not unique to children who were unsuccessful in training, parental anxiety about the toilet training was cited as a significant negative influence on all children's experience and progress in toilet training.

Rapid Toilet Training

In 1971, Azrin and Foxx developed the behaviorally based RTT approach, which garnered strong empirical support. The authors published the book *Toilet Training in Less Than a Day* to disseminate these effective procedures to the lay public. This approach offered a more structured method of toilet training and was parent-directed, as opposed to the child-directed approaches of the 1950s and 1960s (Kiddoo, 2012). One of the benefits to this approach was that toilet training could be achieved within a very short time period (e.g., several hours to several days). Once a child was physically and psychological ready, based on the presence of prerequisite skills, children underwent RTT that broadly included increased fluid intake, scheduled toileting, positive reinforcement, and overcorrection for accidents. Azrin and Foxx demonstrated the effectiveness of this intensive toilet training procedure in both typically developing children and in children and adults with intellectual and developmental disabilities that exhibited urinary incontinence (Kiddoo, 2012; LeBlanc et al., 2005; Warzak Focino, Sandberg, & Gross, 2016).

Treatment

The original treatment package included the following components: (1) scheduled toileting; (2) positive reinforcement for in-toilet urination; (3) positive reinforcement for remaining dry between scheduled toileting; (4) increased fluid intake; and (5) overcorrection. In 1973, Azrin and Foxx demonstrated that RTT could be accomplished in less than a day. The study included 34 participants between ages 24–36 months. The results demonstrated that participants achieved toilet training within an average of 3.9 h and that these gains were maintained at 4-month follow-up. In a second study with 49 children who demonstrated readiness skills (e.g., compliance), children achieved toilet training in an average of 4.5 h.

Positive reinforcement for in-toilet urination was given through providing access to edibles (e.g., preferred foods) and praise. In this seminal study, individuals who received these differential reinforcement procedures had fewer accidents than those who did not receive differential reinforcement. Positive reinforcement for remaining dry involved what the authors termed a "dry pants inspection." Dry pants inspections were used to teach children to remain dry between scheduled toiletings. Children's hands were placed on the crotch of their pants and were given verbal feedback regarding whether they were wet or dry. Positive reinforcement was delivered if children were dry and corrective feedback was given if they were wet. The purpose of the dry pants inspection was to help children associate the sensation of being wet with going to the bathroom.

Overcorrection was used whenever accidents occurred. This component was restitutional in nature and involved children participating in cleaning up the accident. Overcorrection is viewed as a punishment procedure, and more recent variations have included positive practice as a treatment component instead of overcorrection. Overall, research on Azrin and Foxx's behavioral toilet training approach has shown that when this method is systematically applied, typically developing children and children with developmental disabilities show an accelerated rate of becoming independently trained relative no treatment (i.e., maturational) approaches. These effects are most notable when dry pants inspections and professional assistance are included as a component of toilet training (Luxem & Christopherson, 1994).

Professional Use

Although the procedure was pioneered for typically developing children, RTT has been more widely studied in individuals with intellectual and developmental disabilities (see Kroeger & Sorensen-Burnworth, 2009 for a review of this literature). There is minimal research on the use of RTT in typically developing children. Although it is strongly supported by the literature, physicians typically do not recommend the RTT approach for either typically developing children or children with developmental delays, and instead recommend a more passive, child-directed approach that takes approximately 3–6 months for children to become fully toilet trained (Warzak et al., 2016). Some authors speculate that physicians do not recommend these procedures, despite the evidence for the effectiveness of RTT, because RTT is perceived as very involved and difficult for parents to implement without assistance from a trained professional (Warzak et al., 2016). Polaha et al. (2002) surveyed 103 pediatricians about current practices regarding recommendations for toilet training typically developing children and physician acceptability of the intensive RTT approach. The results indicated that the majority of physicians (72%) favored a gradual, passive approach, indicating "child interest in the toilet" as the top criteria children must demonstrate before beginning toilet training. Overall, the participants had an unfavorable opinion of intensive toilet training procedures (i.e., only 29% of physicians endorsed the use of RTT).

Benefits and Drawbacks

The benefits to the child-directed approach include that it is popular among parents and that parent–child conflict can be minimized because parents place few demands on children. Passive approaches also require fewer resources, are less intensive, and require less patient education and less professional support compared with intensive, behavioral toilet training (i.e., RTT). Drawbacks to a passive approach include minimal evidence to support the long-term effectiveness of the passive approach. Additionally, the length of training time is longer and children do not become toilet trained until they are older (i.e., delayed toilet training). There is also concern that children who train later may contribute to the spread of disease in day care centers and could contribute to a larger public health problem (Polaha et al., 2002).

In contrast, there are a number of benefits to RTT, the main benefit being how quickly children become toilet trained. This approach is also associated with decreased long-term parent and child stress, as well as improved hygiene in day care settings. Drawbacks include the intensity with which the procedure must be implemented and the need for professional support. Child compliance is also an important factor that needs to be assessed before implementing intensive toilet training, to minimize negative emotional effects for the parent and the child. There is also evidence that without professional support, typically developing children do not maintain gains at 10-week follow-up (Polaha et al., 2002).

When Azrin and Foxx published their book *Toilet Training in Less Than a Day* in 1974, the book was intended for a lay audience. That is, it was meant for parents to read and independently implement the RTT procedures with their children on their own. There was no intention or recommendation that parents consult with a professional or implement under supervision of a professional (Matson & Ollendick, 1977).

This approach came under scrutiny of some clinicians and researchers who questioned the effectiveness of parent implementation and also posed questions about negative side effects of parent-implemented RTT. Kimmel (1974) expressed reservations regarding the utility of the book for parents performing toilet training on their own. He listed several precautions including the need for research support of the contention that parents using the book alone could train their child, the impressions that not many mothers would be able to develop the self-control and manage the disciplined, subtle guidance required by the method by only reading the book and possible unforeseen emotional consequences from parents using this method.

Matson and Ollendick (1977) were among those authors who had reservations about the utility of this self-help book. They conducted a research study to evaluate (1) the effectiveness of the RTT procedure; (2) the amount of time to acquisition (compared with the results demonstrated by Azrin and Foxx); and (3) any potential side effects in a group of parents who used the RTT book alone compared with a group of parents who implemented the RTT book and supervision with a behavioral psychologist. Parents included in the study were parents of children without a developmental disability. Five parents and their children (ages 20–26 months) were randomly assigned to the book-only condition and five parents were assigned to the book plus supervision condition. The authors found that training was more effective and there were fewer emotional side effects when implementing RTT (for the mother and the child) in the book plus supervision condition compared with the book-only condition. Two of the five children in the book-only condition achieved toilet training compared with four of the five children in the book plus supervision condition. Emotional side effects of RTT implementation included tantrums and avoidance behavior. However, all mothers reported these behaviors across conditions. Many of these behaviors were attributed to the positive practice and/or graduated guidance for remaining seated components of the procedure. Mothers reported feeling uncomfortable and several sought to terminate training early, one parent terminated participation prematurely due to her own reaction to her child's tantrums. Overall, the authors concluded that the RTT book only, without professional supervision is not a sufficient approach for toilet training most children. Instead, they recommend that the use of RTT be implemented under the supervision of a professional (Matson & Ollendick, 1977).

Evidence

In 2006, the Agency of Healthcare Research and Quality published a systematic review evaluating the evidence for methods of toilet training. Within this review, only three studies included typically developing children and none of these studies directly compared the two most common approaches: Brazelton and Azrin and Foxx's methods (Kiddoo, 2012). However, the results from a randomized trial with 71 children comparing the Spock method to the RTT method showed that children who received the RTT procedure achieved successful toilet training (i.e., decreased accidents, increased voiding in the toilet, increased self-initiations) at a faster rate than those who received the Spock method (Kiddoo, 2012).

Recent Variations to Rapid Toilet Training

Principles of operant and classical conditioning have been used to modify the RTT method. Operant conditioning has included positive reinforcement to reward dryness, and when children have accidents, their behavior (i.e., wetness) is punished or positive reinforcement is withdrawn (Kiddoo, 2012). Warzak and colleagues conducted a study to adapt Azrin and Foxx's RTT procedures for typically developing children within a primary care setting. The authors included practiced sittings on the toilet and positive reinforcement for appropriate eliminations and omitted positive practice as a corrective procedure (2016).

Although behavioral approaches to toilet training, such as Azrin and Foxx's RTT approach, have demonstrated efficacy in a variety of populations and for young children, the approach involves a number of intensive components. Greer, Neidert, and Dozier (2016) conducted a component analysis of toilet training procedures recommended for young children. They evaluated the combined and sequential effects of the following components: (1) putting the child in underwear instead of a diaper; (2) dense toileting schedules; and (3) differential reinforcement for remaining dry. The authors evaluated the effects of each component on increasing urinary elimination, decreasing urinary accidents, and increasing self-initiations and/or independent requests to sit on the toilet. There were a total of 20 children (mean age = 26 months), and the study was conducted in a childcare center with teachers as the interventionists. Children were included if they showed slow progress with "low-intensity" (i.e., child-directed) toilet training, showed readiness for toilet training (e.g., compliance, ability to remain seated for several minutes), parents expressed interest, and teachers recommended the child be included in the study. Children were either given all components together or were sequentially presented with the treatment components. The authors used a nonconcurrent multiple baseline design across subjects in which implementation of the treatment package or the first component was staggered across subjects.

The results demonstrated that two out of six children who received the entire package showed clear and immediate improvements in overall toileting performance, as defined by increased urinary eliminations in the toilet, decreased number of accidents, and increases in self-initiations to use the toilet. Two of the four children improved in overall toileting performance from the underwear component, and four of six improved in overall toileting performance when underwear was added as the second or third component of intervention. Zero out of eight children who experienced the dense schedule or differential reinforcement following baseline showed improvements in overall toileting performance. However, three of six children showed improved appropriate elimination when differential reinforcement was used in conjunction with underwear. Based on these results, the authors concluded that the underwear component of the intervention was the most successful component and that self-initiations only improved for children who were not exposed to a dense (e.g., every 30 min) sit schedule (Greer et al., 2016).

Problems with Toileting Training Approaches

Researchers and clinicians discuss the potential for negative emotional and physiological side effects that can take place when toilet training children. Adverse events that are often discussed in the toilet training process include refusals, withholding stool, encopresis, hiding when defecating, and urinary disorders of elimination (Kiddoo, 2012). From a cost-benefit perspective, there are a number of reasons why early, behavioral toilet training procedures are preferable. In addition to the added financial cost of diapers, there are also health risks related to delayed toilet training such as dermatitis, infections spread through stool and diarrhea, and public health hazards in child care settings to the point that child care facilities often require children to be toilet trained before they can attend day care. Additionally, family events such as a new child entering the family and parents returning to work may precipitate the need to toilet train children at younger ages (Luxem & Christopherson, 1994).

A common question from parents is the age at which they should begin toilet training. A recent change in common practice among families has occurred. This was evidenced by a study conducted by Bakker and Wyndaele (2000) who investigated the timing of initiation and practices of toilet training over the past six decades. Of those participants who were 60 years old (i.e., likely trained their children in the 1940s and 1950s), daytime toilet training was initiated in 88% of children before they were 18 months old. However, only 20% of parents who were aged 20–40 years old (i.e., likely trained their children in the 1990s) initiated daytime toilet training with their children before they were 18 months old. These authors indicate that among the changes in toilet training practices throughout history is the age at which toilet training is typically initiated.

This trend may lead to harmful consequences. Findings from two recent studies indicated higher incidence of incontinence and urinary tract infections when children were trained later in development (Bakker et al., 2002; Taubman, Blum, & Nemeth, 2003). One group of researchers found that more adverse effects can take place when toilet training begins after 18 months (Bakker et al., 2002), whereas another group of authors suggested that adverse effects are more likely when toilet training begins after 42 months (Taubman et al., 2003). In another study, researchers found that toilet training at a younger age (18–26 months) was associated with a longer training interval but significantly fewer adverse effects (Blum, Taubman, & Nemeth, 2004).

Joinson et al. (2009) used regression analysis to investigate the association between age of initiating toilet training and the development of bladder control and to determine whether initiating toilet training after 24 months was associated with increased odds of daytime urinary accidents in school-aged children. The sample included a cohort of over 8000 children ages 4.5–9 years old from the Avon Longitudinal Study of Parents and Children in the United Kingdom. The authors found that beginning training after 24 months was associated with higher odds of daytime wetting, delayed acquisition of daytime bladder control, or relapse in daytime wetting when compared with children whose toilet training was initiated between 15 and 24 months. The authors concluded that there is evidence to suggest that toilet training before 24 months is associated with achieving and maintaining daytime urinary continence (Joinson et al., 2009).

Conclusion

In general, toilet training is considered an early child milestone and approaches to toilet training date back to early civilizations. There are a variety of methods used to toilet train children and most of these approaches emphasize the importance of readiness skills, including physiological and psychological factors, in the child (Kiddoo, 2012). There are some differences in the various toilet training approaches that have been used in the past and currently. These differences can be seen in the ages recommended to begin toilet training, cultural variations in toilet training approaches, and parental expectations and beliefs about appropriate toilet training methods.

Pediatricians tend to be the primary resources parents seek guidance from when toilet training their children. Currently, the AAP (2011) recommends that child care centers be involved in the toilet training process including identifying when a child is ready to begin toilet training, assisting parents in developing a training strategy, and implementing the procedures outlined in the training strategy. The AAP also recommends the use of incentives to encourage toilet training skills (Greer et al., 2016). Despite a paucity of evidence to support the effectiveness of child-directed approaches, the AAP favors this method of toilet training on the basis of expert opinion (Kiddoo, 2012).

Although there is empirical evidence to suggest behavioral approaches to toilet training are effective in a variety of child populations, the acceptability of these procedures among parents and pediatricians is poor, and therefore, not widely used. One reason for this is the potential for negative effects when conducting intensive, behavioral toilet training (i.e., RTT) without support from a trained professional. Perhaps with the recent shift toward psychologists working in primary care settings, there will also be more opportunities for families to implement efficient, effective behavioral toilet training through the support of psychologists in integrate primary care settings. Additional empirical investigation is needed to determine the best methods for toilet training typically developing children. There is limited information available regarding the long-term effects (positive and negative) of specific toilet training methods; however, there is some evidence to suggest that children who toilet train late may experience a higher likelihood of developing elimination disorders than those who toilet train earlier in development (Kiddoo, 2012).

References

Ainsworth, M. (1967). *Infancy in Uganda: Infant care and the growth of love*. Oxford, UK: Johns Hopkins Press.

American Academy of Pediatrician. (2011). *Toilet training*. Retrieved from: https://www2.aap.org/sections/scan/practicingsafety/Modules/ToiletTraining/ToiletTraining.pdf

Andrews, C. (2016). *Ancient Roman daily life: Ten ancient Roman facts, figures, and features you never knew you needed to know*. Retrieved from http://www.explore-italian-culture.com/ancient-roman-daily-life-2.html

Antony, M. M., & Roemer, L. (2011). Behavior therapy: Traditional approaches. In S. B. Messer, A. S. Gurman, S. B. Messer, & A. S. Gurman (Eds.), *Essential psychotherapies: Theory and practice* (3rd ed.pp. 1–36). New York, NY: Guilford Press.
Azrin, N. H., & Foxx, R. M. (1971). A rapid method of toilet training the institutionalized retarded. *Journal of Applied Behavior Analysis, 4*, 89–99.
Azrin, N. H., & Foxx, R. M. (1974). *Toilet training in less than a day*. New York, NY: Simon & Schuster.
Bakker, E., Van Gool, J. D., Van Sprundel, M., et al. (2002). Results of a questionnaire evaluating the effects of different methods of toilet training on achieving bladder control. *British Journal of Urology International, 90*, 456–461.
Bakker, E., & Wyndaele, J. J. (2000). Changes in the toilet training of children during the last 60 years: The cause of an increase in lower urinary tract dysfunction? *British Journal of Urology International, 86*, 248–252.
Beck, J. (2016). *Roman plumbing: Overrated*. Retrieved from http://www.theatlantic.com/health/archive/2016/01/ancient-roman-toilets-gross/423072/
Berk, L. B., & Friman, P. C. (1990). Epidemiologic aspects of toilet training. *Clinical Pediatrics, 29*, 278–282.
Blum, N. J., Taubman, B., & Nemeth, N. (2004). Why is toilet training occurring at older ages? A study of factors associated with later training. *Journal of Pediatrics, 145*, 107–111.
Brazelton, T. B. (1962). A child-oriented approach to toilet training. *Pediatrics, 29*, 121–128.
Davis, A., & Havinghurst, R. J. (1946). Social class and color differences in child-rearing. *American Sociological Review, 11*, 698–710.
de Vries, M. W., & de Vries, M. R. (1977). Cultural relativity of toilet training readiness: A perspective from East Africa. *Pediatrics, 60*(2), 170–177.
Engelhart, K. (2014). The powerful history of potty training. *The Atlantic*. Retrieved from: http://www.theatlantic.com/health/archive/2014/06/the-surprisingly-political-history-of-potty-training/371512/
Fulton, J. F. (1926). *Muscular contraction and the reflex control of movement*. Oxford, UK: Williams and Wilkins.
Greer, B. D., Neidert, P. L., & Dozier, C. L. (2016). A component analysis of toilet-training procedures recommended for young children. *Journal of Applied Behavior Analysis, 49*, 69–84.
Harrison, M. (2013). *A brief history of potty training*. Retrieved from: http://www.reachme.co.nz/Articles-Blogs/Parenting/A-brief-history-of-potty-training.aspx
Huschka, M. (1942). The child's response to coercive bowel training. *Psychosomatic Medicine, 4*, 301–308. Reprinted in *Contemporary Psychopathology*, S. Silvan, (Ed.) Harvard University Press.
Joinson, C., Heron, J., Von Gontard, A., Butler, U., Emond, A., & Golding, J. (2009). A prospective study of age at initiation of toilet training and subsequent daytime bladder control in school-age children. *Journal of Developmental and Behavioral Pediatrics, 30*, 385–393.
Keen, D., Brannigan, K. L., & Cuskelly, M. (2007). Toilet training for children with autism: The effects of video modeling. *Journal of Developmental and Physical Disabilities, 19*, 291–303.
Kiddoo, D. A. (2012). Toilet training children: When to start and how to train. *Canadian Medical Association Journal, 184*, 511–512.
Kimmel, H. D. (1974). Review of "toilet training in less than a day: How to do it.". *Journal of Behaviour Therapy and Experimental Psychiatry, 5*, 113–114.
Kroeger, K. A., & Sorensen-Burnworth, R. (2009). Toilet training individuals with autism and developmental disabilities: A critical review. *Research in Autism Spectrum Disorders, 3*, 607–618.
LeBlanc, L. A., Carr, J. E., Crossett, S. E., Bennett, C. M., & Detweiler, D. D. (2005). Intensive outpatient behavioral treatment of primary urinary incontinence of children with autism. *Focus on Autism and Other Developmental Disabilities, 20*, 98–105.
Lowenthal, B. (1996). Teaching basic adaptive skills to young children with disabilities. *Early Child Development and Care, 115*, 77–84.

Luxem, M., & Christopherson, E. (1994). Behavioral toilet training in early childhood: Research, practice, and implications. *Developmental and Behavioral Pediatrics, 15*, 370–378.
Matson, J. L., & Ollendick, T. H. (1977). Issues in toilet training normal children. *Behavior Therapy, 8*, 549–553.
Montgomery, J. C. (1947). Toilet education. *American Journal of Orthopsychiatry, 17*(4), 590–593.
Ojha, H., & Pramanick, M. (1992). Religio-cultural variation in childrearing practices. *Psychological Studies, 37*(1), 65–72.
Paradox, P. (2016). Potty training around the world. *Our everyday life.* Retrieved from: http://oureverydaylife.com/potty-training-around-world-3451.html
Polaha, J., Warzak, W. J., & Dittmer-McMahon, K. (2002). Toilet training in primary care: Current practice and recommendations from behavioral pediatrics. *Developmental and Behavioral Pediatrics, 23*, 424–429.
Radford, J., & Anderson, M. (2003). Encopresis in children on the autistic spectrum. *Early Child Development and Care, 173*(4), 375–382.
Schulze, P. A., Harwood, R. L., Schoelmerich, A., & Leyendecker, B. (2002). The cultural structuring of parenting and universal developmental tasks. *Parenting: Science and Practice, 2*(2), 151–178.
Sears, R. R., Maccoby, E. M., & Levin, H. (1957). *Patterns of child rearing*. Evanston, IL: Row, Peterson & Co.
Spock, B. (1968). *The common sense book of baby and child care, 3rd edition*. New York, NY: Hawthorn.
Stadtler, A. C., Gorski, P. A., & Brazelton, T. B. (1999). Toilet training methods, clinical interventions, and recommendations. American Academy of Pediatrics. *Pediatrics, 103*(6 Pt 2), 1359–1368.
Stendler, C. B. (1950). Sixty years of child training practice. *The Journal of Pediatrics, 36*, 122–136.
Taubman, B., Blum, N. J., & Nemeth, N. (2003). Stool toileting refusal: A prospective intervention targeting parental behavior. *Archives of Pediatrics and Adolescent Medicine, 157*, 1193–1196.
Trainham, G., & Montgomery, J. C. (1946). Developmental factors in learning bowel and bladder control. *American Journal of Nursing, 46*(12), 841.
Varkevisser, C. M. (1973). *Socialization in a changing society: Sukuma childhood in rural and urban Mwanza*. Tanzania. Den Haag: Center for the Study of Education.
Wagoner, L. C. (1933). Elimination. In *The development of learning in young children* (pp. 224–233). New York, NY: McGraw-Hill.
Warzak, W. J., Focino, S. S., Sandberg, S. A., & Gross, A. C. (2016). Advancing continence in typically developing children: Adapting the procedures of Foxx and Azrin for primary care. *Journal of Developmental and Behavioral Pediatrics, 37*, 83–87.
Watson, J. B. (1919). *Psychology, from the standpoint of a behaviorist*. Philadelphia, PA: Lippincott.
Woolley, H. T. (1931). Eating, sleeping, and elimination. In C. Murchinson & C. Murchinson (Eds.), *A handbook of child psychology* (pp. 28–70). Worcester, MA: Clark University Press.

Complications and Side Effects Associated with a Lack of Toileting Skills

Russell Lang, Laurie McLay, Amarie Carnett, Katherine Ledbetter-cho, Xiaoning Sun, and Giulio Lancioni

The majority of children in the United States acquire both bowel and urination toileting skills around 3 years of age following training by parents, daycare staff, and other typical caregivers (Brazelton et al., 1999). Unfortunately, despite the provision of typical toileting instruction, not all children acquire the skills necessary to identify the need to void, obtain access to the toilet, and then use the toilet appropriately. Toileting skill deficits are generally transient and treatable, but in cases where highly specialized toilet training is required, or when bowel or urinary incontinence is related to anatomic or pathophysiological problems, toileting deficits have been associated with a number of adverse health effects as well as psychological and social challenges. This chapter first provides an overview of medical problems and operant behavior that can affect functional voiding and the immediate- and long-term side effects of such problems. Next, the psychological and

R. Lang, PhD, BCBA-D (✉) • X. Sun
Department of Special Education, Clinic for Autism Research Evaluation and Support, Texas State University, San Marcos, TX, USA
e-mail: russlang@txstate.edu

L. McLay
University of Canterbury, College of Education, Health, and Human Development, Christchurch, New Zealand
e-mail: laurie.mclay@canterbury.ac.nz

A. Carnett
Department of Educational Psychology, University of North Texas, Denton, TX, USA

K. Ledbetter-cho
Department of Special Education, Clinic for Autism Research Evaluation and Support, Texas State University, San Marcos, TX, USA

The University of Texas at Austin, Austin, TX, USA

G. Lancioni
University of Bari, Bari, Italy

J.L. Matson (ed.), *Clinical Guide to Toilet Training Children*, Autism and Child Psychopathology Series, DOI 10.1007/978-3-319-62725-0_2

social ramifications of poor toileting skills are considered. Implications of the adverse side effects for practitioners involved in the remediation of toileting deficits and directions for future research and implications are discussed throughout.

Medical and Operant Factors Related to Dysfunctional Voiding and Toilet Training

A number of abnormal voiding patterns can adversely affect the toilet training process. Dysfunctional voiding is a term used to refer to problems controlling both bowel and bladder function; for example, withholding behavior, infrequent elimination, constipation, and incontinence (Berry, 2005; Chase, Homsy, Siggard, Sit, & Bower, 2004). Although dysfunctional voiding problems are often transient and are not usually attributed to an underlying organic cause, it is important to be aware of gastrointestinal (GI) and urinary tract issues that may impact the voiding process (Cook, Talley, Benninga, Rao, & Scott, 2009; Issenman, Filmer, & Gorski, 1999; Rasquin et al., 2006). If not adequately addressed, these problems can effect bowel and bladder continence and delay the achievement of independent toileting.

Fecal or Bowel Voiding Dysfunction GI problems refer to issues that affect the GI tract (e.g., the stomach, small and large intestines, rectum). Two of the most common GI problems are constipation and chronic diarrhea, but these may also include abdominal pain, gastritis, and/or food intolerance. GI problems that affect defecation are often referred to as functional defecation disorders (FDD) and include constipation, diarrhea, and irritable bowel syndrome (IBS).

According to Rome III criteria (Hyman et al., 2006; Rasquin et al., 2006), some of the core diagnostic features of functional constipation (FC) include: (a) the occurrence of two or fewer defecations in the toilet per week; (b) a minimum of one episode of fecal incontinence per week; (c) a history of painful or hard bowel movements; (d) the presence of a large fecal mass in the rectum; and (e) a history of large diameter stools, which may obstruct the toilet (Wang et al., 2013). Constipation is a relatively common and often chronic childhood problem with estimates suggesting that problems with constipation are responsible for 25% of outpatient visits to pediatric gastroenterologists (Levine & Bakow, 1976; Loening-Baucke, 1993). In considering treatment for constipation, it is important to distinguish FC from the less common, functional fecal retention, which consists of repetitive attempts to avoid defecation because of fears associated with doing so (Rasquin-Weber et al., 1999).

Diarrhea is a GI problem that may cause a loss of bowel continence and may impede the acquisition of toileting skills. In the majority of cases, symptoms of diarrhea do not last more than a few days, and the loss of continence or delay in toilet training effects are likely temporary. However, chronic nonspecific diarrhea (CNSD) is more persistent. CNSD is considered the most common cause of prolonged diarrhea in children who are otherwise healthy (Issenman, Hewson, Pirhonen, Taylor, & Tirosh 1987). CNSD includes repeated bouts of diarrhea, which continue for over

3 weeks and usually affect children under 3 years of age (Cohen, Hendricks, Mathis, Laramee, & Walker, 1979). CNSD is defined as diarrhea in children under 4 years of age and IBS in children 5–18 years of age (Baber, Anderson, Puzanovova, & Walker, 2008).

Those affected by IBS may experience a variety of symptoms including: (a) abdominal discomfort or pain that is associated with an improvement following defecation; (b) a change in frequency of defecation and/or appearance of stool following the onset of symptoms; and (c) an absence of inflammatory, anatomic, metabolic, or neoplastic processes that may explain the presence of these symptoms (Hyman et al., 2006; Wang et al., 2013). A diagnosis is typically applied when ongoing bowel upset cannot be explained by an alternative underlying pathology. These include Crohn's disease, ulcerative colitis, and coeliac disease, all of which can result in GI problems and, although rare, can occur during childhood and dramatically influence toilet training outcomes or efficiency (Read, 2012).

As noted, it is uncommon for GI problems to be the result of functional, anatomic, or organic issues. Rather, these are often attributed to idiopathic, transient, or relatively benign causes, such as a restricted or imbalanced diet (Issenman et al., 1987), food intolerances (Moukarzel, Lesicka, & Ament, 2002), and/or the malabsorption of nutrients (Guarino et al., 2012); side effects from medications such as diuretics, sedatives, muscle relaxants, and nerve blockers (Frauman & Brandon, 1996); viral or bacterial infections (bacterial gastroenteritis, rotavirus, Norwalk virus, or *Escherichia coli* infection), and chronic illness (Frauman & Brandon, 1996; Frauman & Myers, 1994). Children with physical disabilities (e.g., cerebral palsy, muscular atrophy) may also be at greater risk of incontinence (Murphy, Boutin, & Ide, 2012) due to a lack of mobility, or being confined to a particular position for long periods of time.

Urinary Voiding Dysfunction Urinary voiding dysfunction describes a pattern of urinating that is abnormal for the child's age and may include issues with the frequency and urgency of voiding, enuresis, an intermittent urine stream, or straining to void. Among the most common urinary voiding issues are overactive bladder, dysfunctional voiding, underactive bladder, and constipation. There are a number of possible causes for these dysfunctions, and if not addressed, they have the potential to have a significant impact on the toilet training process.

Overactive bladder is characterized by symptoms in which an individual has a frequent urgent need to urinate, urge incontinence, or nocturia. Children who experience an overactive bladder may also demonstrate holding techniques (e.g., squatting on the floor) to avoid urination. Conversely, infrequent voiding or an underactive/lazy bladder is a syndrome that is characterized by infrequent urination. Children may be diagnosed with this condition if they eliminate three or fewer occasions over a 24-h period, or if they do not eliminate for 12 h. Children with this condition may develop enlarged bladder capacity experience minimal urge to void and may exhibit incomplete and infrequent voiding (Berry, 2005).

Dysfunctional voiding describes a problem in which children are unable to relax the urethra and pelvic floor muscles during elimination. Dysfunctional voiding is likely caused by involuntary contraction of the pelvic floor muscles or urethral sphincter during voiding. Children who experience dysfunctional voiding may exhibit posturination dribbling, incontinence, attempts to withhold urination (e.g., pelvic holding), and recurrent urinary tract infections (UTI; Berry, 2005; Hellerstein & Linebarger, 2003). Typically, children with urinary dysfunction or uncomplicated enuresis do not have increased incidence of urologic disease, show normal physical, psychiatric, and neurological development, and normal urinalysis and urine culture (Rushton, 1993). As with GI problems, symptoms of urinary voiding dysfunction, including nocturnal enuresis, are usually transient, and are the result of a temporary and highly treatable problem. This can include UTIs, infection of the vulva or vagina (e.g., vulvovaginitis), irritants, moisture around the vulva, and yeast infections (Caldwell, Hodson, Craig, & Edgar, 2005).

In rare cases, urinary problems may be the result of metabolic or nephrological disorders (e.g., kidney disease, diabetes) or there may be an underlying functional anatomic problem (Caldwell et al., 2005; Rushton, 1993). For example, in children with an underactive bladder, the pelvic floor muscles become overactive, which results in discoordination between the bladder, rectum, and pelvic floor muscles (Kajiwara Inoue, Usui, Kurihara, & Usui, 2004). This discoordination can cause the bladder muscle contraction to become weak or absent. As a result, children with this condition tend to strain in an attempt to void (Berry, 2005; Schulman 2004).

Although it is generally accepted that enuresis occurs when the nocturnal bladder volume exceeds capacity due to normal delays in development (Issenman et al., 1999), it is estimated that up to 1/3 of children with enuresis may experience detrusor over activity and reduced bladder capacity while asleep (Yeung et al., 2002). Neurogenic bladder is another condition that can negatively affect urinary voiding functions, particularly in those with spinal cord, neurological, or nerve problems. Neurogenic bladder can occur as the result of diseases (e.g., multiple sclerosis), but it can also occur in people with disabilities such as cerebral palsy and spina bifida (Murphy et al., 2012). In situations in which functional anatomic, neurological, metabolic, or nephrological problems are suspected, further assessment may be required if planning to commence toilet training.

Operant Voiding Dysfunction It is important to note that behaviors that impede voiding and toilet skill acquisition may be learned (operant) behaviors (Hellerstein & Linebarger, 2003) that serve operant functions. There are a variety of reasons why children may learn to withhold voiding. For example, a child may engage in withholding to escape or avoid unsanitary toileting conditions or if the toileting process has been associated with pain (perhaps due to a previous medical condition) or some other aversive stimuli (Kistner, 2009). Over time, withholding of stool or urine can become a chronic, habitual response that can negatively impact voiding patterns and complicate toilet training efforts.

Anatomical and Physiological Side Effects and their Impact on Toilet Training Soiling, withholding, and constipation can result in a number of medical ailments that greatly impact children's physical well-being. If untreated, these medical ailments may exacerbate the voiding problem and result in increased difficulties with toilet training. For example, as a consequence of constipation, many children experience physical discomfort. This can include pain while defecating (Partin, Hammill, Fischel, & Partin, 1992; Van den Berg, Benninga, & Lorenzo, 2006), abdominal pain (Loening-Baucke, 2005; Loening-Baucke & Swidsinski, 2007), and anal fissures (i.e., superficial cracking or tear around the anus). In response to pain while defecating, many children may learn to withhold stool and avoid use of the toilet, further worsening constipation and its side effects. In rare cases, habitual stool withholding can lead to "functional" megacolon. Functional megacolon is characterized by overdistention of the colon (large intestine) and insensitivity around the rectum (Partin et al., 1992). Functional megacolon results in severe constipation, abdominal pain, fecal obstruction, and fecal soiling. Kelly (1996) estimate that in 80–90% of cases, fecal incontinence is the result of chronic constipation with fecal impaction and consequent overflow soiling.

Children with urinary or fecal incontinence that results in frequent soiling may experience skin problems, such as perineal dermatitis (Driver, 2007) or perineal infections. Anal fistulae (i.e., a small occlusion between the end of the bowel and the skin around the anus) may then occur as the result of the infection (Wang et al. 2013). Though this is relatively uncommon, it can result in intense pain, particularly during defecation.

Constipation directly affects bowel function and may also impact urinary function. Withholding stool and constipation are common risk factors for nocturnal enuresis, fecal incontinence, and daytime incontinence, as children may have a lack of control over these functions when constipated (Berry, 2005; Cooper et al., 2002). This may be the result of the fecal mass obstructing the urinary outflow system, which can prevent complete elimination of the bladder, and/or the fecal mass may put pressure on the bladder, which can prevent complete relaxation of the muscles controlling the bladder or result in irritation (Cooper et al., 2002; Kasirga, Akil, Yilmaz, & Polat, 2006). Therefore, treating constipation may have the secondary benefit of reducing urinary tract problems (Schulman, 2004).

UTIs are the most common of all bacterial infections afflicting children (Hoberman et al., 1993; Stull & LiPuma, 1991). The relationship between GI problems, urinary voiding dysfunction, and UTIs is well established (Berry, 2005; Koff, Wagner, & Jayanthi, 1998). Constipation can result in the retention of urine in the bladder or obstruction of the urinary tract (Kajiwara et al., 2004; Loening-Baucke, 1997), which can lead to the proliferation of bacteria. Constipation can cause fecal pathogens to colonize the perineal area, which can, in turn, colonize the urinary tract. UTIs result in painful urination and, if untreated, may result in kidney infections (Cooper et al., 2002). On rare occasions, recurrent UTIs result in vesicoureteral reflux (VUR; Cooper et al., 2002). VUR involves a retrograde flow of urine between the bladder and the ureters and kidneys (Elder et al., 1997). Children with unstable bladder, infrequent voiding, and recurret UTIs are at increased risk of developing this problem, which may result in kidney infection, scarring, and other complications (Shah & Upadhyay, 2005).

If dysfunctional voiding patterns are not treated, problems with bowel and bladder function can persist into adulthood (Bongers, van Wijk, Reitsma, & Benninga, 2010; Bower, Sit, & Yeung, 2006). Many of those affected by voiding problems have a history of fecal soiling, constipation, and UTIs (Bower et al., 2006). Research suggests that symptoms associated with FDD (e.g., constipation) are thought to persist into adulthood in 25–30% of children (Bongers, et al., 2010; Procter & Loader, 2003). Intervention for voiding problems can reduce the risk of ongoing problems (Loenig-Baucke, 1993).

The extent to which GI and urinary voiding problems impact toilet training likely depends on the pervasiveness, severity, and cause of the problem. For most children with voiding problems, the underlying cause is easily and quickly treated and is unlikely to have a long-term impact on toilet training. In such cases, delaying the onset of toilet training or briefly returning to diapers until the issue is remediated may be all that is necessary. For children with functional anatomic problems, or learned responses that may impact voiding function, the implications for toilet training need to be more carefully considered. For example, as a result of constipation, a "lazy bladder," or reduced sensitivity to the urge to void, children may eliminate at a much lower frequency than would normally be expected. As a result, it may be difficult to develop a toileting schedule in which regular practice opportunities are provided and the children are reinforced for in-toilet elimination. This decreases the likelihood that children will be able to be reinforced for in-toilet elimination. In such cases, it is important to explore ways of increasing the frequency of in-toilet elimination and subsequent practice opportunities (e.g., augmenting the children's fluid or dietary fiber intake). It is important to note here that consultation with a medical professional is necessary when implementing liquid or food alterations that may complicate or exacerbate underlying medical problems. For example, because some fruit juices can exacerbate diarrhea, it may be unwise to autonomously decide to increase fruit juice intake in an effort to occasion more urination practice opportunities.

Children who are constipated may also experience painful voiding. As a result, children may learn to withhold, and the toilet or toileting process may become aversive through conditioning (e.g., Christophersen, 1991). Although stool withholding is not uncommon, children who withhold stool are at increased risk of having difficulties acquiring independent toileting skills (Blum, Taubman, & Nemeth, 2004; Taubman & Buzby, 1997). Children who initially resist stool toilet training are also more likely to engage in chronic patterns of soiling and are more likely to require more time (past 42 months of age) to achieve independent toileting. This problem may be exacerbated in those with secondary or overflow encopresis that often results from constipation (Issenman et al., 1999; Taubman & Buzby, 1997). There is a risk that these symptoms may be perceived as toileting "accidents" by caregivers during toilet training, complicating instructional contingencies (e.g., overcorrection and reinforcement) placed on behaviors presumed to be operant and reducing the effectiveness of behavioral intervention.

Children who are experiencing incontinence due to an overactive bladder or chronic diarrhea may also experience a number of toileting accidents during the toilet training process. It is therefore important to carefully gather information about the child's voiding schedule (i.e., the times of day that the child is likely to urinate). This information can be used to determine the frequency and timing of daytime practice opportunities in order increase the likelihood of in-toilet voiding and decrease the likelihood of accidents. For these children, it may also be necessary to avoid bladder irritants and consultation with a medical professional prior to the onset of training is advisable.

If, as a result of medical screening ruling out anatomical or physiological causes, voiding dysfunction appears to a learned behavior, then it is important to assess the environmental context of the behavior (antecedents), the consequences that may be affecting the child's ability to void in the toilet, and ultimately the function of stool or urine withholding. Functional behavioral assessment is a tool that can be used to formulate an intervention that addresses the hypothesized function of the voiding dysfunction (e.g., Tsutomu & Fumiyuki, 2011). If learned withholding behavior is not adequately addressed, it may directly result in GI problems such as constipation, or other medical ailments, all of which may further impact the toilet training process.

Finally, there are many causes of GI and urinary voiding problems that may need to be addressed when planning toilet training programs. For example, for children with mobility problems and associated GI issues, it may be necessary to explore strategies that promote regular bowel motions. It may also be necessary to consider barriers to independent toileting such as bathroom access, undressing, sitting comfortably on the toilet, and self-cleaning (Sansome, 2011). The impact that medication, medical history, infection or disease, and diet may have on the child's GI or urinary tract should also be evaluated.

Psychological or Social Side Effects Associated with Limited Toileting Skills

Failure to acquire hygienic toileting behavior may increase risks for a variety of psychological and social challenges, such as bullying, teasing, and social exclusion (Baeyens et al., 2006; Shreeram, He, Kalaydjian, Brothers, & Merikangas, 2009; Wolfe-Christensen, Veenstra, Kovacevic, Elder, & Lakshmanan, 2012). In addition to externalizing comorbidities, risks for internalizing comorbidities such as sadness, anxiety, and stress may also increase (Reiner, & Gearhart, 2006). These psychological and social difficulties have been associated with additional adversity (e.g., more restrictive residential and educational placements) that is likely to negatively impact an individual's well-being across the life span (Tai, Tai, Chang, & Huang, 2015).

Potential social side effects include negative social repercussions (e.g., stigmatization or social teasing/ridicule) or lack of social opportunities (Chase et al., 2004; Despande & Caldwell, 2012; Kistner, 2009). For example, Butler and Heron (2008) reported children view bed-wetting as a social problem rather than health-related problem and found that children 9 years old were aware of negative social ramifications of bed-wetting, such as social teasing and exclusion. In a review of the literature related to nocturnal enuresis, Schulpen (1997) reported that most children were concerned with their ability to participate in social actives (e.g., sleepovers and school trips), and almost half of the children perceived intolerance by their family and reported being teased by siblings. Further, Philips and colleagues (2015) reported that children with fecal incontinence had significantly more exposure to stressful life events (e.g., bullying, punishment by a parent during toilet training, child abuse) when compared to other children.

With regards to the school environment, parents express frustration when schools have more restricted access to toilets or different toileting procedures than the child's home, particularly when children who have some toileting success at home fail to generalize to school settings (Garman & Ficca, 2012; Palmer, Athanasopoulos, Lee, Takeda, & Wyndaele, 2012). Har and Croffie (2010) identified conditions involving limited toileting skills that tend to result in teasing, bullying, and/or social exclusion in school. These adverse social consequences have in turn been linked to child mental health risks (e.g., reduce feelings of self-worth) and, more concretely, delayed academic progress.

Although some studies have reported rates of psychological issues within the normal limits (Hirassing, van Lerdam, Bolk-Bennin & Bosch, 1997; Robinson, Butler, Holland, & Doherty-Williams, 2003), the majority of current research reports issues associated with psychological side effects for children who struggle with enuresis and fecal incontinence (von Gontard & Hollmann, 2004; Van Hoecke, Fruyt, De Clercq, Hoebeke, & Vande Walle, 2006; Wolfe-Christensen et al., 2012). For example, von Gontard and Hollmann (2004) analyzed somatic and behavioral symptoms associated with functional enuresis and encopresis. The authors reported that 65% of the children (n = 167) with enuresis and encopresis were reported by their parents to have severe behavioral problems. Specifically, children that were encopretic were reported to have a significantly higher rate of externalizing behavioral disorders, such as conduct disorder. In other studies, children with both types of enuresis (night and day) were found to have a higher rate of psychological problems compared to children who have more isolated occurrences of accidents (Joinson, Heron, Emond, & Butler, 2007; Theunis, Van Hoecke, Paesbrugge, Hoebeke, & Vande Walle, 2002; Van Hoecke et al., 2006). Further, Wolfe-Christensen and colleague's (2012) findings indicate that the severity levels of voiding dysfunction and/or enuresis are related to the severity of psychosocial difficulties.

Comorbidity of psychological issues can include anxiety, depression (Cox, Morris, Borowitz, & Sutphen, 2002), reduced self-esteem (Joinson et al., 2007), and attention-related issues (Cox et al., 2002). Wolfe-Christensen and colleagues (2012) reported that 19% of children with urology issues (n = 600) had been diagnosed with at least one psychological disorder, and 26 of these children had more than one. Further, approximately 15% were found to have clinically significant psychosocial difficulties.

Poor self-esteem in children with urological issues has also been reported in the literature (Theunis et al., 2002). In a review, Redsell and Collier (2001) concluded there is an increased likelihood of behavioral problems purportedly related to self-esteem for children with nocturnal enuresis (bedwetting). The authors hypothesized that if bedwetting and low self-esteem were causal, there would be a likely reduction of these psychological problems when instances of bedwetting were reduced. Children who have both nocturnal and diurnal enuresis are reported to experience more distress and have lower self-esteem than children who only have nocturnal enuresis (Feehan, McGee, Stanton, & Silva, 1990; Schulpen, 1997). Further, Schonwald, Sherritt, Stadtler, and Bridgemohan (2004) evaluated temperament profiles of children who were classified as difficult to toilet train and found them to have difficult temperament (e.g., less adaptive, more negative in mood, less persistent) compared to other children.

For some children, psychological issues related to anxiety are reported (Cox et al., 2002; von Gontard, Moritz, Thome-Granz, & Equit, 2015, Reiner & Gearhart, 2006). For example, von Gontard and colleagues (2015) found that symptoms of anxiety and depression were higher among children with any subtype of incontinence (12.8%) and children with any subtype of functional GI disorder (21.4%) when compared to children without any subtype of incontinence (7.7%).

Several studies have reported toileting deficits more often in children with attention deficit hyperactivity disorder (ADHD; Baeyens et al., 2006; von Gontard, Mortiz, Thome-Granz, & Freitag, 2011; Van Hoeck et al., 2006; Shreeram et al., 2009). Night wetting was reported to occur more often in children with ADHD (21.9%) compared to day wetting (6.5%; Robson et al., 1999). Mellon and colleagues (2013) reported approximately 9.8% ($n = 35$) of children (mean age 6.7 years) with ADHD had a comorbidity of enuresis compared to the control group where approximately 4.7% of children met the criteria for enuresis ($n = 34$). Shreeram and colleagues (2009) reported that 12.5% of children (ages 8–11) with nocturnal enuresis had a comorbidity of ADHD compared to 3.6% of children without nocturnal enuresis. Approximately 25% of children with diurnal urinary incontinences (Joinson, Heron, & von Gontard, 2006) and approximately 9% of children with fecal incontinence (Joinson, Heron, & von Gontard, 2006 or Joinson, Heron, Butler, & von Gontard, 2006) were reported to have a comorbidity of ADHD.

Health-Related Quality of Life A number of studies have looked at the effect of voiding problems on children's quality of life (Clarke et al., 2008; Rajindrajith et al., 2013; Wang et al., 2013). Health-related quality of life (HRQoL) is a concept that is used to capture dimensions of emotional, physical, psychological, and social functioning. HRQOL, including physical dimensions, is often rated lower in children with FC or fecal incontinence (Clarke et al., 2008; Peeters, Noens, Kuppens, & Benninga, 2016; Rajindrajith Devanarayana, Weerasooriya, Hathagoda, & Benninga, 2013; Wang et al., 2013). Furthermore, those with fecal incontinence and constipation have been found to have lower HRQoL scores than those with constipation alone (Rajindrajith et al., 2013). The impact of functional voiding problems and associated medical ailments on children's well-being underscores the importance of toilet training and the extent to which such factors may impact training outcomes.

Conclusion

Children can be affected by a variety of medical issues related to voiding and toilet training. The impact these anatomical and/or physiological problems may have on the toileting training process depends on the cause, trajectory, and persistence of the problem. The current body of literature also identifies a number of psychological conditions that tend to be found in children who struggle with enuresis and fecal incontinence; the most commonly reported comorbidity is ADHD, followed by anxiety and depression. Further research is needed to examine how these comorbidities relate to intervention procedures and to identify more efficient or efficacious interventions suitable for children with these conditions. Although research has identified some social side effects, further research is needed to determine the extent to which a lack of toileting skills may impede a child's opportunities to participate in social environments. Regardless of the cause or type of toileting deficit, early intervention is necessary in order to minimize the short- and long-term impact on children's physical health, psychological, and social-emotional well-being.

References

Baeyens, D., Roeyers, H., D'Haese, L., Pieters, F., Hoebeke, P., & Walle, J. (2006). The prevalence of ADHD in children with enuresis: Comparison between a tertiary and non tertiary care sample. *Acta Paediatrica, 95*, 347–352.

Baber, K. F., Anderson, J., Puzanovova, M., & Walker, L. S. (2008). Rome II versus Rome III classification of functional gastrointestinal disorders in pediatric chronic abdominal pain. *Journal of Pediatric Gastroenterology and Nutrition, 47*, 299–302.

Berry, A. (2005). Helping children with dysfunctional voiding. *Urologic Nursing, 25*, 193–202.

Blum, N. J., Taubman, B., & Nemeth, N. (2004). During toilet training, constipation occurs before stool toileting refusal. *Pediatrics, 113*, 520–522.

Bongers, M. E., van Wijk, M. P., Reitsma, J. B., & Benninga, M. A. (2010). Long-term prognosis for childhood constipation: Clinical outcomes in adulthood. *Pediatrics, 126*, 156–162.

Bower, W. F., Sit, F. K., , & Yeung, C. K. (2006). Nocturnal enuresis in adolescents and adults is associated with childhood elimination symptoms. The Journal of Urology, 176, 1771–1775.

Brazelton, T. B., Christopherson, E. R., Frauman, A. C., Gorski, P. A., Poole, J. M., Stadtler, A. C., & Wright, C. L. (1999). Instruction, timeliness, and medical influences affecting toilet training. *Pediatrics, 103*, 1353–1358.

Butler, R., & Heron, J. (2008). An exploration of children's views of bed-wetting at 9 years. *Child: Care, Health and Development, 34*, 65–70.

Caldwell, P. H. Y., Hodson, E., Craig, J. C., & Edgar, D. (2005). Bedwetting and toileting problems in children. *The Medical Journal of Australia, 182*, 190–195.

Chase, J. W., Homsy, Y., Siggaard, C., Sit, F., & Bower, W. F. (2004). Functional constipation in children. *The Journal of Urology, 171*, 2641–2643.

Christophersen, E. R. (1991). Toileting problems in children. *Pediatric Annals, 20*, 240–244.

Clarke, M. C. C., Chow, C. S., Chase, J. W., Gibb, S., Hutson, J. M., & Southwell, B. R. (2008). Quality of life in children with slow transit constipation. *Journal of Pediatric Surgery, 43*, 320–324.

Cohen, S. A., Hendricks, K. M., Mathis, R. K., Laramee, S., & Walker, W. A. (1979). Chronic nonspecific diarrhea: Dietary relationships. *Pediatrics, 64*, 402–407.

Cook, I. J., Talley, N. J., Benninga, M. J., Rao, S. S., & Scott, M. M. (2009). Chronic constipation: Overview and challenges. *Neurogastroenterology and Motility, 21*, 1–8.
Cooper, C. S., Hoebeke, P., Vande Wall, J., Bishop, W. P., Bower, W. F., & Austin, J. C. (2002). Current management of dysfunctional voiding. *Dialogues in Pediatric Urology, 25*, 1–8.
Cox, D. J., Morris, J. B., Borowitz, S. M., & Sutphen, J. L. (2002). Psychological differences between children with and without chronic encopresis. *Journal of Pediatric Psychology, 27*, 585–591.
Deshpande, A. V., & Caldwell, P. H. (2012). Medical management of nocturnal enuresis. *Pediatric Drugs, 14*, 71–77.
Driver, D. S. (2007). Perineal dermatitis in critical care patients. *Critical Care Nurse, 27*, 42–46.
Elder, J. S., Peters, C. A., Arant Jr., B. S., Ewalt, D. H., Hawtrey, C. E., Hurwitz, R. S., …, & Hasselblad, V. (1997). Pediatric vesicoureteral reflux guidelines panel summary report on the management of primary vesicoureteral reflux in children. The Journal of Urology, 157, 1846–1851.
Feehan, M., McGee, R., Stanton, W., & Silva, P. (1990). A 6-year follow-up of childhood enuresis: Prevalence in adolescence and consequences for mental health. *Journal of Pediatrics and Child Health, 26*, 75–79.
Frauman, A. C., & Brandon, D. H. (1996). Toilet training for the child with chronic illness. *Pediatric Nursing, 22*, 469–472.
Frauman, A. C., & Myers, J. T. (1994). Cognitive, psychosocial, and physical development in infants and children with end-stage renal disease. *Advances in Renal Replacement Therapy, 1*, 49–54.
Garman, K., & Ficca, M. (2012). Managing encopresis in the elementary school setting the school nurse's role. *The Journal of School Nursing, 28*, 175–180.
Guarino, A., Lo Vecchio, A., & Canani, R. B. (2012). Chronic diarrhoea in children. *Best Practice and Research Clinical Gastroenterology, 26*, 649–661.
Har, A. F., & Croffie, J. (2010). Encopresis. *Pediatrics in Review, 31*, 368–374.
Hellerstein, S., & Linebarger, J. S. (2003). Voiding dysfunction in pediatric patients. *Clinical Pediatrics, 42*, 43–49.
Hirasing, R. A., van Leerdam, F. J., Bolk-Bennink, L. B., & Bosch, J. D. (1997). Bedwetting and behavioral and/or emotional problems. *Acta Paediatrica, 86*, 1131–1134.
Hoberman, A., Chao, H. P., Keller, D. M., Hickey, R., Davis, H. W., & Ellis, D. (1993). Prevalence of urinary tract infection in febrile infants. *Journal of Pediatrics, 123*, 17–23.
Hyman, P. E., Milla, P. J., Benninga, M. A., Davidson, G. P., Fleisher, D. F., & Taminiau, J. (2006). Childhood functional gastrointestinal disorders: Neonate/toddler. *Gastroenterology, 130*, 1519–1526.
Issenman, R. M., Filmer, R. B., & Gorski, P. A. (1999). A review of bowel and bladder control development in children: How gastrointestinal and urologic conditions relate to problems in toilet training. *Pediatrics, 103*, 1346–1352.
Issenman, R. M., Hewson, S., Pirhonen, D., & Taylor, W. (1987). Are chronic digestive complaints the result of abnormal dietary patterns? *American Journal of Diseases of Children, 141*, 679–682.
Joinson, C., Heron, J., Butler, U., & von Gontard, A. (2006). Psychological differences between children with and without soiling problems. *Pediatrics, 117*, 1575–1584.
Joinson, C., Heron, J., Emond, A., & Butler, R. (2007). Psychological problems in children with bedwetting and combined (day and night) wetting: A UK population-based study. *Journal of Pediatric Psychology, 32*, 605–616.
Joinson, C., Heron, J., & von Gontard, A. (2006). Psychological problems in children with daytime wetting. *Pediatrics, 118*, 1985–1993.
Kajiwara, M., Inoue, K., Usui, A., Kurihara, M., & Usui, T. (2004). The micturition habits and prevalence of daytime urinary incontinence in Japanese primary school children. *Journal of Urology, 167*, 1069–1073.
Kasirga, E., Akil, I., Yilmaz, O., & Polat, M. (2006). Evaluation of voiding dysfunctions in children with chronic functional constipation. *Turkish Journal of Pediatrics, 48*, 340–343.

Kelly, C. (1996). Chronic constipation and soiling in children: A review of the psychological and family literature. *Child Psychology and Psychiatry Review, 1*, 59–66.
Kistner, M. (2009). Dysfunctional elimination behaviors and associated complications in school-age children. *The Journal of School Nursing, 25*, 108–116.
Koff, S. A., Wagner, T. T., & Jayanthi, J. R. (1998). The relationship among dysfunctional elimiation syndromes, primary vesicoureteral reflex and urinary tract infections in children. *The Journal of Urology, 160*, 1019–1022.
Levine, M. D., & Bakow, H. (1976). Children with encopresis: A study of treatment outcome. *Paediatrics, 58*, 845–897.
Loening-Baucke, V. (1993). Constipation in early childhood: Patient characteristics, treatment, and long-term follow-up. *Gut, 34*, 1400–1404.
Loening-Baucke, V. (1997). Urinary incontinence and urinary tract infection and their resolution with treatment of chronic constipation of childhood. *Pediatrics, 100*, 228–232.
Loening-Baucke, V. (2005). Prevalence, symptoms, and outcome of constipation in infants and toddlers. *Journal of Pediatrics, 146*, 359–363.
Loening-Baucke, V., & Swidsinski, A. (2007). Constipation as a cause of acute abdominal pain in children. *The Journal of Pediatrics, 151*, 666–669.
Mellon, M. W., Natchev, B. E., Katusic, S. K., Colligan, R. C., Weaver, A. L., Voigt, R. G., & Barbaresi, W. J. (2013). Incidence of enuresis and encopresis among children with attention-deficit/hyperactivity disorder in a population-based birth cohort. *Academic Pediatrics, 13*, 322–327.
Moukarzel, A. A., Lesicka, H., & Ament, M. E. (2002). Irritable bowel syndrome and nonspecific diarrhea in infancy and childhood: Relationship with juice malabsorption. *Clinical Pediatrics, 41*, 145–150.
Murphy, K. P., Boutin, S. A., & Ide, K. R. (2012). Cerebral palsy, neurogenic bladder, and outcomes of lifetime care. *Developmental Medicine and Child Neurology, 54*, 945–950.
Palmer, M. H., Athanasopoulos, A., Lee, K. S., Takeda, M., & Wyndaele, J. J. (2012). Sociocultural and environmental influences on bladder health. *International Journal of Clinical Practice, 66*, 1132–1138.
Partin, J. C., Hamill, S. K., Fischel, J. E., & Partin, J. S. (1992). Painful defecation and fecal soiling in children. *Pediatrics, 89*, 1007–1009.
Peeters, B., Noens, I., Kuppens, S., & Benninga, M. A. (2016). Toilet training in children with a functional defecation disorder and concomitant symptoms of autism spectrum disorder. *Research in Autism Spectrum Disorders, 26*, 91–98.
Philips, E. M., Peeters, B., Teeuw, A. H., Leenders, A. G., Boluyt, N., Brilleslijper-Kater, S. N., & Benninga, M. A. (2015). Stressful life events in children with functional defecation disorders. *Journal of Pediatric Gastroenterology and Nutrition, 61*, 384–392.
Procter, E., & Loader, P. (2003). A 6-year follow-up study of chronic constipation and soiling in a specialist pediatric service. *Child: Care, Health, and Development, 29*, 103–109.
Rajindrajith, S., Devanarayana, N. M., Weerasooriya, L., Hathagoda, W., & Benninga, M. A. (2013). Quality of life and somatic symptoms in children with constipation: A school-based study. *Journal of Pediatrics, 163*, 1069–1072.
Rasquin, A., Di Lorenzo, C., Forbes, D., Guiraldes, E., Hyams, J. S., Staiano, A., & Walker, L. S. (2006). Childhood functional gastrointestinal disorders: Child/adolescent. *Gastroenterology, 30*, 1527–1537.
Rasquin-Weber, A., Hyman, P. E., Cucchiara, S., Fleisher, D. R., Hyams, J. S., Mills, P. J., & Stalano, A. (1999). Childhood functional gastrointestinal disorders. *Gut, 45*, 1160–1168.
Read, N. (2012). Irritable bowel syndrome in children explained. *Community Practitioner, 85*, 40–41.
Redsell, S. A., & Collier, J. (2001). Bedwetting, behaviour and self-esteem: A review of the literature. *Child: Care, Health and Development, 27*, 149–162.
Reiner, W. G., & Gearhart, J. P. (2006). Anxiety disorders in children with epispadias-exstrophy. *Urology, 68*, 172–174.

Robinson, J. C., Butler, R. J., Holland, P., & Doherty- Williams, D. (2003). Self-construing in children with primary mono-symptomatic nocturnal enuresis: An investigation of three measures. *Scandinavian Journal of Urology and Nephrology*, *37*, 124–128.

Robson, W. L. (1999). Enuresis treatment in the US. *Scandinavian Journal of Urology and Nephrology*, *202*, 56–60.

Rushton, H. G. (1993). Evaluation of the enuretic child. *Clinical Pediatrics*, *32*, 14–18.

Sansome, A. (2011). Bladder and bowel management in physically disabled children. *Paediatrics and Child Health*, *21*, 454–458.

Schonwald, A., Sherritt, L., Stadtler, A., & Bridgemohan, C. (2004). Factors associated with difficult toilet training. *Pediatrics*, *113*, 1753–1757.

Schulman, S. L. (2004). Voiding dysfunction in children. *Urologic Clinics of North America*, *31*, 481–490.

Schulpen, T. W. J. (1997). The burden of nocturnal enuresis. *Acta Paediatrica*, *86*, 981–984.

Shah, G., & Upadhyay, J. (2005). Controversies in the diagnosis and management of urinary tract infections in children. *Pediatric Drugs*, *7*, 339–346.

Shreeram, S., He, J. P., Kalaydjian, A., Brothers, S., & Merikangas, K. R. (2009). Prevalence of enuresis and its association with attention-deficit/hyperactivity disorder among US children: Results from a nationally representative study. *Journal of the American Academy of Child & Adolescent Psychiatry*, *48*, 35–41.

Stull, T. L., & LiPuma, J. J. (1991). Epidemiology and natural history of urinary tract infections in children. *Medical Clinics of North America*, *75*, 287–297.

Tai, T. T., Tai, B. T., Chang, Y. J., & Huang, K. H. (2015). Parents have different perceptions of bed-wetting than children from six to 15 years of age. *Acta Paediatrica*, *104*, 466–472.

Taubman, B., & Buzby, M. (1997). Overflow encopresis and stool toileting refusal during toilet training: A prospective study on the effect of therapeutic efficacy. *The Journal of Pediatrics*, *131*, 768–771.

Theunis, M., Van Hoecke, E., Paesbrugge, S., Hoebeke, P., & Vande Walle, J. (2002). Self-image and performance in children with nocturnal enuresis. *European Urology*, *41*, 660–667.

Tsutomu, K., & Fumiyuki, N. (2011). Effectiveness of parent-implemented interventions based on functional assessment of toilet skills in young children with autism. *Japanese Journal for Behavior Analysis*, *25*, 153–164.

Van den Berg, M. M., Benninga, M. A., & Lorenzo, C. (2006). Epidemiology of childhood constipation: A systematic review. *The American Journal of Gastroenterology*, *101*, 2401–2409.

Van Hoecke, E., De Fruyt, F., De Clercq, B., Hoebeke, P., & Vande Walle, J. (2006). Internalizing and externalizing problem behavior in children with nocturnal and diurnal enuresis: A five-factor model perspective. *Journal of Pediatric Psychology*, *31*, 460–468.

von Gontard, A., & Hollmann, E. (2004). Comorbidity of functional urinary incontinence and encopresis: Somatic and behavioral associations. *The Journal of Urology*, *171*, 2644–2647.

von Gontard, A., Moritz, A. M., Thome-Granz, S., & Equit, M. (2015). Abdominal pain symptoms are associated with anxiety and depression in young children. *Acta Paediatrica*, *104*, 1156–1163.

von Gontard, A., Moritz, A. M., Thome-Granz, S., & Freitag, C. (2011). Association of attention deficit and elimination disorders at school entry: A population based study. *The Journal of Urology*, *186*, 2027–2032.

Wang, C., Shang, L. Zhang, Y., Tian, J., Wang, B., Yang, X., …, & Xu, Y. (2013). Impact of functional constipation in health-related quality of life in preschool children and their families in Xi'an, China. PloS One, 8, e77273.

Wolfe-Christensen, C., Veenstra, A. L., Kovacevic, L., Elder, J. S., & Lakshmanan, Y. (2012). Psychosocial difficulties in children referred to pediatric urology: A closer look. *Urology*, *80*, 907–913.

Yeung, C. K., Sit, F. K. Y., To, L. K. C, Chiu, H. N., Sihoe, J. D. Y., Lee, E., & Wong, C. (2002). Reduction in nocturnal functional bladder capacity is a common factor in the pathogenesis of refractory nocturnal enuresis. *BJU International*, *90*, 302–307.

Risk Factors

K.A. Kroeger, Stephanie Weber, and Jennifer Smith

Risk Factors

Risk factors are inherent to any activity in life. Toileting is a natural life activity. Therefore, it is logical to assume that there are risk factors natural to toilet training. The World Health Organization defines a risk factor as "any attribute, characteristic or exposure of an individual that increases the likelihood of developing a disease or injury" (World Health Organization, 2017). In reference to the current topic, risk factors pose as barriers to delaying successful toilet training or ultimately preventing successful toilet training from being achieved. In training toileting, continence, where an individual must be able to recognize the sensation for elimination, and mastery of the entire chain of behaviors accompanying a toilet visit including traveling, excreting, washing, and redressing must be present in order to achieve independent and appropriate toileting skills (Kroeger & Sorensen-Burnworth, 2009). Risks to successful toileting behavior are inherent across those areas of continence and toileting behavior. This chapter explores continence potential risk factors related to child and caregiver characteristics, environmental challenges, and cultural barriers. Directions for future research endeavors and considerations not yet addressed by the current empirical body are also presented as additional areas of potential risk.

K.A. Kroeger (✉) • S. Weber • J. Smith
Kelly O'Leary Center for Autism Spectrum Disorders, Division of Developmental and Behavioral Pediatrics, Cincinnati Children's Hospital Medical Center, University of Cincinnati College of Medicine, ML 4002, 3333 Burnet Avenue, Cincinnati, OH 45229, USA
e-mail: Kimberly.Kroeger-Geoppinger@cchmc.org

J.L. Matson (ed.), *Clinical Guide to Toilet Training Children*, Autism and Child Psychopathology Series, DOI 10.1007/978-3-319-62725-0_3

Child Factors

Risk factors related to child characteristics are vast and, while not a comprehensive list, include factors related to developmental concerns, special healthcare needs, developmental delays, intellectual disabilities, chronic illnesses, comorbid psychiatric diagnoses, phobias, noncompliance, behavioral disorders, stand-alone symptoms, such as anxiety, and personality traits, such as temperament or birth order. Each of these factors alone could present risk and, in combination of one or more, potentially limit achievement of continence.

Children with Special Healthcare Needs The federal Maternal and Child Health Bureau (MCHB) defines the population of children with special healthcare needs (CSHCN) as "those who have (or are at increased risk for) a chronic physical, developmental, behavioral or emotional condition and who also require health and related services of a type or amount beyond that required by children generally" (2012). In order to ascertain that children who fall within the category of special healthcare needs receive the necessary intervention for remediation of skills that are less than expected of their typical age-matched peers, the MCHB defined the category broadly and across developmental domains. In light of this qualifying definition, researchers have discussed risk potentials and include overall disruptive behaviors (and "difficult" temperament described children) as baseline qualifiers for inclusion of CSHCN and worthy of consideration for readiness in terms of approaching developmental milestones, such as toileting (Howell, Wysocki, & Steiner, 2010; Macias, Roberts, Saylor, & Fussel, 2006). The American Academy of Pediatrics makes strong statements against forcing children to initiate a training program prior to being behaviorally, emotionally, or developmentally ready (Stadtler, Gorski, & Brazelton, 1999). Research determining "readiness" for toileting is scarce, and professional opinion currently guides those readiness parameters. Previous literature on toilet training various populations of children describes a number of behaviors to identify if a child is ready to train. These include asking to use a potty chair, removing and putting clothing back on, demonstrating interest in using the toilet and imitation of adults using the toilet, and communicating in some way when soiled or wet or when in need of voiding (Schum, McAuliffe, Simms, Walter, Lewis, & Pupp, 2001; van Nunen, Kaerts, Wyndaele, Vermandel, & Hal, 2015). While it is generally agreed upon that "toileting readiness" should be assessed and determined before beginning the training, especially for CSHCN, exactly what those readiness behaviors are have yet to reach consensus.

It is noted that for CSHCN, some children experience toileting readiness earlier or later than other children of the same chronological age. In preparing to train CSHCN, delayed readiness is considered (Macias et al., 2006). Delays in readiness to train may be related to a variety of developmental factors including physical development, for example, as in the case of children with spina bifida, psychological development, such as attention deficit hyperactivity disorder, or cognitive delays, such as intellectual disability. Howell and colleagues (2010) further the concept of readiness for CSHCN by discussing the topic in regard to children being "neurophysiologically ready" (p. 262) and note factors that would make a child completely independent in toileting including having the capability to follow adults' instructions, maintaining dry pants for 2 h or more, demonstrating the interest and ability to stay dry, potentially imitating others who remain dry, and physically manipulating clothing and sitting on the toilet. It should be noted that the standards for CSHCN as outlined by these authors are obviously similar to the standards for typical children who do not meet special needs qualifications. Given that some CSHCN may never be "neurophysiologically ready," such children and individuals may never accomplish independent toileting due to developmental delays in or across key areas of development, such as motor planning (Howell et al., 2010). However, as "toilet trained" is defined by continence in conjunction with mastery of the chain of behaviors that goes along with the bathroom trip, it might be that children, who do not become fully toilet trained, do indeed master a specific one or set of toileting behaviors, contributing still to an improved quality of life. Such that the child with spina bifida may need assistance with getting to the bathroom, but is otherwise continent and able to communicate the need "to go," the child with ADHD may remain daytime toilet trained, but struggle with nocturnal enuresis ongoing, and the child with intellectual disability may be continent and able to complete the chain of bathroom behaviors, but may not be able to communicate the need "to go." Regardless of complete readiness, the authors of this chapter believe in the importance of attempting to train CSHCN as improvement in quality of life factors for child and family could be achieved with mastery of even a specific toileting behavior, if not the entire chain.

In continuing the topic of readiness, researchers agree upon the importance of psychological readiness for children prior to toilet training (Brazelton, 1962; Foxx & Azrin 1973), mostly typically described as the ability to cooperate with training and the ability to follow a finite number of instructions. Psychological readiness is twofold: one, to reduce the potential for parent-child power struggles and, two, to assure the child is able to respond to simple directions. Also, readiness of physical factors, such as reflex sphincter control and motor skills, is important for independence in training (Vermandel, Van Kampen, Van Gorp & Wyandaele, 2008). Still other researchers suggest readiness factors include an IQ score of 20 or higher (Lohmann, Eyman & Lask, 1967), regular urinary and bowel voiding (Lowenthal, 1996), and ability to void in a large amount (Azrin & Foxx, 1971; Richmond, 1983). Many factors, across development and across children, should be reviewed when considering initiation of toilet training, especially for children who do not meet age-appropriate developmental markers. Given the more broad lists above or the more specific areas here, readiness should be considered, even though consensus has not been established on what true skill "readiness" is required for successful training. Toileting, as a mastered skill, is critical for independent living, meaning that incontinence is a significant quality of life barrier for individuals with special healthcare needs and developmental disabilities (Kroeger & Sorensen, 2010). Hence, readiness behaviors should be assessed and, if lacking, subsequently targeted for intervention in order to prepare CSHCN for toilet training. This is especially important as the general early intervention research body demonstrates that the earlier children demonstrate acquisition of such (toileting) behaviors, the more opportunity they have to participate in typical community events and mainstream educational placements (LeBlanc, Carr, Crossett, Bennett, & Detweiler, 2005).

Developmental Issues, Delays, and Disabilities As the diagnoses suggest, children displaying one or more developmental issues are likely to be delayed in development, including typical benchmark milestones, such as toileting. Delays in development, specifically delays in cognitive development, have been presented as a particular noteworthy risk factor for toilet training in the literature (Brazelton, 1962; Brazelton et al., 1999; Ellis, 1963). Children who fall within the overarching umbrella of "children with special healthcare needs" should be followed particularly closely given that they are already considered to be a vulnerable population and at risk for marginalization. Incontinence brings a diminished quality of life for those who experience it due to stigma, reduced self-confidence, personal hygiene issues, and limitations on engagement with others in one's environment (Kircaali-Iftar, Ulke-Kurkcuoglu, Cetin, & Unlu, 2009). Therefore, the combination of developmental issues and ongoing incontinence poses particular threat to the individual's self-esteem, social opportunities, and school and vocational placements. These factors are even more important when considering the improved quality of life that may result upon successful toilet training for children with delayed development. Teaching toileting skills is both challenging and highly advantageous for caregivers of children with delayed development (Kircaali-Iftar et al., 2009). Therefore, while obtaining continence in individuals with developmental disabilities may require extended training time or the presence of more systematic teaching protocols, pursuit of this developmental milestone holds significance in increasing both the child and family's quality of life, perhaps especially in light of the life-long implication of the developmental delay.

Extended time in training for individuals with developmental disabilities is a commonplace notion that general and developmental pediatrics alike often counsel families, assumedly from reviewing the general literature on toileting training (e.g., Bettison, 1986; Brazelton et al., 1999). However, upon closer inspection, it appears that the current body of research would challenge that generally held belief and posit that extended training time is not always required and that some children with developmental disabilities (particularly autism) actually train quicker than typically developing children in some instances. Studies on single case studies and small sample, controlled studies with individuals with developmental disabilities cite completion training times in less than 2 weeks (Azrin & Foxx, 1971; Kroeger & Sorensen, 2010), 1 month or less (Bainbridge & Myles, 1999; Cicero & Pfadt, 2002; LeBlanc et al., 2005; Post & Kirkpatrick, 2004), 2–3 months (Hagopian, Fisher, Piazza, & Wierzbicki, 1993; Luiselli, 1994, 1997; Wilder, Higbee, Williams, & Nachtwey, 1997), and 4–10 months (Keen et al., 2007; Luiselli, 1994, 1996a). These findings counter the commonplace belief that toilet training takes longer with children with developmental disabilities and perhaps even instill hope in that the diagnosis of autism is often associated with significant deficits, perhaps leading to the belief that toilet training is unobtainable – but now is potentially obtainable and in relatively reasonable amounts of time. However, before making recommendation to families of children with developmental disabilities, two caveats should be kept in mind when considering time of training: (1) these studies used highly specific protocols for training and were supervised variously by professionals, and (2) these were small sample studies as opposed to large, controlled population studies. Recommendations should be made to reflect that while there is promise that the presence of a developmental disability may not pose as much of a risk factor to training as originally suspected, the higher the likelihood of training in a timely manner will be influenced by the direct involvement of professional supervision and/or specific, detailed protocols for implementation.

An additional risk factor to this specific population exists in that even after trained and independent in toileting, regression of skill could occur. It is not likely that the individuals will regress to lose *all* toileting behavior but more likely that an individual might lose a specific toileting behavior, such as communicating the need "to go" or self-initiating to use the bathroom. Dalrymple and Ruble (1992) generated survey results that indicated 30% of individuals with autism who were toilet trained regressed in training at some later point in time, while Hyams and colleagues (1992) additionally noted regression in reference to self-initiation in a review of long-term follow-up of toilet training in developmental disabilities. Kroeger and Sorensen (2010) suggest to engage the parents as primary trainers so that they have the training tools necessary to problem-solve toileting issues that may arise once trained and to ultimately prevent backslide or subsequent regression. Treating clinicians should continue to monitor once children are reportedly trained to be sure that regression is not occurring and to recommend to families to intervene sooner rather than later if accidents start to occur as it is may be the beginning of a backslide in skills, rather than an isolated incident. Therefore, while a diagnosis of a developmental disability carries inherent risk to continence, evidence exists that training within normal parameters is possible, but again the ongoing issue of continence carries additional risk in that the threat of regression may remain for some individuals.

Chronic Illnesses Children suffering from childhood chronic illnesses are at threefold risk. First, it might be that simply having a chronically ill child is enough to make a parent reticent to pursue toilet training for a number of reasons including sympathy for the child, perceived ability to train based on illness, and reduced resources including parent's stamina, focus, and time (Brazelton et al., 1999; Frauman & Brandon, 1996). Second, beyond any attributed sympathy is the additional risk associated with chronic care, including reduced parent one-on-one time due to increase coordination of care time for the illness and medical follow-up, and financial strain and potential loss of family income, leading to increased caregiver-associated risks (Turchi et al., 2009). Third, children with chronic illnesses may also have inherent risk factors affecting the ability to achieve continence, including organic functioning (e.g., renal transplant, kidney disease), ongoing prescribed medications such as diuretics or diarrhea-inducing antibiotics and/or steroids, or the opposite-effect medications such as muscle relaxants and constipating narcotic pain relievers or related and associated developmental cognitive or motoric delays (Brazelton et al., 1999; Frauman & Brandon, 1996; Frauman & Myers, 1994). The associated risks are pervasive within children with acute long-term or chronic illnesses. Regardless of risk factor at play, it is generally recognized that despite the chronic illness, such children should still attempt toilet training and at seemingly similar age (before the age of 4) as typically developing, healthy children (Brazelton et al., 1999). Toilet training is a developmental milestone and becomes self-reinforcing once learned, and extended use of diapers has additional hygiene and risk factors that would be best eliminated by effective toilet training.

Comorbid Psychiatric Symptoms and Diagnoses As suspected, coexisting psychological symptoms are likely to act as potential barriers to successful toilet training. Children with both internalizing and externalizing psychiatric disorders are more likely to experience issues in the area of continence, and more so, even children with subclinical features are at higher risk than the general population for toileting difficulties (von Gontard, Baeuns, Van Hoecke, Warzak, & Bachman, 2011; Zinc, Freitag, & von Gonard, 2008). If left untreated, the unresolved toileting issue then places the child at further risk for additional associated psychological issues including reduced quality of life, chronic stress, and reduced self-esteem and sense of self-worth, not to mention the lingering associated physical hygiene risks.

Children presenting with all types of incontinence are more likely to be diagnosed with a comorbid psychological disorder (von Gontard et al., 2011). The highest co-occurring childhood disorder is attention deficit hyperactivity disorder (ADHD), where diagnosed children are more likely to be difficult to train and treat, likely to wet more frequently and problematic toileting patterns more likely to persist (Baeyens et al., 2006). Clinicians working with children diagnosed with ADHD should be particularly aware of this increased risk and monitor ongoing in order to intervene in a timely manner to reduce the long-term negative associated outcomes. Additionally, sharing with parents this coexisting tendency between ADHD and toileting difficulties may help to alleviate parental distress (who may place the toileting burden of blame elsewhere, such as on themselves or the child) and lead to a shortened lag time between problem presentation and obtaining targeted treatment.

Other externalizing and behavioral disorders with increased risk for enuresis include (but not limited to) oppositional defiant disorder and conduct disorder and internalizing or emotional disorders such as depressive and anxiety disorders. For children who do not meet full diagnostic criteria though, inherent risk still exists for those who present at the subclinical level. The global coexistence of behavior problems and toileting issues is high, and children with incontinence issues are two to four times more likely to present with such issues; children with the highest associated rate of behavior problems are those with fecal incontinence (Law, Yang, Coit, & Chan, 2016; von Gontard et al., 2011). Additional subclinical issues that present as risk factors include noncompliance, fears, and nonclinical anxiety and low self-esteem. Given the wide range of associated comorbid diagnoses, as well as associated isolated psychological symptoms, clinicians would benefit from generally assessing for underlying toileting issues initially and periodically thereafter, as secondary enuresis or encopresis can present even once trained, especially with the onset of significant life stressors. With earlier identification of toileting issues in these populations at risk and implied earlier intervention, the subsequent outcomes may be less intensive, pervasive, or enduring for children and their families.

Temperament Temperament is often characterized as the pattern of differences in individuals' emotions, reactivity to the environment, and behavioral and emotional self-regulation (Putnam, Sanson, & Rothbart, 2002; Thomas, Chess & Birch, 1970). Despite there being various theories on this topic, a child's temperament is widely agreed to emerge shortly after birth, has biological foundations, can be influenced by the environment, and remains consistent throughout childhood (Saudino, 2005). As discussed by Thomas and colleagues (1963), children can be described on a continuum of "difficultness" and can be identified as "easy," "slow to warm," or "difficult" based on key variables such as child's mood, adaptability, activity level, attention span and persistence, intensity of reaction, and other factors (Thomas, Chess, Birch, Hertzig, & Korn, 1963; Thomas et al., 1970). Literature on the influence of temperament has been inconsistent in regard to toilet training, though the key categories of rhythmicity (i.e., regularity of hunger, excretion, sleep, and wakefulness), approach withdrawal (i.e., response to a new object or person), attention span and persistence, and general mood are important factors to a child's participation and successful completion of toilet training as a developmental milestone (Thomas et al., 1970).

Difficult temperament has been suggested as a risk factor in toilet training (Blum, Taubman & Osborne, 1997). Schonwald, Sherritt, Stadtler and Bridgemohan (2004) presented the first study to demonstrate a "positive correlation among difficult toilet training, constipation, and temperament" (p. 1755). These researchers used parent report on the *Carey-McDevitt Behavioral Style Questionnaire* and the *Parenting Scale* to examine differences between a group of children identified as "difficult to train (DTT)" and a comparison group. They found children in the comparison group were more likely to have "easy" temperament cluster ratings than the DTT group. Though DTT children were not rated as significantly more "difficult" or "slow to warm up," they were significantly rated as less adaptable, less persistent, lower in approach, and with more negative mood than comparison children (Schonwald et al., 2004). Schum et al. (2001) examined the impact of temperament on toilet training using *The Toddler Temperament Scale* (1- to 2-year-olds) and *Behavioral Style Questionnaire* (3-year-olds). These researchers did not find significant differences when comparing the easy and difficult temperament clusters. They were surprised to find that children who were less rhythmic were more likely to have completed toilet training, which suggested that less predictable child behavior led to successful toileting (Schum et al., 2001). These findings are counter to what is known about child development overall; therefore, findings should be replicated before making global statements about the relationship between routines and toileting. Blum, Taubman and Osborne (1997) used the same temperament measures as Schum and colleagues (2001) and examined temperament on stool toileting refusal but did not find statistically significant results on any of the nine temperament subscales. While research has been mixed in regard to the impact of a child's temperament on toilet training success, these individual child factors cannot be ignored when determining a toilet training approach or likelihood of success. Such factors though should be loosely interpreted and suggested more as guidelines on how to problem-solve pitfalls of temperament and not presented as hard fact to families attempting toilet training as it may delay attempts to toilet train simply for fear of temperamental influence on outcome.

Additionally, it should be noted that the research on temperament and toilet training has limitations related to recall bias and small sample sizes (Joinson, Heron, Gontard, Butler, Golding & Emond, 2008). The studies described reviewing temperament utilized small samples of children referred to clinics that specialized in treatment for children with toileting difficulties. Given that these caregivers were seeking support for difficult to train children, bias in reporting on assessment measures must be considered when examining these results. More research on children without clinical levels of toileting problems is necessary to further delineate the impact of child's temperament on toilet training.

Clinicians who undertake toilet training work with parents and children should consider the implications of temperament on the process. Clinicians may consider recommending toilet training methods that align with the child's temperament. For instance, the more structured Azrin and Foxx (1971) intensive method may be encouraged for children with easier temperaments, whereas the child-centered approach may be considered for children with more difficult or slow-to-warm temperaments (see Chapter "Applications of Operant-Based Behavioral Principles to Toilet Training" for detailed description of training methods). Zweiback (1998) suggested the importance of determining a child's activity level prior to approaching training. If a child is overly active, he/she may not be ready for frequently scheduled sits requiring him/her to remain on the toilet or "potty chair" for longer than a minute or two. Children with predictable rhythmicity may be more successful with toileting use at regular intervals. A child's attention span is important to consider when training to best predict the reminders he/she may need to leave preferred activities to use the toilet since young children may have difficulty shifting attention when focused on a task or activity. Intensity is a temperamental factor that may lead a child to protest toilet training and lead to more work on the part of the parent to engage and reinforce the child for appropriate attempts (Zweiback, 1998).

Caregiver Factors

Caregivers are inherent to the toilet training process in that they are the "keepers" of children, and even if not the primary trainers, such as with children who attend daycare full time during the week, they are the ones the children return home to and are ultimately responsible for the completion of training in order to be fully "toilet trained." Given the expansiveness of the toilet training literature, it is surprising to find that parent variables are not better studied than would be suspected. Perhaps this lesser studied area is due to the fact that most typical children are toilet trained at one point or another, and therefore, the reason to study parent factors is null. There is more work that focuses on children with special needs, and these studies are more likely to question the impact of incontinence rather that the success or risk factors. Nonetheless, it would be hard to find a professional anywhere within the field of child development who would argue that caregiver factors are irrelevant in toilet training.

General Caregiver Traits One trend that is consistent in parent factors is the increase in age of onset toilet training. In the early to mid-twentieth century, toilet training was initiated at or before 18 months of age, whereas during the latter half of the twentieth century, training onset was closer to 2 to 3 years of age and currently nearer to 3 years of age with 30 months of age on average for onset (Bakker & Wyndaele, 2000; van Nunen et al., 2015; Schum, Kolb, McAuliffe, Simms, Underhill, & Lewis, 2002). Perhaps parenting over the century took into consideration its own assessment of risk and determined that delays in age would be beneficial in increasing the likelihood of initial training success.

Specific parent correlated risk factors generally focus on parenting style, as well as parent mental health. While we previously noted that psychological symptoms are more likely to be present in children with toileting difficulties, it appears that the presence of maternal depression or anxiety around the time of toilet training of the child also poses risk for development of toileting difficulties (Joinson et al., 2008). The phase of toilet training should be of clinical discussion in mothers of toddlers who present for treatment both in order to reduce maternal stress and related psychological correlates and to also decrease the risk of subsequent toileting problems in their toddlers. While studied and hypothesized, it was not found that parenting style in general presents as a risk factor for incontinence (Schonwald et al., 2004), although it is still held that unusual harshness and parental rigidity could lead to toileting difficulties regardless (Joinson et al., 2008). Interestingly, researchers have hypothesized that single parenthood would be a risk factor associated with delayed toileting and related toileting difficulties given the potential for reduced resources; however, research demonstrates the converse in that single parents are more likely to be successful in toilet training (Schum et al., 2001). Possible explanation for this relationship might lie in those same potential resources. That is, increased motivation to reduce family costs by eliminating the use of diapers and increased training plan consistency by the default of one parent and not an additional spouse having conflicting feelings or ideas on how to train effectively could be the same reasons single parents are more successful.

Parents of CSHCN Parents of incontinent children with developmental disabilities and related special (healthcare) needs report higher personal stress and distress likely related to the toileting problems presented by their children than parents of toilet-trained children without CSHCN (Macias et al., 2006). Given theories of persistent distress and the noted relationship between maternal stress and subsequent toileting difficulties, it is suggested that families of CSHCN be provided with additional resources and support in order to reduce the potential for risk and increase the likelihood of initial and maintained success with toilet training. It could be deduced then that continence training not only increases quality of life factors for the child by increasing associated hygiene factors and access to activities and placements but also increases the quality of life for the parents by reducing stress and subsequently for other family members such as siblings as corollary recipients of the distress. Toilet training, and protecting against the risk of incontinence, could then be one source of long-term stress reduction for families with individuals with pervasive developmental disorders and CSHCN.

Environmental Factors

Environmental factors posing risk are wide reaching and are as close as the child's physical and immediate environment and as far reaching as cultural climate and beliefs. Within the more immediate environment, risk is possible in physical settings, such as the child with spina bifida who lives in a second-floor-only bathroom home, to access to medical resources for tough to train children, such as those who may live in rural areas, to support from childcare or daycare settings for working parents, and to children living in multiple households and multi-generational caregivers. Likewise, clinicians may disregard cultural variables and potentially alienate families from seeking help, make over, or under assumptions about a particular race or class of families, or ultimately search out the literature for toileting answers and find that the research itself may pose risk by sample bias and reporting.

Cultural Climate Parental beliefs and attitudes regarding the age at which to start toilet training play a primary role in the process of toilet training. These beliefs and attitudes may vary according to cultural factors. The *Fundamentals of Toilet Training* study by Schum and colleagues (2001) examined the influence of child demographics compared to family demographics on the status of toilet training (not started training, in training, and training complete) in typically developing children. A majority of participants were Caucasian (76%), while 14% were African-American, and 10% were reported as from an "other" racial group. African-American children were found to start and complete toilet training much earlier than Caucasian children and children from other racial groups. The 50th percentile for starting toilet training was 21 months for African American children, compared to 29.5 months for Caucasian children. The 50th percentile for completing toilet training was 30 months for African American children, compared to 39 months for Caucasian children. Whereas only 4% of Caucasian parents reported that it was important for a child to be toilet trained by 2 years of age, 50% of African American parents reported this as an important developmental milestone for this chronological age.

Similarly, Horn, Brenner, Rao and Cheng (2006) examined differences in parental beliefs about the appropriate age at which to start toilet training in relation to various factors including race, family income, and parental education and age. A majority of respondents were African-American (59.4%) or Caucasian (32.4%) and were female (85.3%). Other racial groups including "Asian or Pacific Islander," "American Indian or Alaskan Native," and "others" were included in a single "other" category due to accounting for only 8.1% of total respondents. Parents reported a range of 6–48 months for when toilet training should be initiated, with the average age reported at 20.6 months. Caucasian parents reported a later age when initiation should occur (25.4 months), compared to African-American parents who reported an initiation age of 18.2 months and parents from "other" groups reporting an initiated age of 19.4 months on average. Hence, when counseling on toileting to the general population, population estimates are appropriate markers to cite with attention paid to racial differences; however, when counseling on individual cases, minority status should be considered when providing recommendations, with full awareness of potential population bias.

Role of Socioeconomic Status As indicated by Horn et al. (2006) and Schum et al. (2001), parents from different races have differing attitudes and beliefs regarding the age at which toilet training should be initiated. Horn and colleagues (2006) found that parents with higher incomes (above $50,000 per year) reported beliefs that toilet training should begin around 2 years of age, compared to 18 months of age reported by parents with lower incomes. It has been speculated that the cost of disposable diapers and disposable, pull-on style absorbent pants is a factor that impacts toilet training beliefs and practices of parents with lower incomes. Socioeconomic status (SES) is a factor that intersects with race and culture. It is unclear where such differences in attitudes and beliefs should be attributed as previous studies comparing toilet training in families from different races have been confounded by socioeconomic status (SES). One of the limitations of the Schum et al. (2001) study was the comparison between predominantly Caucasian children from suburban areas and urban African American children from lower-SES families (from Milwaukee) with the complete rule out of Hispanic children whose families did not speak English. Given these major study limitations, economic and cultural factors must be taken into account when examining child-rearing beliefs and practices such as toilet training. This factor is especially true in light of the fact that pediatricians and other professional providers often treat patients from different cultural backgrounds than their own, and, in turn, families seek guidance from such medical providers in primary care settings when concerns arise regarding typical childhood processes such as toileting. Practitioners should proceed with culturally competent recommendations that reflect awareness that "typical childhood processes" have different parameters and expectations for any given race or SES bracket.

Research Sample Bias as a Risk A majority of research studies conducted on toilet training include samples that are predominantly educated Caucasian parents in suburban settings, reflecting significant sample bias. It is critical that research on toilet training and other child-rearing practices reflect the racially, ethnically, and economically diverse population in which we live today. Therefore, when reviewing the body of research for at-risk, minor, and/or impoverished patient consultation, recommendations should be made with caution given the potential for population bias and for the potential of such patient populations to be susceptible to majority/ medical authority influences, for either positive or negative outcomes.

Professionals' Beliefs Perhaps one of the most subtle, yet powerful, risk factors is the belief of the childcare professionals themselves. Preschool teachers, daycare workers, program coordinators, and developmental specialists are key players for today's young children, providing extensive time spent with the majority of children (US Census Bureau, 1994), as well as sources of comfort and counsel for parents and viable resources of parenting recommendations simply by the nature of their roles. Ritblatt and colleagues compared parents' and childcare professionals' practices and attitudes on toilet training for typical children (Ritblatt, Obegi, Hammons, Ganger, & Ganger, 2003). They found that childcare professionals are significantly more likely to recommend a later age to initiate toilet training, have higher expectations for toileting readiness behaviors, display more endorsement for positive preparation for training, and demonstrate higher tolerance for and child education around accidents. Professionals should be aware of their own preconceptions in attitude and higher expectation for toileting readiness and training routines, especially if they have children in their care for extended hours of the day whose parents are ready to start training at an earlier age. Likewise, parents should be aware that they might not be met with support and agreement if attempting to solicit help (in initiating toilet training) from childcare providers if those providers are not in agreement with the child's readiness to train.

Noncustodial Caregivers Related to professional care providers are noncustodial caregivers that spend a significant amount of time with today's young. If not in formal daycare settings, the majority of youth with working parents spend their time in their own homes with babysitters or nannies, in relatives' homes (or living within a multi-generational home themselves) or in shared childcare provider homes. As with professional childcare providers, these additional sources of care may have differing opinions on how and when to toilet train from the child's parents or guardian. Differing opinions on training readiness lead to potential risk of giving the child mixed messages, differential reinforcement, and to the potential for different consequences across levels of training leading to delayed time in training to a host of toileting difficulties.

Conclusions

Perhaps one of the most pervasive topics in risk alludes to the concept of child "readiness" and the potential of risk to falter or fail in toileting. For as pervasive as this concept is throughout the literature, there is little to no true empirical evidence to support what actual readiness is nor support for the behaviors or cognitions recommended to be present at the time of initiating training. This paucity in the research body is more interesting given the "age" of toileting research – nearly 50 years ago, the seminal Foxx and Azrin studies were published for toilet training adults with intellectual disabilities. Fifty years is a long time to talk about toilet training, both typical children and CSHCN, and create multiple, detailed problem-solving protocols to train the hardest-to-train children without ever evaluating the true readiness criteria referred to in publications ubiquitously. Future research would benefit from evaluating the various recommended readiness behaviors, both in true readiness (i.e., Do children display them prior to successful continence training?) and parental and caregiver beliefs (i.e., Do parents feel the need for these behaviors to be present or assume that they already are regardless of true demonstration of target skill?). Findings might suggest that such readiness behaviors are indeed required and likely to lead to success; alternatively, they might find that such suggested readiness behaviors actually act as prohibitors to training certain children under the guise of the risk of not being ready.

Awareness of risk factors are important for a number of reasons: (1) to make families aware of potential risk and prevent for feelings of failure and related psychological correlates if training is not completed and (2) to give families at risk needed additional resources and support in order to increase the likelihood of successful toilet training. As outlined, there are endless sources of potential risk to continence. Hopefully though, it is highlighted that while risk is evident, it should not be debilitating and instead should act as a prompt to provide additional support and resources as necessary in order to increase the likelihood of those carrying risk potential to ultimately be toilet trained and without residual difficulty. Most importantly, clinicians should be aware of these areas of risk (and areas of non-risk as shown that some suspected risk factors are indeed not, or even protective factors instead) as patients present at their offices for counsel on when and if to initiate training, to seek help in problem-solving toileting difficulties and to be encouraged to try again after a failed attempt to train their child. To quote Carmelo Anthony, a popular basketball player of the time, who risks traumatic brain injury each time he steps onto the court, "Life is a risk." As clinicians, guidance and informed decision-making are the best guards against risk in the long run for counseling families who are considering toilet training for their child.

References

Azrin, N. H., & Foxx, R. M. (1971). A rapid method of toilet training the institutionalized retarded. *Journal of Applied Behavior Analysis, 4*, 89–99.

Baeyens, D., Roeyers, H., D'Haese, L., Pieters, F., Hoebeke, P., & Vande Walle, J. (2006). The prevalence of ADHD in children with enuresis: Comparison between a tertiary and non-tertiary care sample. *Acta Paediatricia, 95*, 347–352.

Bainbridge, N., & Myles, B. S. (1999). The use of priming to introduce toilet training to a child with autism. *Focus on Autism and Other Developmental Disabilities, 14*, 106–109.

Bakker, E., & Wyndaele, J. J. (2000). Changes in the toilet raining of children during the last 60 years: The cause of an increase in lower urinary tract dysfunction? *British Journal of Urology, 86*, 248–252.

Bettison, S. (1986). Behavioral approaches to toilet training for retarded persons. *International Review of Research in Mental Retardation, 14*, 319–350.
Blum, N. J., Taubman, B., & Osborne, M. L. (1997). Behavioural characteristics of children with stool toileting refusal. *Pediatrics, 99*, 5–53.
Brazelton, T. B. (1962). A child-oriented approach to toilet training. *Pediatrics, 99*, 5–35.
Brazelton, T. B., Christophersen, E. R., Frauman, A. C., Gorski, P. A., Poole, J. M., Stadtler, A. C., & Wright, C. L. (1999). Instruction, timeliness and medical influences affecting toilet training. *Pediatrics, 103*, 1353–1358.
Cicero, F. R., & Pfadt, A. (2002). Investigation of a reinforcement-based toilet training procedure for children with autism. *Research in Developmental Disabilities, 23*, 319–331.
Dalrymple, N. J., & Ruble, L. A. (1992). Toilet training and behaviors of people with autism: Parent views. *Journal of Autism and Developmental Disorders, 22*, 265–275.
Ellis, N. R. (1963). Toilet training the severely defective patient: An S-R reinforcement analysis. *American Journal of Mental Deficiency, 68*, 98–103.
Frauman, A. C., & Brandon, D. H. (1996). Toilet training for the child with chronic illness. *Pediatric Nursing, 22*, 469–472.
Frauman, A. C., & Myers, J. T. (1994). Cognitive, psychosocial and physical development in infants and children with end-stage renal disease. *Advanced Renal Replacement Therapy, 1*, 49–54.
Foxx, R. M., & Azrin, N. H. (1973). *Toilet training persons with developmental disabilities: A rapid program for day and nighttime independent toileting*. Harrisburg, PA: Help Services Press.
von Gontard, A., Baeyens, D., Van Hoecke, E., Warzak, W. J., & Bachmann, C. (2011). Psychological and psychiatric issues in urinary and fecal incontinence. *The Journal of Urology, 185*, 1432–1437.
Hagopian, L. P., Fisher, W., Piazza, C. C., & Wierzbicki, J. J. (1993). A water-prompting procedure for the treatment of urinary incontinence. *Journal of Applied Behavior Analysis, 26*, 473–474.
Horn, I. B., Brenner, R., Rao, M., & Cheng, T. L. (2006). Beliefs about the appropriate age for initiating toilet training: Are there racial and socioeconomic differences? *The Journal of Pediatrics, 149*(2), 165–168.
Howell, D. M., Wysocki, K., & Steiner, M. J. (2010). Toilet training. *Pediatric in Review, 31*, 262–263.
Hyams, G., McCoull, K., Smith, P. S., & Tyrer, S. P. (1992). Behavioural continence training in mental handicap: A 10-year follow-up study. *Journal of Intellectual Disability Research, 36*, 551–558.
Joinson, C., Heron, J., von Gontard, A., Butler, U., Golding, J., & Emond, A. (2008). Early childhood risk factors association with daytime wetting and soiling in school-age children. *Journal of Pediatric Psychology, 33*, 739–750.
Keen, D., Brannigan, K. L., & Cuskelly, M. (2007). Toilet training for children with autism: The effects of video modelling. *Journal of Developmental and Physical Disabilities, 19*, 291–303.
Kircaali-Iftar, G., Ulke-Kurkcuoglu, B., Cetin, O., & Unlu, E. (2009). Intensive daytime toilet training of two children with autism: Implementing and monitoring systematically guarantees success. *International Journal of Early Childhood Special Education, 1*, 117–126.
Kroeger, K. A., & Sorensen, R. (2010). A parent training model for toilet training children with autism. *Journal of Intellectual Disability Research, 54*, 556–567.
Kroeger, K. A., & Sorensen-Burnworth, R. (2009). Toilet training individuals with autism and other developmental disabilities: A critical review. *Research in Autism Spectrum Disorders, 3*, 607–618.
LeBlanc, L. A., Carr, J. E., Crossett, S. E., Bennett, C. M., & Detweiler, D. D. (2005). Intensive outpatient behavioral treatment of primary urinary incontinence of children with autism. *Focus on Autism and Other Developmental Disabilities, 20*, 98–105.

Law, E., Yang, J. H., Coit, M. H., & Chan, E. (2016). Toilet school for children with failure to toilet train: Comparing a group therapy model with individual treatment. *Journal of Developmental and Behavioral Pediatrics, 37*, 223–230.
Lohmann, W., Eyman, R. K., & Lask, E. (1967). Toilet training. *American Journal of Mental Deficiency, 71*, 551–557.
Lowenthal, B. (1996). Teaching basic adaptive skills to young children with disabilities. *Early Child Development and Care, 115*, 77–84.
Luiselli, J. K. (1994). Toilet training children with sensory impairments in a residential school setting. *Behavioral Interventions, 9*, 105–114.
Luiselli, J. K. (1996). A case study evaluation of a transfer-of-stimulus control toilet training procedure for a child with pervasive developmental disorder. *Focus on Autism and Other Developmental Disabilities, 11*, 158–162.
Luiselli, J. K. (1997). Teaching toilet skills in a public school setting to a child with pervasive developmental disorder. *Journal of Behavior Therapy and Experimental Psychiatry, 28*, 163–168.
Macias, M. M., Roberts, K. M., Saylor, C. F., & Fussel, J. J. (2006). Toileting concerns, parenting stress, and behavior problems in children with special health care needs. *Clinical Pediatrics, 45*, 415–422.
van Nunen, K., Kaerts, N., Wyndaele, J. J., Vermandel, A., & Hal, G. V. (2015). Parents' views on toilet training (TT): A quantitative study to identify the beliefs and attitudes of parents concerning TT. *Journal of Child Health Care, 19*, 265–274.
Post, A. R., & Kirkpatrick, M. A. (2004). Toilet training for a young boy with pervasive developmental disorder. *Behavioral Interventions, 19*, 45–50.
Putnam, S. P., Sanson, A., & Rothbart, M. K. (2002). Child temperament and parenting. In M. Bornstein (Ed.), *Handbook of parenting* (2nd ed.). Mahwah, NJ: Erlbaum.
Richmond, G. (1983). Shaping bladder and bowel continence in developmentally retarded preschool children. *Journal of Autism and Developmental Disorders, 13*, 197–204.
Ritblatt, S. N., Obegi, A. D., Hammons, B. S., Ganger, T. A., & Ganger, B. C. (2003). Parents' and child care professionals' toilet training attitudes and practices: A comparative analysis. *Journal of Research in Childhood Education, 17*, 133–146.
Saudino, K. J. (2005). Behavioral genetics and child temperament. *Journal of Developmental and Behavioral Pediatrics, 26*, 214–223.
Schonwald, A., Sherritt, L., Stadtler, A., & Bridgemohan, C. (2004). Factors associated with difficult toilet training. *Pediatrics, 113*, 1753–1757.
Schum, T. R., Kolb, T. M., McAuliffe, T. L., Simms, M. D., Underhill, R. L., & Lewis, M. (2002). Sequential acquisition of toilet-training skills: A descriptive study of gender and age differences in normal children. *Pediatrics, 109*, 1–7.
Schum, T. R., McAuliffe, T. L., Simms, M. D., Walter, J. A., Lewis, M., & Pupp, R. (2001). Factors associated with toilet training in the 1990s. *Ambulatory Pediatrics, 1*(2), 79–86.
Stadtler, A. C., Gorski, P. A., & Brazelton, T. B. (1999). Toilet training methods, clinical interventions, and recommendations. *Pediatrics, 103*, 1359–1361.
Thomas, A., Chess, S., & Birch, H. G. (1970). The origin of personality. *Scientific American, 223*, 102–109.
Thomas, A., Chess, S., Birch, H. G., Hertzig, M. E., & Korn, S. (1963). *Behavioral individuality in early childhood*. New York, NY: University Press.
Turchi, R. M., Berhane, Z., Bethell, C., Pomponio, A., Antonelli, R., & Minkovitz, C. S. (2009). Care coordination for CSHCN: Associations with family-provider relations and family/child outcomes. *Pediatrics, 124*, 5428–5434.
U.S. Census Bureau. (1994). *Who's minding our preschoolers?* Washington, D.C.: Department of Commerce.
U.S. Department of Health and Human Services, Health Resources and Service Administration (HRSA), Maternal and Child Health Bureau. (2012). Who are children with special health care needs (CHSCN). *Child and Adolescent Health Measurement Initiative*.. Retrieved from www.childhealthdata.org

Vermandel, A., Van Kampen, M., Van Gorp, C., & Wyndaele, J. J. (2008). How to toilet train healthy children? A review of the literature. *Neurourology and Urodynamics*, *27*, 162–166.
Wilder, D. A., Higbee, T. S., Williams, W. L., & Nachtwey, A. (1997). A simplified method of toilet training adults in residential settings. *Journal of Behavior Therapy and Experimental Psychiatry*, *28*(3), 241–246.
World Health Organization. (2017). *Health topics: Risk factors*. Geneva: World Health Organization. Retrieved from http://www.who.int/topics/risk_factors/en/
Zink, S., Freitag, C. M., & von Gonard, A. (2008). Behavioral comorbidity differences in subtypes of enuresis and urinary incontinence. *Journal of Urology*, *179*, 295–298.
Zweiback, M. (1998). *Keys to toilet training*. New York, NY: Barron's Educational Series.

Normal Developmental Milestones of Toileting

Claire O. Burns and Johnny L. Matson

Introduction

Many parents hold different perceptions regarding when children should begin and complete toilet training. Although there is no exact age at which parents ought to initiate toilet training, many children follow similar developmental trajectories. The extant literature on toilet training indicates that the average age in the United States is between 24 and 36 months (American Academy of Pediatrics, 2009), and the majority of children do not achieve successful toilet training before 24 months of age (Largo, Molinari, Siebenthal, & Wolfensberger, 1999; Mota & Barros, 2008b; Stehbens & Silber, 1971). Researchers have also found that toilet training is usually begun later than it has been in the past (Bakker & Wyndaele, 2000; Blum, Taubman, & Nemeth, 2004; Schum et al., 2001). This may be reflective of a move toward more focus on child readiness (Berk & Friman, 1990) and less emphasis on specific age milestones. The American Academy of Pediatrics (2009) suggests that this is a positive shift, as children become more self-sufficient as they get older, so the older children are at the initiation of training the more quickly they are likely to achieve successful toilet training.

The current chapter reviews the extant literature on current toilet training milestones and the ages at which these targets are typically met. These include prerequisite skills for toilet training, or "readiness" skills, as well as differences between urine and bowl control and daytime and nighttime control. The authors also address some of the current fads in toilet training methods and attempt to dispel common misconceptions. In particular, the idea that toilet training can be completed early in infancy, before children have either the physiological or psychological abilities necessary to attain this skill, is evaluated.

C.O. Burns, BS (✉)
Louisiana State University, Department of Psychology, Baton Rouge, LA 70830, USA
e-mail: Cburn26@lsu.edu

J.L. Matson
Department of Psychology, Louisiana State University, Baton Rouge, LA 70803, USA
e-mail: johnmatson@aol.com

J.L. Matson (ed.), *Clinical Guide to Toilet Training Children*, Autism and Child Psychopathology Series, DOI 10.1007/978-3-319-62725-0_4

Definitions of "Toilet Trained"

There is a lack of consensus within the field as to what exactly constitutes "toilet trained" (Vermandel, Van Kampen, Van Gorp, & Wyndaele, 2008). Therefore, discrepant measures are often used to define successful toilet training across research studies. Researchers have used criteria such as absence or very low rates of accidents (Foxx & Azrin, 1973), staying consistently dry (Schum et al., 2002), urinating or defecating on the toilet (Smeets, Lancioni, Ball, & Oltva, 1985), and communication of need (e.g., reaching/grabbing responses; Smeets et al., 1985). There are also inconsistent requirements for how long a child must be dry (e.g., day, week, month) or how infrequently accidents must occur in order for the child to be considered toilet trained. The ambiguity regarding the definition of toilet training makes it difficult to interpret the current literature on the topic, as researchers have found different results for particular criteria. For the purposes of integrating the literature for the current chapter, any criterion that indicates a socially significant amount of success is considered "toilet trained"; however, this success should be achieved independently, without the direct assistance of a parent or caregiver.

Toileting Readiness

Signs of toileting readiness are generally factors that are related to physical (e.g., musculature, reflex sphincter control) or psychological abilities (e.g., understanding of toileting-related words, interest in toilet training, verbal and nonverbal indication of soiled diaper; Vermandel et al., 2008). The American Academy of Pediatrics proposed that some of these factors include physiological and motor skills. Certain cognitive, social, emotional, and language skills are also involved. This is consistent with the aspects of physical and emotional readiness proposed by Brazelton in his child-oriented approach (1962) as well as the readiness tests used by Azrin and Foxx (i.e., bladder control, physical readiness, and instructional readiness; 1974). Most children possess some physiological readiness factors (i.e., the digestive system and bladder are developed enough to postpone bowel movement and urination) at approximately 18 months of age. However, most children lack the cognitive abilities and more advanced physiological development necessary until around 24 months of age (American Academy of Pediatrics, 2009).

Physiological Maturity

Certain physical processes are necessary for children to possess in order to have sufficient control over their bladder and bowel movements. Researchers have found that from birth to age 3, the number of voiding events decreases while bladder capacity increases (Jansson, Hanson, Hansom, Hellström, & Sillén, 2000). Micturition, or the ejection of urine from the urinary bladder, involves the following steps: (1) filling of the bladder, (2) desire to expel the contents of the bladder, (3) delaying expulsion, (4) initiating bladder contraction and sphincter relaxation, (5) control of flow of urine during expulsion, and (6) refilling of the bladder (Berk & Friman, 1990). The delayed elimination phase is the target of toilet training efforts, as it allows for the bladder control necessary to achieve successful toileting behavior. Each of the steps in the micturition cycle involves a certain amount of muscle control, particularly of the detrusor and sphincter muscles (Berk & Friman, 1990). Some control of these muscles may develop in children as young as 9 months old, but voluntary control of sphincter muscles usually does not fully develop until 12–18 months of age (Brazelton, 1962). A similar timeline has also been found for bowel control, which indicates that both of these processes rely on physical maturation (Largo et al., 1999).

Motor skills are also necessary for toilet training. Gross motor skills (e.g., the ability to walk to and sit on the toilet; Brazelton, 1962), as well as fine motor skills (e.g., the ability to take on and off necessary articles of clothing and effectively clean themselves), contribute to the ability to use the toilet (American Academy of Pediatrics, 2009; Azrin & Foxx, 1974). These capabilities give children the physical autonomy to use the toilet independently.

Psychological Maturity

In addition to physiological maturity, several psychological factors are involved in toilet training. One of these variables is cognitive abilities, as children must be able to make the association between the urge to eliminate and the act of using the toilet. It is also necessary for the child to avoid becoming distracted so that the he or she is able to complete the toileting process. Cognitive processes such as symbolic thought, problem solving, and memory are also thought to be involved in toileting skills (American Academy of Pediatrics, 2009).

Emotional maturity should also be considered, as it enhances the drive for independence as well as social readiness (American Academy of Pediatrics, 2009). Brazelton (1962) specifically emphasized the importance of impulse control and how it is induced by social and emotional abilities. Brazelton cited social factors such as the desire to please parents and imitate socially appropriate behavior of adult models, as well as the emotional drive to develop autonomy, as important influences on impulse control. Lastly, language skills are relevant to the toileting process, as children must have the receptive language skills necessary to understand an explanation of how to use the toilet and what steps are necessary (Azrin & Foxx, 1974). Expressive language can also facilitate this process so that children can communicate their need to use the toilet or express any discomfort they may be having (American Academy of Pediatrics, 2009). The development of these internal psychological processes is crucial to the progression of toilet training.

General Timeline of Readiness Skills

As previously discussed, certain readiness skills (e.g., understands words related to toileting and verbal or nonverbally indicates that they have to go) emerge earlier than others (e.g., tells before having to urinate; Schum et al., 2002). While these skills can be broadly separated into two types of development (i.e., physiological and psychological) and six types of skills (i.e., physiological, motor, cognitive, emotion, social, and language), there are specific abilities within these domains that tend to emerge around the same time. The American Academy of Pediatrics (2009) suggests that the simultaneous achievement of certain skills represents the following age-related developmental milestones for toddlers:

Before 12 months of age: Infants develop a general association between cause and effect. They also begin to recognize and be positively reinforced by social attention and praise.

12–18 months: Physiological skills emerge such as the physical awareness that they need to eliminate, as well as gross motor skills such as walking. Cognitively, children become able to associate the sensation of needing to eliminate with the physical act of elimination. They also begin to develop the early verbal communication skills. With regard to social and emotional development, the inclination to imitate increases and children start to desire more independence.

18–24 months: Children begin to be able to control the sphincter muscles for short periods of time, and their memories and goal-oriented cognition increase. Receptive language skills as well as verbal language development also progress, so children are better able to understand explanations and communicate expressively. Emotional desire for self-mastery and social desire to please parents and receive praise also intensify.

24–36 months: Children's fine motor skills develop to the point where they are able to manipulate clothing, which is necessary to independently use the toilet. Their memories improve and they are able to better remember toileting routines. Emotional and social development also progress, furthering their desire for competence, independence, and social reinforcement. By 3 years old, many children possess the necessary skills to be considered successfully toilet trained.

These guidelines represent a range of ages for certain developmental milestones; however, more advanced toileting development continues into childhood. Children over 3 develop more mature digestive systems and muscular control, which decreases the likelihood of accidents. Attention abilities also continue to increase, and children become less easily distracted and more likely to complete tasks (American Academy of Pediatrics, 2009).

These recommendations are consistent with the findings of several researchers. For example, Gesell and Amatruda (1941, cited from Berk & Friman, 1990) estimated that at 18 months of age children may have the ability to briefly delay urination, though not for long periods of time, and may not be able to communicate their need to urinate until 24 months. They also posited that at 36 months of age children can use the toilet independently. This is in accordance with the findings of MacKeith and colleagues (1974, cited from Berk & Friman, 1990), who suggested that children can nonverbally indicate that their diaper needs to be changed at 15 months, verbally request changing between 18 and 24 months, and communicate their need to urinate at 24 months. They also proposed that by 36 months of age children are able to delay urination for long enough to reach a toilet, though completely appropriate toileting behavior may not be achieved until 48 months of age. Relatedly, Brazelton (1962) found that the average age that children first successfully used the toilet was 27.7 months and that 80.3% were fully trained by 36 months of age. These ranges represent general ages for the acquisition of these skills, but as mentioned previously, there are no specific and concrete ages at which children should be "ready" to toilet train, just as there is no definitive age at which children should be expected to achieve successful toilet training.

Stages of Toilet Training

Once children have achieved the prerequisite readiness skills for toileting, they begin to progress through the stages of toilet training. The term "toilet trained" encompasses continual control over bladder and bowel movements; however, there are several milestones in successful toileting. The general progression of these stages is nighttime bowel control, then daytime bladder and bowel control, and lastly nighttime bladder control (American Academy of Pediatrics, 2009).

For daytime training, some children may attain bladder control earlier than bowel control, and vice versa. A possible explanation for this discrepancy is that for some children it is easier to urinate into the toilet than defecate; however, it is easier to postpone bowel movements (American Academy of Pediatrics, 2009). Therefore, children sometimes begin urinating in the toilet at a younger age but achieve successful bowel training earlier. Other children may attain both aspects of daytime training simultaneously. For example, Brazelton (1962) found that 12.3% achieved bowel training first, 8.2% achieve bladder training first, and 79.5% achieved both simultaneously. This is similar with Bloom and colleagues' (1993) estimate that the 28 months was the average age for both daytime bladder and bowel control. Further, Largo and colleagues (1999) found that by age 3, 53% of males and 84% females were daytime bladder trained and 54% of males and 82% of females were bowel trained. The results across these studies indicate that bowel training and daytime bladder training occur at roughly the same time.

There is substantial evidence that nighttime bladder control occurs significantly later than daytime bladder control. Multiple researchers have estimated daytime bladder training to be around 28 months (Bloom et al., 1993; Brazelton, 1962). However, Brazelton (1962) found that the average age for nighttime training was 33.3 months. The results of a study conducted by Largo and colleagues indicated that 53% of males and 84% of females were daytime bladder trained at 36 months of age, but only 23% of males and 42% of females were nighttime bladder trained.

Additionally, the results of a longitudinal study on bladder control by Jansson and colleagues (2005) found that the average age for daytime dryness was 3.5 years and for nighttime dryness was 4 years. Although it is possible for children to attain nighttime bladder control at the same time as daytime bladder control, most children do not achieve nighttime bladder control until several months or more after daytime training (Stadtler, Gorski, & Brazelton, 1999).

Several factors have been suggested to contribute to late completion of toilet training. These include physiological factors such as constipation, as well as psychological factors such as adaptability and temperament (Schonwald, Sherritt, Stadtler, & Bridgemohan, 2004). One particularly common issue is stool refusal, where the child is considered toilet trained for urination but does not defecate in the toilet for at least 1 month. Stool refusal can lead to constipation and painful bowel movements (Taubman, 1997). These concerns are discussed in greater detail in other chapters but are worth noting as they may interfere with normal developmental milestones of toileting.

Age at Initiation Versus Completion

Researchers have posited contradictory opinions regarding whether the age when children begin toilet training is related to the age at which children achieve successful toilet training. Blum and colleagues (2004) found that age at initiation significantly predicted age at completion, with parents who began training earlier reporting success at a younger age. Specifically, children who were toilet trained before 42 months of age on average began initial training at 20.6 months and began intensive training around 28 months. Those who did not achieve toilet training until after 42 months of age on average began toilet training around 22.3 moths and intensive training around 31.9 months. These results and the findings of other researchers suggest that earlier age of initiation may lead to earlier completion (Rugolotto, Sun, Calò, & Tatò, 2008).

However, the results of other studies offer conflicting results that suggest that toilet training at a young age is not associated with earlier training (Berk & Friman, 1990). For example, Largo and colleagues (1999) found that neither age at initiation of training nor intensity of training was related to age at successful bladder or bowel control. These researchers also investigated whether early toilet training and frequent prompting facilitate the development of bowel control. Their findings indicated that bladder control is not effectively improved by these methods, as there was not a significant difference in progress at age 18 months between children that began toilet training near the beginning of the first year of life (i.e., 1–6 months of age) and those who began toilet training near the end of the first year (i.e., 8–12 months of age; Largo & Stutzle, 1977).

Similarly, Matson and Ollendick (1977) found that children who began training before 24 months of age required a longer training duration than those who began after 24 months, despite the fact that all children passed a readiness test.

This is consistent with the findings of Foxx and Azrin (1973) that when the same toilet training method was used, children aged 26–36 months completed toilet training in less time than those 20–25 months old. These results indicate that older children are able to toilet train faster than younger children (in general those under 2 years of age).

Overall, much of the literature supports the concept that a physical maturation process leads the development of bowel and bladder control, and it is therefore unlikely that control can be attained at a very young age by beginning training earlier or using a more intensive approach (Largo et al., 1999; Largo, Molinari, von Siebenthal, & Wolfensberger, 1996). While this does not necessarily imply that there are no differences in age at completion based on when a child begins training, it does offer evidence that training at a very young age (i.e., before 12 months of age) is unlikely to yield lasting benefits in terms of earlier successful toilet training.

Factors Related to Age of Training

Although many professionals emphasize the importance of readiness factors and a child-centered approach, there is also research that suggests that external factors play a significant role in toilet training. For example, Schum and colleagues (2001) found that demographic variables (e.g., age, gender, race) were more closely related to toileting success than readiness factors (i.e., cognitive development and temperament). Although the influence of age has already been explored, researchers have also found noteworthy trends regarding considerations such as gender, race, and culture.

Gender, Race, and Socioeconomic Status

There are specific gender differences that have been observed in toilet training. Specifically, researchers have found that females tend to achieve successful toilet training earlier than males (Mota & Barros, 2008b; Oppel, Harper, & Rider, 1968; Schum et al., 2001). Schum and colleagues (2002) found that the median age for daytime toilet training was 32.5 months for females and 35.0 months for males. Also, the average age at start of the study was 2 months earlier for females than males. This is consistent with the assertion that females develop physically and cognitively faster than males (Schum et al., 2002), but may also be related to parental expectations that girls will achieve toilet training earlier (Stehbens & Silber, 1971; Vermandel et al., 2008).

Race and socioeconomic status have been implicated as factors related to age at initiation of toilet training. Horn and colleagues (2006) found that race and income significantly predicted the age at which parents thought toilet training should begin. Specifically, Caucasian race and higher income were related to later age at toilet training. On average, African American parents believed in initiating training at 18 months of age, while Caucasian parents on average stated 25 months. This is consistent with the results of a study by Schum and colleagues (2001), whose findings indicated that African American children begin and complete toilet training at younger ages than Caucasian children and children of other races. These findings indicate that there may be demographic variables that are related to differences in parental attitudes toward toilet training.

Cross-Cultural Differences

Researchers have also found cross-cultural differences in toileting practices on a multinational scale. Some countries have similar developmental trajectories for toilet training as the United States. For example, a study conducted nearly 30 years ago in Japan found that the average age for toilet training (i.e., no longer wearing diapers) was 27 months and that this was 6 months later than the average age 20 years previously (i.e., 1950s; Takahashi, 1986). Both the average age for completion of toilet training and the fact that this age has increased in recent years are consistent with findings in samples from the United States. Similarly, researchers in Brazil and Sweden have found that the age at toilet training completion has increased in recent years (Mota & Barros, 2008a), which indicates that this trend may indicate a global shift.

Conversely, in some regions such as parts of Asia, Africa, South America, Central America, and Europe, caregivers begin toilet training at much younger ages (Sun & Rugolotto, 2004). Many caregivers in these regions begin some type of training with their child prior to 12 months of age. deVries and deVries (1977) investigated toilet training in East Africa and found that children in a Digo village began toilet training around 2–3 weeks of age and were successfully toilet trained by 5 or 6 months of age. This training system consists of mothers holding their infants in a position thought to encourage elimination. For bladder training, mothers make a "shuus" noise to facilitate an association between the noise and urination. Most children are expected to reliably respond to this stimulus by 4–5 months of age. In regard to bowel movements, mothers hold their infants in a position facing them and using their feet as a "toilet." No verbal stimulus is used, as the position is thought to serve as the stimulus. deVries and deVries posit that this training differs from that undertaken in the Unites States in that the infant is an active participant and the training is less strict and more child-centered (deVries & deVries, 1977). The findings of these studies suggest that cultural influences impact toilet training practices both in terms of age at initiation and the type of training used.

Similar practices were reported from a study conducted in Vietnam, which indicated that 100% of mothers who participated were potty training their children at 12 months of age and 82% had already begun toilet training by 3 months (Duong, Jansson, Holmdahl, Sillén, & Hellstrom, 2010). Relatedly, a comparison of children in Sweden and children in Vietnam indicated that 98% of Vietnamese children who participated had completed toilet training by 24 months, while only 5% of Swedish children had begun toilet training at that age (Duong, Jansson, Holmdahl, Sillén, & Hellström, 2013). However, the training methods and the definitions of toilet training are often much different than those previously described in this chapter, as the training primarily involves caregiver response to the infants cues that he or she is about to eliminate. Therefore, successful training is more often defined as no longer wearing diapers than as independent use of a toilet.

Birth Order

While less extensively researched than other factors, there is some evidence that birth order may play a role in age at training completion. For instance, Brazelton (1962) suggested that first children tended to achieve daytime training around 1–2 months later and nighttime training 1–7 months later than their younger siblings. Other researchers, such as Taubman and colleagues (1997), found that the presence of siblings was not associated with age at toilet training, but was associated with stool toileting refusal, which was more common in children with younger siblings. Although the impact of birth order is not well established, future research on this topic may help to clarify whether parental expectations and practices are influenced by the presence of siblings.

"Diaperless Babies" and Elimination Communication

The Theory

The preceding sections outline the prerequisite skills to toilet training, many of which are not attained until well after infancy; however, there is a great deal of publicity in the media regarding parents who advocate for beginning toilet training at much younger ages. There have been multiple books and articles published recently describing the trend of raising infants without using diapers (Boucke, 2003; Bruno, 2012; Gross-Loh, 2007; Hartocollis, 2013; Kelley, 2005). This method is often referred to as "elimination communication," and parents who subscribe to this technique begin toilet training as early as a few weeks after birth.

The concept behind elimination communication is that infants are aware of their elimination urges and it is possible for parents to recognize their infant's cues (Bauer, 2006; Kelley, 2005). Parents work to identify physical or verbal signals that their child is about to eliminate. They then take steps to prepare the child for elimination, such as holding them over the toilet or placing a bowel or other receptacle under the child. Once parents have identified their child's cues, they pair these with their own verbal prompts (e.g., "sss," "grunting") in an effort to get the child to associate the parent's cue with elimination. They then use these cues to prompt their child to use the toilet at appropriate times (i.e., while being held over the toilet; Gross-Loh, 2007; Hartocollis, 2013). Parents of one child even claimed that the 6-month old infant toilet trained herself, as she said reportedly "boo boo" to indicate that she needed to use the toilet and refused to eliminate until her parents put her on the toilet (Sheldrick, 2012).

The proposed advantages of this technique for families include financial (e.g., reduced need to buy diapers), environmental (less waste), and social (a closer relationship between infant and parent; Kelley, 2005) benefits. The suggested benefits for the child include earlier understanding of toileting habits and a potentially easier transition to independent toileting (Sun & Rugolotto, 2004). However, as previously discussed, there is evidence that earlier training may not necessarily be related to earlier toileting completion. Nevertheless, this ideology has encouraged the trend of "diaper-free" infants.

Advocates for the elimination communication method also cite practices in countries other than the United States. Parents state that comparable techniques are customary in parts of Africa, South America, and Asia (Gross-Loh, 2007), and the method is similar to the one described earlier that is in practice in East Africa (deVries & deVries, 1977). Although limited, some researchers have investigated the results of elimination communication. Sun and Rugolotto (2004) found that a child being raised in a Western family setting attained bowel movement control at approximately 5 months of age. However, it should be noted that this was with the assistance of his mother, who had learned to recognize and differentiate his cues for defecation from those for hunger or fatigue. The authors reported that the child was not able to clearly communicate his defecation need or to stay dry during the day until 2 years of age. This case study stressed the role of the mother and her ability to pick up on and respond to the infants' elimination cues, rather than the infant's independent ability to communicate his needs.

In a similar study, Rugolotto and colleagues (2008) found that children whose parents began toilet training when the children was under 6 months old completed toilet training at a younger age. Ninety percent of respondents in this study reported that their child displayed elimination signals, and all participants began toilet training prior to 12 months of age. However, many of the participants from this study were obtained through an infant potty training mailing list, and therefore, the sample may be overly representative of parents who subscribe to early toilet training methods. Also, daytime dryness was defined as the child urinating in a receptacle either independently or with assistance. This suggests that some of the participants were not able to independently use the toilet, which is inconsistent with other definitions of successful toilet training.

While many parents endorse this method and assert that it enhances their bond with their child, many experts in the field are skeptical. In a 2005 New York Times article, the main proponents of the method were parents, whereas researchers questioned its feasibility in terms of parent availability as well as its overall effectiveness (Kelley, 2005). Other researchers have also expressed the concern that the procedures for these types of trainings may not be practical for most mothers due to the large investment of time and effort (Smeets et al., 1985). Relatedly, the general literature on the topic consists of parenting blogs and books published by parents who advocate for the method. There is little published research on elimination communication and toilet training in infants, as well as a lack of endorsement from professionals in medical fields. This indicates that the majority of the information on this technique is based off of anecdotal evidence rather than empirical research.

There are also physical concerns with this method. Some experts caution parents against toilet training at too young an age. One potentially negative aspect is the fact that it may be physiologically healthier for infants to engage in unconstrained elimination, as training children to attempt to control their bladder and bowel movements can result in chronic holding (Hodges, 2012). Chronic holding is related to a variety of toileting issues, such as constipation and urinary tract infections (Issenman, Filmer, & Gorski, 1999).

The reports of success of this method also warrant discussion of the definition of "toilet training." In regard to this type of training, Berk and Friman (1990) raised the question of whether training is considered complete when "caregivers can anticipate and respond to children's need to eliminate" or whether it is complete when children can respond when a parent asks them if they need to use the toilet. Relatedly, Smeets and colleagues (1985) found that a similar program was successful in teaching infants under 12 months of age to indicate when they had to eliminate; however, the researchers stated that the skill that was successfully trained did not meet the criteria used by most child care professionals. Based on the criteria commonly used by researchers, "toilet trained" typically constitutes some level of ability to independently communicate the need to eliminate or use the toilet without help (Mota & Barros, 2008a). Berk and Friman (1990) emphasized the importance of the clinician's role in helping parents to distinguish between "independent performance" and "interactional performance." The elimination communication method represents an interactional performance because parents are taught to identify their child's signals and help the child to associate their signals to toileting behaviors. However, they cautioned against encouraging parents to expect independent performance from their infants. By most researchers and clinicians' definitions, the results of the elimination communication method typically do not represent true control over the bladder or bowel, but rather the caregiver's ability to successfully get their child to a toilet or receptacle in time.

Although it is likely that infants display certain cues when there is an impending bladder or bowl movement and quite possible that parents can learn to pick up on and respond to these cues, overall the extant literature does not support the idea that infants under 12 months can be trained to control their urination or bowel movements. Parents who are interested in exploring this method should be informed that these techniques more accurately represent parent training than child training. This practice therefore reflects the parents' ability to recognize and respond to when their child is going to urinate or have a bowel movement and does not necessarily represent the child's own ability to recognize his or her bodily cues and respond appropriately. Even if infants do learn to associate their physical need to eliminate, there are more complex developmental abilities, such as motor skills and cognitive understanding of directions, that are necessary for true toilet training.

Conclusion

Toilet training is a process that requires physiological, behavioral, and emotional development on the part of the child, as well as sufficient support provided by parents or caregivers. Overall, the extant literature supports the practice of beginning toilet training around 24 months of age and predicts that many children become successfully toilet trained by 36 months and almost all by 48 months. Researchers also suggest that beginning toilet training at a very young age (i.e., before 12 months) usually does not significantly influence the age at completion (Largo et al., 1999) or the amount of time needed to successfully toilet train the child (Foxx & Azrin, 1973; Matson & Ollendick, 1977). There is no exact time to begin toilet training or specific age at which children should be expected to be toilet trained, as individual differences also play a role in acquisition of skills.

According to parent-report questionnaires, many parents do not discuss concerns they have about toilet training with professionals and are more likely to confer with relatives or friends (Stephens & Silber, 1974). Therefore, it is recommended that clinicians consult with parents regarding any questions they may have about toilet training, as healthcare professionals can provide parents with evidence-based recommendations (American Academy of Pediatrics, 2009; Stadtler et al., 1999).

References

American Academy of Pediatrics. (2009). *The American academy of pediatrics guide to toilet training*. Bantam: Random House Publishing Group.

Azrin, N., & Foxx, R. M. (1974). *Toilet training in less than a day*. New York, NY: Simon and Schuster.

Bakker, E., & Wyndaele, J. J. (2000). Changes in the toilet training of children during the last 60 years: The cause of an increase in lower urinary tract dysfunction? *BJU International*, *86*(3), 248–252. http://doi.org/10.1046/j.1464-410x.2000.00737.x.

Bauer, I. (2006). *Diaper free: The gentle wisdom of natural infant hygiene*. New York, NY: Plume.

Berk, L. B., & Friman, P. C. (1990). Epidemiologic aspects of toilet training. *Clinical Pediatrics*, *29*(5), 278–282. http://doi.org/10.1177/000992289002900505.

Bloom, D. A., Seeley, W. W., Ritchey, M., & McGuide, G. (1993). Toilet habits and continence in children: An opportunity sampling in search of normal parameters. *The Journal of Urology*, *149*(5), 1087–1090.

Blum, N. J., Taubman, B., & Nemeth, N. (2004). Why is toilet training occurring at older ages? A study of factors associated with later training. *The Journal of Pediatrics*, *145*(1), 107–111. http://doi.org/10.1016/j.jpeds.2004.02.022.

Boucke, L. (2003). *Infant potty basics: With or without diapers ... The natural way*. Lafayette, CO: White-Boucke Publishing.

Brazelton, T. B. (1962). A child-oriented approach to toilet training. *Pediatrics*, *29*(1), 121–128.

Bruno, D. (2012). Potty training Chinese style: With a diaper-free child, look for potted plants. *Christian Science Monitor*. Retrieved from http://www.csmonitor.com/The-Culture/Family/2012/1123/Potty-training-Chinese-style-With-a-diaper-free-child-look-for-potted-plants?cmpid=gigya-mail deVries, M. W., & deVries, M. R. (1977). Cultural relativity of toilet training readiness: A perspective from East Africa. *Pediatrics, 60*(2), 170–177.

Duong, T. H., Jansson, U.-B., Holmdahl, G., Sillén, U., & Hellstrom, A.-L. (2010). Development of bladder control in the first year of life in children who are potty trained early. *Journal of Pediatric Urology, 6*(5), 501–505. http://doi.org/10.1016/j.jpurol.2009.11.002.

Duong, T. H., Jansson, U.-B., Holmdahl, G., Sillén, U., & Hellström, A.-L. (2013). Urinary bladder control during the first 3 years of life in healthy children in Vietnam – A comparison study with Swedish children. *Journal of Pediatric Urology, 9*(6, Part A), 700–706. http://doi.org/10.1016/j.jpurol.2013.04.022.

Foxx, R. M., & Azrin, N. H. (1973). Dry pants: A rapid method of toilet training children. *Behaviour Research and Therapy, 11*(4), 435–442. http://doi.org/10.1016/0005-7967(73)90102-2.

Gross-Loh, C. (2007). *The diaper-free baby: The natural toilet training alternative*. New York, NY: Regan.

Hartocollis, A. (2013, April 18). Baby's Latest: Going Diaperless, at Home or Even in the Park. *The New York Times*. Retrieved from http://www.nytimes.com/2013/04/19/nyregion/babys-latest-going-diaperless-at-home-or-even-in-the-park.html

Hodges, S. (2012, April 17). A Doctor Responds: Don't Potty Train Your Baby. Retrieved August 19, 2016, from http://www.huffingtonpost.com/steve-hodges-md/potty-training_b_1424826.html

Horn, I. B., Brenner, R., Rao, M., & Cheng, T. L. (2006). Beliefs about the appropriate age for initiating toilet training: Are there racial and socioeconomic differences? *The Journal of Pediatrics, 149*(2), 165–168. http://doi.org/10.1016/j.jpeds.2006.03.004.

Issenman, R. M., Filmer, R. B., & Gorski, P. A. (1999). A review of bowel and bladder control development in children: How gastrointestinal and urologic conditions relate to problems in toilet training. *Pediatrics, 103*(Supplement 3), 1346–1352.

Jansson, U. B., Hanson, M., Hansom, E., Hellström, A. L., & Sillén, U. (2000). Voiding pattern in healthy children 0 to 3 years old: A longitudinal study. *The Journal of Urology, 164*(6), 2050–2054. http://doi.org/10.1016/S0022-5347 (05)66963-7.

Jansson, U. B., Hanson, M., Sillén, U., & Hellström, A. L. (2005). Voiding pattern and acquisition of bladder control from birth to age 6 years: A longitudinal study. *The Journal of Urology, 174*(1), 289–293. http://doi.org/10.1097/01.ju.0000161216.45653.e3.

Kelley, T. (2005, October 9. A fast track to toilet training for those at the crawling stage. *The New York Times*. Retrieved from http://www.nytimes.com/2005/10/09/nyregion/a-fast-track-to-toilet-training-for-those-at-the-crawling-stage.html

Largo, R. H., Molinari, L., Siebenthal K von, & Wolfensberger, U. (1999). Development of bladder and bowel control: Significance of prematurity, perinatal risk factors, psychomotor development and gender. *European Journal of Pediatrics, 158*(2), 115–122. http://doi.org/10.1007/s004310051030.

Largo, R. H., Molinari, L., von Siebenthal, K., & Wolfensberger, U. (1996). Does a profound change in toilet-training affect development of bowel and bladder control? *Developmental Medicine and Child Neurology, 38*(12), 1106–1116. http://doi.org/10.1111/j.1469-8749.1996.tb15074.x.

Largo, R. H., & Stutzle, W. (1977). Longitudinal study of bowel and bladder control by day and at night in the first six years of life. II: The role of potty training and the child's initiative. *Developmental Medicine and Child Neurology, 19*(5), 607–613. http://doi.org/10.1111/j.1469-8749.1977.tb07994.x.

Matson, J. L., & Ollendick, T. H. (1977). Issues in toilet training normal children. *Behavior Therapy, 8*(4), 549–553. http://doi.org/10.1016/S0005-7894(77)80184-6.

Mota, D. M., & Barros, A. J. D. (2008a). Toilet training: Methods, parental expectations and associated dysfunctions. *Jornal de Pediatria, 84*(1), 9–17. http://doi.org/10.2223/JPED.1752.

Mota, D. M., & Barros, A. J. D. (2008b). Toilet training: Situation at 2 years of age in a birth cohort. *Jornal de Pediatria, 84*(5), 455–462. http://doi.org/10.1590/S0021-75572008000600013.

Oppel, W. C., Harper, P. A., & Rider, R. V. (1968). The age of attaining bladder control. *Pediatrics, 42*(4), 614–626.

Rugolotto, S., Sun, M., Calò, D., & Tatò, L. (2008). Toilet training started during the first year of life: A report on elimination signals, stool toileting refusal and completion age. *Minerva Pediatrica, 60*(1), 27–35.

Schonwald, A., Sherritt, L., Stadtler, A., & Bridgemohan, C. (2004). Factors associated with difficult toilet training. *Pediatrics, 113*(6), 1753–1757.

Schum, T. R., Kolb, T. M., McAuliffe, T. L., Simms, M. D., Underhill, R. L., & Lewis, M. (2002). Sequential acquisition of toilet-training skills: A descriptive study of gender and age differences in normal children. *Pediatrics, 109*(3), e48–e48. http://doi.org/10.1542/peds.109.3.e48.

Schum, T. R., McAuliffe, T. L., Simms, M. D., Walter, J. A., Lewis, M., & Pupp, R. (2001). Factors associated with toilet training in the 1990s. *Ambulatory Pediatrics, 1*(2), 79–86. http://doi.org/10.1367/1539-4409(2001)001<0079:FAWTTI>2.0.CO;2.

Sheldrick, G. (2012, April 7). The baby who can talk at 6 months. Retrieved August 19, 2016, from http://www.express.co.uk/news/uk/313128/The-baby-who-can-talk-at-6-months

Smeets, P. M., Lancioni, G. E., Ball, T. S., & Oltva, D. S. (1985). Shaping self-initiated toileting in infants. *Journal of Applied Behavior Analysis, 18*(4), 303–308. http://doi.org/10.1901/jaba.1985.18-303.

Stadtler, A. C., Gorski, P. A., & Brazelton, T. B. (1999). Toilet training methods, clinical interventions, and recommendations. *Pediatrics, 103*(Supplement 3), 1359–1361.

Stehbens, J. A., & Silber, D. L. (1971). Parental expectations in toilet training. *Pediatrics, 48*(3), 451–454.

Stephens, J. A., & Silber, D. L. (1974). Parental expectations vs outcome in toilet training. *Pediatrics, 54*(4), 493–495.

Sun, M., & Rugolotto, S. (2004). Assisted infant toilet training in a western family setting. *Journal of Developmental & Behavioral Pediatrics, 25*(2), 99–101.

Takahashi, E. (1986). Investigation of the age of release from the diaper environment. *Pediatrician, 14*(Suppl 1), 48–52.

Taubman, B. (1997). Toilet training and toileting refusal for stool only: A prospective study. *Pediatrics, 99*(1), 54–58. http://doi.org/10.1542/peds.99.1.54.

Vermandel, A., Van Kampen, M., Van Gorp, C., & Wyndaele, J.-J. (2008). How to toilet train healthy children? A review of the literature. *Neurourology and Urodynamics, 27*(3), 162–166. http://doi.org/10.1002/nau.20490.

Theories of Toileting

Xinrui Jiang and Johnny L. Matson

Introduction

The acquisition of independent toileting is a critical developmental milestone and is an event that every parent faces when raising a child. The failure in achieving or maintaining control of eliminative functions can be distressing to both the child and the parents. In addition to the physical discomfort and reduced personal hygiene, children may also experience limitations in participation in activities, loss of sense of self-control, and reduced self-confidence (Cicero & Pfadt, 2002; McCartney & Holden, 1981). The concern of the parents can lead to a heightened level of stress (Macias, Roberts, Saylor, & Fussell, 2006; Plant & Sanders, 2007) and conflicts may arise between family members regarding appropriate treatment of the child.

Independent toileting is not only dependent on learning the set of complex skills related to this process (e.g., postponement of voiding, undressing, and redressing) but also on the maturation of the individual attempting to master these skills. While the former component bears similar meanings to different individuals, the latter component is subject to change across time (Berk & Friman, 1990; Kaerts, 2013; van Nunen, Kaerts, Wyndaele, Vermandel, & Hal, 2015) and cultures (Abramovitch & Abramovitch, 1989; Hindley, Filliozat, Klackenberg, Nicolet-Meister, & Sand, 1965; Schulze, 2000; Schulze, Harwood, Schoelmerich, & Leyendecker, 2002).

X. Jiang (✉) • J.L. Matson
Department of Psychology, Louisiana State University, Baton Rouge, LA 70803, USA
e-mail: xjian16@lsu.edu; johnmatson@aol.com

J.L. Matson (ed.), *Clinical Guide to Toilet Training Children*, Autism and Child Psychopathology Series, DOI 10.1007/978-3-319-62725-0_5

Enuresis and Encopresis

There are two common forms of elimination disorders, namely, enuresis and encopresis. The word enuresis derives from the Greek word "enourein" which means "to void urine." As defined in the Diagnostic and Statistical Manual of Mental Disorders, Fifth Edition (DSM-5), it involves "repeated voiding of urine into inappropriate places" in children at or above the age of 5. It can occur during the day or at night and can be divided into two types, primary enuresis and secondary enuresis. While primary enuresis is applied to individuals who have never established urinary continence, secondary enuresis is used to describe the development of disturbance after a period of continence (American Psychiatric Association [APA], 2013).

Encopresis was initially coined by Weissenberg in 1926, referring to soiling in inappropriate situations (Feeney, 2005). In DSM-5, it is defined as "repeated passage of feces into inappropriate places" with or without accompanying constipation in children that are at least 4 years old (APA, 2013). Similar to enuresis, encopresis can also take the primary or secondary form.

While the above definitions are sufficient for the purpose of this chapter, when closer examinations of different elimination disorders are required, one should refer to the taxonomy proposed by the International Children's Incontinence Society (ICCS) for enuresis and urinary incontinence (Austin et al., 2014; Nevéus et al., 2006) and the ROME-III categorizations for functional gastrointestinal disorders including constipation (with and without fecal incontinence) and fecal incontinence without constipation (Rasquin et al., 2006). These criteria have proven to be more reflective of existing research data and provide more precise categorizations for research and clinical purposes (Alpaslan, Koçak, Avci & Güzel, 2016; Equit, Klein, Braun-Bither, Gräber, & von Gontard, 2013; von Gontard, 2013).

To account for the etiology of incontinence, several theories have been proposed and these can be divided into three main categories: behavioral theories, physiological and biochemical explanations, and also propositions regarding the effects of psychological disturbance. Behavioral theories are based on the principles of learning and conditioning and regard incontinence as the result of a failure to learn. Treatments based on behavioral theories using classical and operant conditioning have been widely adopted and consistently demonstrated their effectiveness (Chopra, 1973; Hundziak, Maurer, & Watson, 1965; LeBlanc, Carr, Crossett, Bennett, & Detweiler, 2005; Luxem & Christophersen, 1994; Waye & Melnyr, 1973). Sometimes the learning process can be hindered by organic problems (e.g., central nervous system lesions, structural problems of the urinary system). In the presence of these problems, researchers should also take a physiological and biochemical perspective, as assessments and treatments for the interfering physiological or medical conditions should be considered and carried out. In addition to organic problems, psychological disturbances can also interfere with one's learning of toileting skills. In fact, the most widely held etiological theory regarding toileting used to be that of emotional disturbance (Walker, Kenning, & Faust-Capanille, 1989). In more recent studies, however, researchers have been putting more emphasis on the first two categories. Some also alluded to a combination of these theoretical models may better account for some instances of toileting related conditions.

Behavioral/Learning Theories

To successfully master independent toileting, children must acquire cognitive control over the reflexes involved in this process, including the postponement of voiding and the control over sphincter relaxation and bladder contraction (Berk & Friman, 1990). To gain cognitive control, a wide range of prerequisite skills must be developed or learned in gradual stages (Azrin & Foxx, 1989; Brazelton, 1962). While most individuals are expected to achieve physical (e.g., voluntary control of sphincter muscles) and psychological (e.g., desire to control impulses to defecate and urinate) readiness within a certain period of time, learning theories postulate that individual differences are present. Specifically, some individuals might have more difficulties than others in learning these skills, in the same way that some people may experience difficulties learning how to swim or how to ride a bike (Mash & Barkley, 2006).

Based on the principles of learning and conditioning, behavioral toileting programs have been developed and were demonstrated to be effective within various populations, including adults with intellectual disabilities (Azrin, Sneed, & Foxx, 1973) and Alzheimer's disease (Lancioni et al., 2011), children with autism (Cicero & Pfadt, 2002; Eikeseth, Smith, Jahr, & Eldevik, 2002), intellectual disabilities (Edgar, Kohler, & Hardman, 1975), and constipation (Wassom & Christophersen, 2014). The core components of behavioral theories are classical conditioning and operant conditioning. This section will introduce each of these core components and relevant constructs.

Classical Conditioning

Classical conditioning occurs through the pairing of a conditioned stimulus (CS; usually a neutral stimulus that does not yet readily produce a certain response) and an unconditioned stimulus (US; usually a stimulus that already produces a reliable response/unconditioned response [UR]). After this pairing is established through repetition, the presence of the CS will serve as a predictor of the US and subsequently elicits the conditioned response (CR), which is the same as or similar to the UR (Clark, 2004). The term "conditioned" is used to indicate that this response is "learned" and "unconditioned" indicates the behavior is innate and "not learned" (Clark, 2004).

Ivan Pavlov The most widely known development of classical conditioning stemmed from the work of Ivan Pavlov, a Russian physiologist in the 1880s. At that time, Pavlov and his colleagues' work focused on digestion, including the investigations of the gastric and salivary functions in dogs. The subjects (dogs) were constrained and fed, their production of saliva and gastric juices were collected and measured by special devices. Salivation and the production of gastric fluids were thought to be the innate reflex response to the tasting of foods, however, Pavlov observed that the presence of the experimenter, the sound of experiment equipment, or another neutral stimulus that was repeatedly paired with food, was enough to make the dogs salivate even without the presence of food; this phenomenon was reported as "psychic secretion." Pavlov and colleagues concluded that salivation, a reflexive response, can be produced as the result of two types of stimuli: those that produce salivation without previous training (i.e., food or US), and those which were learned to predict the presence of food (e.g., experimenter, or CS; Fontaine, 2008; Kimble, 1967).

Edwin Twitmyer At around the same time, although having received little attention, another researcher in the United States, Edwin Twitmyer, also made the discovery of classical conditioning in his study of "knee-jerk" reflex in human. In his doctoral dissertation, Twitmyer proposed studying the variability of the patellar tendon reflex with two forms of augmentations, namely, the ringing of a bell right before and squeezing of the hands at the tapping of a hammer on the patellar tendon. In one incidence the hammer failed to fall after the ringing of the bell, despite this, the participant was still observed to kick both legs, in Twitmyer's words, "without the usual blow of the hammers on the tendons." He then followed up with this observation by repeating this "accident" and found that the same response could be elicited in all participants, specifically, the knee jerk was produced by a stimulus (i.e., bell or CS) other than the usual one (i.e., tapping of the tendon or US; Fernberger, 1943; Twitmyer, 1905).

With the repetition of pairing of the CS and the US, the former gains control of the CR, leading to *acquisition*. This pairing process is influenced by *contiguity* and *contingency* – the temporal relationship between CS and US, and the frequency of their pairing. If US is taken out of the process, the repetition of CS in the absence of US will lead to the *extinction* of CR. While so far we have discussed the effect of CS to be signaling the presence of US/*excitation*, a CS can also function as an indicator of the omission of the US/*inhibition* (Davis & Buskist, 2008; Pierce & Cheney, 2004). Based on classical conditioning, in 1938 at Yale University, Mowrer and Mowrer developed the first conditioning device, an apparatus composed of an iron-sensitive pad and a bell that activates an alarm when the pad detects the presence of urine. This bell-and-pad system was designed to wake the individual who must manually turn off the alarm, go to the bathroom to complete voiding, change the sheet, and then reset the alarm (Mowrer & Mowrer, 1938). They regarded enuresis as a simple faultily trained habit and suggested that through pairing the proprioceptive stimuli from the bladder with the alarm, the individual will gradually learn to wake up when experiencing sensory input from the bladder. The following sections will briefly discuss the above-mentioned constructs in relation to the bell-and-pad method.

Acquisition Often, toilet training using classical conditioning is aimed at training the individual to acquire the connection between the feeling of fullness in the bladder (CS) and the action of waking up (CR) through the repeated paring of the CS with a US (e.g., alarm noise) that naturally leads to the target UR (e.g., wakefulness). Once the connection between CS and CR is established, *acquisition* is said to have taken place (Davis & Buskist, 2008; Pierce & Cheney, 2004).

Contiguity The temporal *contiguity* of the CS and US can affect the effectiveness of the *acquisition* process. In the case of the bell-and-pad method, the US (alarm) takes place shortly after the CS (the feeling of fullness of the bladder). As you can imagine, if there is to be a long delay between CS and US, the *acquisition* might need a longer time or more effort to be achieved (Davis & Buskist, 2008; Pierce & Cheney, 2004).

Contingency In addition to *contiguity*, another factor also plays a role in the establishment of connection between CS and US, namely, *contingency*. It refers to the correlation between CS and US, or the frequency that the two occur together versus apart (Davis & Buskist, 2008; Pierce & Cheney, 2004). Even if the US (alarm) occurs shortly after the CS (fullness of the bladder), if they are not consistently paired together, one may still experience difficulties acquiring their connection.

Extinction With appropriate *contiguity* and *contingency*, CS's *acquisition* of control over the CR can be completed effectively. However, if the *contingency* is broken where the CS (fullness of the bladder) is no longer paired with US (alarm), their connection can be lost and so is the control of the CS (fullness of the bladder) over CR (waking up), this phenomenon is called *extinction* (Davis & Buskist, 2008; Pierce & Cheney, 2004).

Excitation and inhibition In the case of bell-and-pad, the presentation of the CS signifies the occurrence of the US, this relationship is referred to as *excitation*, presentation of the CS "excites" the production of the CR. In other cases, the opposite may apply, where the presentation of the CS "inhibits" the production of the CR, and this is known as *inhibition* (Davis & Buskist, 2008; Pierce & Cheney, 2004).

The initial study of the treatment effect of Mowrer and Mowrer's bell-and-pad system reported that all participants achieved "elimination of enuresis." This success sparked numbers of subsequent studies evaluating the effectiveness of this urine alarm system. Although lower than the initial rate of 100%, these studies demonstrated impressive rates of success in the elimination of bedwetting, ranging from 70% to 90% (Brown, Pope, & Brown, 2011; Doleys, 1977; Friman & Jones, 2005; Ikeda, Koga, & Minami, 2006; Lovibond, 1964). Despite the high success rates, treatments utilizing the bell-and-pad system were reported to have a high relapse (Azrin & Thienes, 1978; Brown et al., 2011; Doleys, 1977; Friman & Jones, 2005) and dropout rate (Azrin & Thienes, 1978; Brown et al., 2011). The high relapse rate may not need to be considered a major drawback as the reinstatement of treatment usually reduced or eliminated the problem (Azrin & Thienes, 1978; Brown et al., 2011; Doleys, 1977; Friman & Jones, 2005). Having said this, the additional training and monitoring do add to the overall effort and time required to achieve success, which may be one of the reasons leading to the high dropout rate. Other reasons that families may prematurely terminate the treatments include the initial long period of time needed to achieve elimination (from weeks to months), the parents' annoyance at being awakened by the alarm (Azrin & Thienes, 1978), frequent breakdowns of the apparatus (Walker et al., 1989), and the efforts parents may need to put in making sure the children are following the protocols consistently.

While the bell-and-pad urinary alarm system was initially conceptualized to a paradigm of classical conditioning, where the tension of the bladder is associated with the awakening alarm, later studies pointed out that this may not be the only factor taking place here, as most children treated with this method learn to sleep throughout the night instead of waking up to go to the bathroom. Some have suggested that operant conditioning also may be a potential underlying mechanism of this learning process. Children learn to retain urine or wake up as avoidance of the aversive alarm or due to the positive reinforcement of dry nights (Ikeda et al., 2006; Walker et al., 1989). We will next discuss the theory of operant conditioning.

Operant Conditioning and Reinforcement

Before the 1940s, classical conditioning was often referred to as the "conditioned reflex," or "conditioning" (Walker et al., 1989). By the 1930s, researchers began to understand the difference between the learning processes based on conditioned reflexes and those contingent on reinforcements, and the latter came to be known as operant or instrumental conditioning (Clark, 2004; Konorski, 1948; Marquis & Porter, 1939; Skinner, 1937). While the learning process in classical conditioning is achieved through the pairing of a US and a CS, in operant conditioning, one's learning is mediated by the relationship between a behavioral response and the consequence. Specifically, the frequency or possibility of the behavior is modified by its consequence (Murphy & Lupfer, 2014).

Edward L. Thorndike Operant conditioning was first extensively studied by Edward L. Thorndike through his observations of the behaviors of cats attempting to escape puzzle boxes. To escape from a puzzle box, a cat must complete one or a set of specific responses (e.g., pulling a cord). With the repetition of trials, Thorndike observed that the time needed by the cats to perform the target action(s) is reduced, the cats "learned" to escape from the puzzle boxes with increased speed. He then generalized his findings into the Law of Effect, which states that responses that produced satisfactory consequences will be more likely to be produced and those that lead to discomforting results will be less likely to occur again (Davis & Buskist, 2008; Thorndike, 1965).

B. F. Skinner Burrhus Frederick Skinner (often known as B. F. Skinner) is often considered the father of operant conditioning. He studied observable behaviors in highly controlled laboratory conditions and created several experiment apparatuses including the operant chambers, in which subjects (animals) can be exposed to carefully designed and controlled stimuli, allowing the observation and recording of specific target behaviors (e.g., rats pressing a lever, pigeons pecking a disk). His findings of what we now know as operant conditioning was first articulated in his book, *The Behavior of Organisms*, published in 1938. Skinner reported that behavior can be modified through its consequences and that different schedules of consequences also produce different effects on the behavior (Davis & Buskist, 2008; Skinner, 1990).

Based on the effect a consequence has on the frequency of the behavior, it can be divided in to *reinforcement* and *punishment*. In addition to the choice of specific reinforcement or punishment, different techniques can be applied when designing the sequence and scheduling of the display of the chosen behavioral modification methods. They include *chaining* of events in a certain order, the use of *prompting* and *shaping* to guide an individual towards a target behavior, and the establishment of independence through *fading* of assistance. These terms are further explained below.

Reinforcement and punishment A consequence that increases the frequency of a behavior is considered a reinforcement and one that decreases the frequency of a behavior is a punishment (Murphy & Lupfer, 2014). The core element of toileting treatments based on operant conditioning is the systematic reinforcement of appropriate toileting behaviors. In correspondence with the cultural and political zeitgeist, positive reinforcements constitute the main choice of behavioral protocols compared to punishment.

Chaining The end goal of toilet training is for the individual to master the entire chain of behaviors associated with going to the toilet: from indicating the need to use the bathroom, to going to the bathroom, to voiding in the toilet, and to washing one's hands. Through the systematic presentation of response cues and contingent reinforcements, behavioral protocols based on operant conditioning may assist individuals in learning the components of or the complete behavioral chain of toileting. In the context of toileting, *forward chaining* is often utilized where the first step of the task (e.g., going to the toilet) is taught at the beginning, and as the individual acquires new skills, additional segments further down the behavior chain are added until the last step of the task (e.g., washing one's hands) and the complete behavioral sequence is presented (Drysdale, Lee, Anderson, & Moore, 2015; Shrestha, Anderson, & Moore, 2013). The sequence of the behavior chain can also be reversed, that the last step of the task is taught first while the initial step is taught last, and this is referred to as *backward chaining*.

Prompting In addition to reinforcement, prompting is also needed at the beginning to guide the individual along the behavioral chain. Common methods used include visual, verbal, and physical prompting (Hyams, McCoull, Smith, & Tyrer, 2008). A visual schedule with each step drawn out for the child is an example of a visual prompt. Verbal prompts are also frequently used to provide verbal guidance, for example, "wash your hands;" and the corresponding physical prompt maybe holding the child's hands over the sink.

Fading To attain the goal of independence so that the child can perform the task without external assistance, the technique of fading is often utilized by gradually removing the prompts until the need for them fade away (Hyams et al., 2008). Fading can take place in two ways with regard to the quantity and quality of the prompts used. Specifically, one can choose to remove prompts by individually omitting each prompt (e.g., removing the physical guidance of holding the child's hands over the sink) or fading the prompt into a less intrusive form (e.g., fading from holding the child's hands to pushing the hands towards the sink).

Shaping Individuals may not be able to perform a target action initially either due to the task being aversive or too complex for the person. For example, some children may dislike sitting on the cold toilet seat or some may not know how to pull up their pants and redress appropriately. In situations like this, the components of the behavioral chain need to be broken down further into successive approximations of the target behavior which are reinforced, gradually guiding an individual towards the end behavior. This process is referred to as *shaping* (Fernald & Fernald, 1999; Skinner, 1953).

Compared to the bell-and-pad method, treatments based on operant conditioning are more individualized, with greater variations produced by differences in any of the constructs described above. Through the systematic reinforcement of appropriate toileting behaviors, treatments based on operant conditioning were shown to be more effective, require shorter training time (from hours to days), and have a lower relapse and dropout rate (Azrin & Foxx, 1971; Azrin et al., 1973; Stover, Dunlap, & Neff, 2008; van Londen, van Londen-Barentsen, van Son, & Mulder, 1995). Since the work of Pavlov, Twitmyer, Thorndike, and Skinner, the studies of behavior have extended from animal behaviors to arrays of complex human behaviors. This branch of scientific study of behavior, known as *experimental analysis of behavior*, is concerned with the controlling and changing of behaviors and related factors. One major application and contribution of the knowledge gained from *experimental analysis of behavior* is the development of applied behavioral analysis (ABA), one of the liveliest fields of applied psychology today. It involves both the application of behavioral principles, including classical conditioning and operant conditioning, into the improvement of socially significant behaviors, and the development of effective behavioral interventions (Baer, Wolf, & Risley, 1968; Davis & Buskist, 2008; Pierce & Cheney, 2004).

Physiological and Biochemical Explanations

While behavioral principles are able to address the observable components of toilet training, successful independent toileting also involves the mastery of a series of processes that behavioral approaches may not be suitable or capable to explain. Specifically, these processes are the functioning of the physical structures (e.g., sphincter and bladder muscles), neural systems (e.g., central nervous system, CNS; peripheral neural system, PNS), and the regulatory endocrine system (Madersbacher, 1990; Stanhewicz & Larry Kenney, 2015). Abnormalities in these processes may hinder or even prohibit one's learning of independent toileting skills. Understanding the physiology and biochemical mechanisms of urination and defecation is essential to select appropriate pharmacological, surgical, and other interventions to remediate related problems and assist one's learning of independent toileting. Our discussion will be divided into two components: (1) the physiological perspective involving the physical structures and the neural systems; and, (2) the biochemical perspective revolving around the neuroendocrine system.

Physiological Perspective

Normal bladder functioning involves coordination of the relaxation and contraction of the detrusor and sphincter (i.e., relaxation of the detrusor and contraction of the sphincter during the urine storage phase; detrusor contraction and sphincter relaxation during voiding). These processes are dependent on the CNS and PNS which govern the control and reflexes of related muscles in correspondence with the sensory input and feedback (Dorsher & McIntosh, 2012). Similarly, normal bowel performance relies on functioning bowel and sphincter structures, the innervations of these structures, and the central and peripheral nervous systems. Mechanisms involved include delivery of contents to the rectum, regulation of rectal capacity and compliance, reception and communication of anorectal sensation, and control of pelvic floor and anal sphincter functioning (Jorge & Wexner, 1993). Structural insufficiencies, impairments to the innervations, as well as deficits in the above-mentioned nervous systems can lead to toileting difficulties. Infections, medical conditions, and certain injuries or surgical procedures are common causes of these disturbances.

In some cases, urinary or fecal incontinence is the consequence of deficits, damage, or surgical trauma to the pelvis. Some of the examples are congenital malformations including anorectal malformation [ARM], Hirschsprung's disease [HD], sacral and presacral abnormalities, and kidney and urinary tract anomalies (Hanneman et al., 2001; Moore, Jackson, Boyko, Scholes, & Fihn, 2008; Wallner et al., 2008). ARM is also known as imperforate anus; it is a wide spectrum of deficits involving the fetal development of the anus and the rectum with varying degrees of anomalies (e.g., rectourethral fistula/ an abnormal hole between the urethra and the rectum, anal stenosis/ narrowing of the anal canal; Holschneider et al., 2005; Peña, 1995). HD is a genetic disorder resulting from missing nerve cells in the large intestine muscles leading to partial to complete obstruction of the passing of stool (Lukac et al., 2016; Romeo et al., 1994). Toileting processes may also be complicated by sacral and presacral abnormalities, including sacral agenesis and abnormal mass in the presacral area. While the former refers to a congenital condition characterized by partial or full absence of the vertebral column and spinal cord, the latter may be congenital or developmental (Cho et al., 2016; Kocaoglu & Frush, 2006; Sharma, 2015). Congenital anomalies of the kidney and urinary tract (CAKUT) represents around 20–30% of prenatal malformations, including a broad range of disorders affecting the kidney(s) and/or lower urinary tract (dos Santos Junior, de Miranda, & Simões e Silva, 2014; Nakai, Asanuma, Shishido, Kitahara, & Yasuda, 2003). In addition to the above-mentioned and other congenital conditions, urinary and fecal incontinence may also be a consequence of physical damage such as pelvic fracture, or a complication of surgical procedures including radical prostatectomy and vaginal prolapse repair (Bartley, Sirls, Killinger, & Boura, 2015; Galiano et al., 2016; Welk et al., 2015). Among these, the more relevant to children is pelvic fracture, which can lead to urethral and/or bladder injuries with incontinence as a common complication (Brandes & Borrelli, 2001; Gomez et al., 2004; Koraitim, Marzouk, Atta, & Orabi, 1996).

Neurological impairments in other relevant structures may also negatively impact one's urinary and fecal functioning. Neurogenic bladder (NB) refers to bladder dysfunctions caused by congenital neurological deficits (e.g., spina bifida) and diseases or lesions of the central and/or peripheral nervous systems (e.g., stroke, diabetic autonomic neuropathy; Dorsher & McIntosh, 2012; Kay et al., 2013). Symptoms may include urinary incontinence, increased frequency and urgency, and overflow or retention of urine. Other commonly reported conditions that are related to NB include cerebral palsy, multiple sclerosis, Parkinson's disease, spinal cord injury, nerve damage caused by surgery, and traumatic brain injury, with 15–90% individuals affected exhibiting NB symptoms (Araki, Kitahara, Oida, & Kuno, 2000; Clayton, Brock, & Joseph, 2010; de Seze et al., 2007; Dorsher & McIntosh, 2012; Duby, Campbell, Setter, & Rasmussen, 2004; Gelber, Good, Laven, & Verhulst, 1993; Havenga, Maas, DeRuiter, Welvaart, & Trimbos, 2000; Masel, 2004; Murphy, Boutin, & Ide, 2012). Many with NB report experiencing negative impact on self-esteem, body image, mental health, independence, and participation in work, home, school, and leisure activities (Fischer, Church, Lyons, & McPherson, 2015). In addition to these impairments and limitations, NB may lead to secondary symptoms affecting the health of the individual, such as renal damage, urinary tract infections, stones in the urinary tract, and hydronephrosis (Dorsher & McIntosh, 2012; Murphy et al., 2012; Rabadi & Aston, 2014; Stephany et al., 2014; Stover, Lloyd, Waites, & Jackson, 1991).

Disturbance of the nervous system also often leads to fecal incontinence and constipation, also referred to as neurogenic bowel dysfunction (NBD; Faaborg et al., 2009; Krogh, Christensen, Sabroe, & Laurberg, 2006). Many of the conditions that are related to NB such as stroke, spina bifida, cerebral palsy, Parkinson's disease, and spinal cord injury, are also shown to be frequently accompanied by NBD (Gor, Katorski, & Elliott, 2016; Hinds, Eidelman, & Wald, 1990; Krogh & Christensen, 2009; Krogh, Ostergaard, Sabroe, & Laurberg, 2007; Lie et al., 2008). Similar to NB, NBD also results in limitations of participation in everyday activities and reduced quality of life (QOL) in many affected individuals (Faaborg et al., 2009; Krogh et al., 2006).

While the above conditionals often require invasive interventions like surgical procedures, noninvasive treatments have also been developed for those without such medical disturbances. One example is retention control training (RTC), which was proposed as a potential treatment for nocturnal enuresis through increasing bladder capacity by urine retention training. This is based on the findings that some children with nocturnal enuresis have relatively smaller bladder capacity, and the hypothesis that through the training in retaining urine these children will be able to increase their bladder capacity, thus enabling them to sleep through the night without the need to urinate. While it has been shown to be effective in eliminating incontinence in some individuals, its effects were very marginal in most cases despite the increased bladder capacity (De Wachter, Vermandel, De Moerloose, & Wyndaele, 2002; Florin & Tunner, 1970; Hamano, Yamanishi, Igarashi, Ito, & Murakami, 2000). This is not to say, however, that RTC lacks clinical value. As pointed out by de Wachter et al. (2002), RTC has the advantage of being noninvasive and risk-free, and that it can be used as first-line treatment for children with smaller bladder capacity; those who do not achieve satisfactory results from RTC can then move onto other treatment methods like a urinary alarm.

Pharmacological methods have also been developed targeting the dysfunctions of the bladder and sphincter muscles. Anticholinergic medications (e.g., oxybutynin) block the binding of acetylcholine to its receptors inhibiting parasympathetic activities, thus reducing bladder contractions and relaxing the smooth muscle leading to increased bladder capacity (Radvanska, Kovács, & Rittig, 2006; Thompson & Lauvetz, 1976). Often referred to as Botox, OnabotulinumtoxinA, a nerve toxin, also produces relaxation of the detrusor smooth muscle through blocking nerve activities; additionally, it also leads to reduction of feeling of fullness or urgency (Apostolidis, Dasgupta, & Fowler, 2006). Similarly, Mirabegron was also found to cause relaxation of the smooth muscle and contributing to increased bladder storage capacity (Radomski, 2014). Tofranil (imipramine) is one of the primary medications used for nocturnal enuresis, although its mechanism is still not clear, it is suggested to ameliorate enuresis symptoms by producing an anticholinergic effect and increasing one's wakefulness (Butler, 2001). Another less studied medication is duloxetine, a selective serotonin and norepinephrine reuptake inhibitor; it was found to be effective in increasing urethral sphincter activity thus improving continence (Norton, Zinner, Yalcin, & Bump, 2002). While varying amount of evidence has accumulated on different medications, these pharmacological approaches have all been able to demonstrate efficacy in the treatment of enuresis (Andersson & Schröder, 2004; Berkenwald, Pires, & Ellsworth, 2016; Bulchandani & Thomson,

2015; Chung, Cheng, & Tse, 2016; Hoebeke et al., 2009; Landman, Van capelle, Kollen, & Steffens, 2009; Poussaint & Ditman, 1965; Radomski, 2014; Tomasi, Siracusano, Monni, Mela, & Delitala, 2001).

Biochemical Perspective

Toileting involves both the production and voiding of urine and feces, disturbances in either process can both lead to toileting difficulties. Our discussion so far has mainly focused on the former, in this section we will focus on the system that is centered around the production process, namely, the neuroendocrine system.

The endocrine system is composed of organs and tissues that function to maintain a stable internal environment by producing and excreting regulatory chemicals called hormones. Under its control are several functions essential to life, including growth, metabolism, the regulation of body temperature, stress response, immune system, reproduction, digestion, and fluid intake and balance (Betts, DeSaix, Johnson, & Johnson, 2013; Sloane, 1994). While the primary sources of water intake come from drinking water, water in foods and beverages, and metabolic water; water output occurs through respiration, perspiration, discharge of feces, with the main passage being the passing of urine (Bossingham, Carnell, & Campbell, 2005). Together with the nervous system, the endocrine system monitors and regulates the production of urine, and the hormones and organs involved in this process include antidiuretic hormone (ADH; also known as vasopressin), pituitary, hypothalamus, and kidney (Bossingham et al., 2005; Stanhewicz & Larry Kenney, 2015; Stout, Kenny, & Baylis, 1999).

Hypothalamus and pituitary The homeostatic mechanisms are monitored and regulated by the autonomic nervous system. As the central automatic structure, the hypothalamus-pituitary complex functions as the bridge connecting the nervous and endocrine systems. Regulated by the input (e.g., osmotic pressure signals of dehydration) from the nervous system, the hypothalamus and the pituitary produce and release hormones (e.g., ADH) that stimulate or inhibit the hormone release of other glands or tissues (e.g., kidney) (Betts et al., 2013; Stanhewicz & Larry Kenney, 2015).

Kidney The kidneys are part of the urinary system and participate in several endocrine pathways. Some of its many functions include producing hormones, filtration of blood, regulation of iron concentrations, elimination of metabolic byproducts and wastes, and production of urine. Each kidney contains millions of urine-forming units, nephrons; and each nephron is composed of a vascular component and a tubular component (Betts et al., 2013; Sloane, 1994).

ADH/vasopressin ADH is one of the hormones produced by the hypothalamus. It is then stored in the pituitary for later release into the bloodstream. Upon detection of dehydration, osmotic signals detected by the hypothalamus lead to the release of ADH from the pituitary. ADH functions to increase the water absorption in the collecting ducts of the kidney, leading to reduced urine production and normalized osmotic pressure (Betts et al., 2013; Stanhewicz & Larry Kenney, 2015).

Dysfunctions of these mechanisms can lead to medical conditions including diabetes insipidus (DI), which is characterized by chronic excessive secretion of highly dilute urine. There are four types of DI each with different pathological mechanisms. The first type is pituitary/central DI, which is due to inadequate production and secretion of ADH. A second form of DI is caused by an impaired ability of the kidney to respond to ADH, and it is called nephrogenic DI. Gestational DI is another type of DI, and it is a result of increased degradation of ADH. Lastly, excessive fluid intake can also lead to a form of GI, nephrogenic DI, which can subsequently lead to suppression of ADH secretion and increased urine production. Hormone therapy using desmopressin, a synthetic replacement for ADH, is a common method used in the treatment of DI, and it has been found to be effective with different degrees for each subtype of DI (Robertson, 2016).

Some studies have suggested that a subgroup of individuals with enuresis exhibit night-time ADH deficiency, which leads to overproduction of urine that exceeds bladder capacity contributing to enuresis at night (Aceto et al., 2003; Mark & Frank, 1995; Pomeranz, Abu-Kheat, Korzets, & Wolach, 2000). Based on this finding hormone replacement therapy using desmopressin has been widely adopted and was found to be effective treating nocturnal enuresis in children and adolescents (Chua et al., 2016; Lottmann & Alova, 2007; Önol, Guzel, Tahra, Kaya, & Boylu, 2015; Stenberg & Lackgren, 1994; Wille, 1994; Yang, Guo, Chang, Yang, & Huang, 2015). A review study conducted by Alloussi et al. (2011) selected and evaluated 99 studies assessing the treatment's outcomes of enuresis using desmopressin. Their findings supported the use of desmopressin both by itself and in combination with other treatment options, including urinary alarm and anticholinergic medications in the treatment of enuresis.

Psychological Disturbances

The last category of etiological theories of toileting focuses on the relationship between psychological factors and one's developing of toileting skills. Psychological issues ranging from subclinical symptoms (e.g., anxiety symptom) to comorbid, clinically relevant psychiatric disorders (e.g., attention-deficit/hyperactivity disorder; ADHD) have been identified and studied by researchers in their relationships to toileting issues including urinary incontinence, fecal incontinence, and constipation. In general, prevalence studies support a positive correlation between psychological conditions with toileting difficulties (von Gontard, Baeyens, Van Hoecke, Warzak, & Bachmann, 2011). Despite that, the presence and direction of a causal relationship between the two have not been established due to the limitations of existing studies, there is a consensus that researchers, parents, pediatricians, urologists and other professionals should have a basic understanding of psychological principles in order to effectively assist those children who experience difficulties learning toileting skills.

Heightened levels of anxiety and depression have been frequently reported in individuals with elimination difficulties. In a population-based study, Equit and colleagues (Equit et al., 2013) collected information from 2079 preschool age children in Germany and found that children with one or more elimination disorders, especially encopresis, acquired significantly higher ratings of anxious/depressed symptoms than those without. This is consistent with the results of other population-based studies conducted by Joinson and colleagues on children around the age of 7 years; they found that children with enuresis, urinary and fecal incontinence compared to those who were continent had a higher rate of depressive symptoms (Joinson, Heron, Butler, von Gontard, & Avon Longitudinal Study of Parents and Children Study Team, 2006; Joinson, Heron, von Gontard, & and the ALSPAC Study Team, 2006). Another study with a smaller sample size and older participants (9–12 years) also found similar results indicating that children with enuresis experience more internalizing symptoms (i.e., withdrawal, anxiety, depression) than those without (E Van Hoecke, Hoebeke, Braet, & Walle, 2004). Similarly, a study on children (6–15 years) with and without encopresis found that encopresis was correlated with more anxiety/depression symptoms (Cox, 2002).

Prominent differences have also been found in externalizing symptoms between children with and without urinary and fecal incontinence. In a series of population-based studies conducted by Joinson and colleagues, it was found that parents of those children who experienced wetting or soiling problems reported higher rates of behavioral problems including attention and activity problems, obsessions and compulsions, oppositional behavior, and conduct problems than those parents of children who did not exhibit daytime wetting (Joinson, Heron, Emond, & Butler, 2007; Joinson, Heron, Butler, et al., 2006; Joinson, Heron, von Gontard, et al., 2006). Similarly, other researchers have also found elevated prevalence of externalizing problems in children with toileting difficulties (Byrd, Weitzman, Lanphear, & Auinger, 1996; Cox, 2002; Redsell & Collier, 2001; von Gontard et al., 2011; von Gontard, Mauer-Mucke, Plück, Berner, & Lehmkuhl, 1999).

Among the externalizing conditions, ADHD is the most common comorbid condition identified (Baeyens, Roeyers, Vande Walle, & Hoebeke, 2005). Studies assessing the prevalence of ADHD in children and adolescents found that individuals with enuresis, urinary incontinence, encopresis, or fecal incontinence exhibited significantly higher rates of ADHD symptoms than those without (Baeyens et al., 2004; Joinson, Heron, von Gontard, et al., 2006; Robson, Jackson, Blackhurst, & Leung, 1997; von Gontard, Moritz, Thome-Granz, & Freitag, 2011). Children with ADHD were also found to be more likely than their peers without ADHD to meet criteria for enuresis and encopresis (Michael W. Mellon et al., 2013; Robson et al., 1997).

While sufficient data has been collected supporting the association between eliminative dysfunctions and psychological disturbances, there is little direct evidence to support the causal relationship between the two. The majority of existing studies accessing the internalizing and externalizing symptoms in individuals with toileting problems have been cross-sectional, thus it is not clear whether emotional and behavioral problems are the cause or the result of toileting disturbances, or a combination of both. Additionally, it has been proposed that there might be potential common risk factors that underline the association between toileting disturbances and psychopathology. One example is the study conducted by Van Hoecke and colleagues (Eline Van Hoecke, Baeyens, Vande Walle, Hoebeke, & Roeyers, 2003) in which they examined 154 children with enuresis and 153 continent children, and found that although those with enuresis exhibited more internalizing and externalizing symptoms, when socioeconomic status (SES) was controlled for, this difference was no longer present. Longitudinal studies are needed to further examine and determine whether there is a causal relationship.

Consistent with the fact that there is little evidence to support the psychological etiology theories of toileting issues, few data exist indicating the treatment effect of psychotherapy to be significantly different from no-treatment controls (De Leon & Mandell, 1966; Werry & Cohrssen, 1965). A predominant treatment method targeting psychological disturbances is hypnosis, which often involves relaxation training and use of suggestions to provide sense of self-control. While many studies have reported significant treatment effects, they are often subjective to limitation due to the use of uncontrolled or single case study designs (Kohen, Olness, Colwell, & Heimel, 1984; Mellon, 2000; Olness, 1975). While no studies have been found that evaluated the effect of treatments of psychological problems on enuresis or encopresis, improvement in toileting functions were found to be correlated with amelioration of emotional disturbances (Longstaffe, Moffatt, & Whalen, 2000; Moffatt, Kato, & Pless, 1987).

Regardless of the nature and direction of the relationship between toileting difficulties and psychological disturbances, the implications of related studies remain significant. Children with psychological disturbances tend to be less compliant and thus, improvements of psychological symptoms may assist the attaining of continence. Due to the high comorbid rate and negative effects of the above-mentioned psychological issues, these concomitant disturbances should be assessed and treated, if needed, in children with toileting difficulties (Equit et al., 2013; von Gontard et al., 2011).

Conclusion

Challenges are faced by many children and their parents in the process of gaining independency in toileting. A significant portion of literature on self-help has been focused on toileting, and researchers have made great efforts to gather scientific evidence to develop effective treatment and intervention methods to facilitate toilet training. While the spotlight was initially taken by theories of psychological disturbances, with the advance in research studies and the accumulation of empirical evidence, behavioral and biological theories quickly took over and treatments based on these theories have received growing attention.

Behavioral theories based on the principles of learning have long been studied in relation to our acquisition of everyday life skills. In the application to toilet training, behavioral theories regard toileting difficulties as a result of failure to learn, more specifically, a lack of or false establishment of appropriate toileting behaviors. Behavioral treatments based on classical conditioning and operant conditioning (e.g., the use of urinary alarm apparatus, reinforcement of proper behaviors) have been widely adopted and were found to be the most effective intervention methods (Azrin et al., 1973; Brown et al., 2011; Cicero & Pfadt, 2002; Edgar et al., 1975; Ikeda et al., 2006; Lancioni et al., 2011; Lovibond, 1964; Wassom & Christophersen, 2014). Despite this success, behavioral theories and treatments are not free of limitations. In addition to high relapse and dropout rates (Azrin et al., 1973; Azrin & Thienes, 1978; Brown et al., 2011; Stover et al., 2008; van Londen et al., 1995), the behavioral approach's reach becomes restricted when there are organic disturbances (e.g., nervous system deficits, physical structure abnormalities) underlying toileting difficulties. While only a small fraction of children with toileting difficulties exhibit these disturbances, addressing organic impairments is necessary to allow advances in learning toileting skills. While lower than behavioral treatments, interventions targeting the biological components of the toileting process, primarily pharmacological treatments (e.g., imipramine, desmopressin) also have demonstrated significant treatment effects (Alloussi et al., 2011; Apostolidis et al., 2006; Butler, 2001).

At this time, there is a lack of evidence supporting the etiological theories of psychological disturbances. However, due to the high comorbid rates of psychological issues (e.g., anxiety, behavioral problems) and toileting problems, and the negative effects these emotional disturbances have on the functioning and learning of affected children, psychological disturbances are to be assessed and attended if needed (Equit et al., 2013; von Gontard, et al., 2011).

Research on the effect of treatments of emotional and behavioral problems on toileting functioning are needed to further examine the nature and direction of their connections. Future studies should also aim to construct and utilize a more precise taxonomy of elimination dysfunctions. This goal is necessitated by studies showing that treatment effects may vary based on the type of underlying disturbances (Alloussi et al., 2011). Inconsistent grouping of elimination disorders and standards of toileting success should also be addressed to allow better between-study comparisons. While behavioral, biological, and psychological theories each revolve around different aspects of toileting, they are not to be taken separately as, when integrated, they might provide better account and treatment effects (Alloussi et al., 2011; Brown et al., 2011; Mellon, 2000). With the ongoing accumulation of new knowledge, researchers should further refine these theoretical structures to reflect the growth in the field and to provide continued guidance for following scientific endeavor. Individuals involved in the training process should also be educated on this knowledge to better facilitate children in their acquisition of toileting independence.

References

Abramovitch, I. B., & Abramovitch, H. H. (1989). Enuresis in cross-cultural perspective: A comparison of training for elimination control in three Israeli ethnic groups. *The Journal of Social Psychology, 129*(1), 47–56. http://doi.org/10.1080/00224545.1989.9711698.

Aceto, G., Penza, R., Coccioli, M. S., Palumbo, F., Cresta, L., Cimador, M., …, & Caione, P. (2003). Enuresis subtypes based on nocturnal hypercalciuria: A multicenter study. *The Journal of Urology*, 170(4 Pt 2), 1670–1673. http://doi.org/10.1097/01.ju.0000091221.55082.17.

Alloussi, S. H., Mürtz, G., Lang, C., Madersbacher, H., Strugala, G., Seibold, J., …, & Alloussi, S. (2011). Desmopressin treatment regimens in monosymptomatic and nonmonosymptomatic enuresis: A review from a clinical perspective. *Journal of Pediatric Urology, 7*(1), 10–20. http://doi.org/10.1016/j.jpurol.2010.04.014.

Alpaslan, A. H., Koçak, U., Avci, K., & Güzel, H. I. (2016). Association between elimination disorders and abusive maternal attitudes. *Journal of Forensic and Legal Medicine, 40*, 22–27. http://doi.org/10.1016/j.jflm.2016.02.004.

American Psychiatric Association. (2013). *Diagnostic and statistical manual of mental disorders: DSM-5*. Arlington, VA: American Psychiatric Association.

Andersson, K.-E., & Schröder, A. (2004). Therapeutic strategies for drug treatment of stress urinary incontinence. *Drug Discovery Today: Therapeutic Strategies, 1*(2), 259–265. http://doi.org/10.1016/j.ddstr.2004.09.006.

Apostolidis, A., Dasgupta, P., & Fowler, C. J. (2006). Proposed mechanism for the efficacy of injected botulinum toxin in the treatment of human detrusor overactivity. *European Urology, 49*(4), 644–650. http://doi.org/10.1016/j.eururo.2005.12.010.

Araki, I., Kitahara, M., Oida, T., & Kuno, S. (2000). Voiding dysfunction and parkinson's disease: Urodynamic abnormalities and urinary symptoms. *The Journal of Urology, 164*(5), 1640–1643. http://doi.org/10.1016/S0022-5347(05)67048-6.

Austin, P. F., Bauer, S. B., Bower, W., Chase, J., Franco, I., Hoebeke, P., …, & Nevéus, T. (2014). The standardization of terminology of lower urinary tract function in children and adolescents: Update report from the standardization committee of the International Children's Continence Society. *The Journal of Urology, 191*(6), 1863–1865.e13. http://doi.org/10.1016/j.juro.2014.01.110.

Azrin, N., & Foxx, R. M. (1989). *Toilet training in less than a day*. New York, NY: Simon and Schuster.

Azrin, N. H., & Foxx, R. M. (1971). A rapid method of toilet training the institutionalized retarded. *Journal of Applied Behavior Analysis, 4*(2), 89–99.

Azrin, N. H., Sneed, T. J., & Foxx, R. M. (1973). Dry bed: A rapid method of eliminating bedwetting (enuresis) of the retarded. *Behaviour Research and Therapy, 11*(4), 427–434. http://doi.org/10.1016/0005-7967(73)90101-0.

Azrin, N. H., & Thienes, P. M. (1978). Rapid elimination of enuresis by intensive learning without a conditioning apparatus. *Behavior Therapy, 9*(3), 342–354. http://doi.org/10.1016/S0005-7894(78)80077-X.

Baer, D. M., Wolf, M. M., & Risley, T. R. (1968). Some current dimensions of applied behavior analysis. *Journal of Applied Behavior Analysis, 1*(1), 91–97. http://doi.org/10.1901/jaba.1968.1-91.

Baeyens, D., Roeyers, H., Hoebeke, P., Verté, S., Van Hoecke, E., & Walle, J. V. (2004). Attention deficit/hyperactivity disorder in children with nocturnal enuresis. *The Journal of Urology, 171*(6), 2576–2579. http://doi.org/10.1097/01.ju.0000108665.22072.b2.

Baeyens, D., Roeyers, H., Vande Walle, J., & Hoebeke, P. (2005). Behavioural problems and attention-deficit hyperactivity disorder in children with enuresis: A literature review. *European Journal of Pediatrics, 164*(11), 665–672. http://doi.org/10.1007/s00431-005-1712-1.

Bartley, J. M., Sirls, L. T., Killinger, K. A., & Boura, J. A. (2015). Secondary surgery after vaginal prolapse repair with mesh is more common for stress incontinence and voiding dysfunction

than for mesh problems or prolapse recurrence. *International Urology and Nephrology*, *47*(4), 609–615. http://doi.org/10.1007/s11255-015-0930-3.
Berkenwald, A., Pires, J., & Ellsworth, P. (2016). Evaluating use of higher dose oxybutynin in combination with desmopressin for refractory nocturnal enuresis. *Journal of Pediatric Urology*, *12*(4), 220.e1–220.e6. http://doi.org/10.1016/j.jpurol.2016.05.029.
Berk, L. B., & Friman, P. C. (1990). Epidemiologic aspects of toilet training. *Clinical Pediatrics*, *29*(5), 278–282. http://doi.org/10.1177/000992289002900505.
Betts, J. G., DeSaix, P., Johnson, E., & Johnson, J. E. (2013). *Anatomy and physiology*. Houston, TX: OpenStax College.
Bossingham, M. J., Carnell, N. S., & Campbell, W. W. (2005). Water balance, hydration status, and fat-free mass hydration in younger and older adults. *The American Journal of Clinical Nutrition*, *81*(6), 1342–1350.
Brandes, S., & Borrelli, J. (2001). Pelvic fracture and associated urologic injuries. *World Journal of Surgery*, *25*(12), 1578–1587. http://doi.org/10.1007/s00268-001-0153-x.
Brazelton, T. B. (1962). A child-oriented approach to toilet training. *Pediatrics*, *29*, 121–128.
Brown, M. L., Pope, A. W., & Brown, E. J. (2011). Treatment of primary nocturnal enuresis in children: A review. *Child: Care, Health and Development*, *37*(2), 153–160. http://doi.org/10.1111/j.1365-2214.2010.01146.x.
Bulchandani, S., & Thomson, A. (2015). Recent advances in urinary incontinence management: Drug review. *Prescriber*, *26*(12), 21–26. http://doi.org/10.1002/psb.1369.
Butler, R. J. (2001). Combination therapy for nocturnal enuresis. *Scandinavian Journal of Urology and Nephrology*, *35*(5), 364–369.
Byrd, R. S., Weitzman, M., Lanphear, N. E., & Auinger, P. (1996). Bed-wetting in US children: Epidemiology and related behavior problems. *Pediatrics*, *98*(3 Pt 1), 414–419.
Chopra, H. D. (1973). Treatment of encopresis in a mongol with operant conditioning. *Indian Journal of Mental Retardation*, *6*(1), 43–46.
Cho, P. S., Bauer, S. B., Pennison, M., Rosoklija, I., Bellows, A. L., Logvinenko, T., …, & Borer, J. G. (2016). Sacral agenesis and neurogenic bladder: Long-term outcomes of bladder and kidney function. *Journal of Pediatric Urology, 12*(3), 158.e1–158.e7. http://doi.org/10.1016/j.jpurol.2015.12.008.
Chua, M. E., Silangcruz, J. M., Chang, S.-J., Williams, K., Saunders, M., Lopes, R. I., …, & Yang, S. S. (2016). Desmopressin withdrawal strategy for pediatric enuresis: A meta-analysis. *Pediatrics, 138*(1), e20160495–e20160495. http://doi.org/10.1542/peds.2016-0495.
Chung, A. S. J., Cheng, J. N. C., & Tse, V. (2016). Psychotropic drugs and their effects on lower urinary tract function: An update. *Current Bladder Dysfunction Reports*, *11*(3), 258–265. http://doi.org/10.1007/s11884-016-0372-5.
Cicero, F. R., & Pfadt, A. (2002). Investigation of a reinforcement-based toilet training procedure for children with autism. *Research in Developmental Disabilities*, *23*(5), 319–331. http://doi.org/10.1016/S0891-4222(02)00136-1.
Clark, R. E. (2004). The classical origins of Pavlov's conditioning. *Integrative Physiological & Behavioral Science*, *39*(4), 279–294. http://doi.org/10.1007/BF02734167.
Clayton, D. B., Brock, J. W., & Joseph, D. B. (2010). Urologic management of spina bifida. *Developmental Disabilities Research Reviews*, *16*(1), 88–95. http://doi.org/10.1002/ddrr.92.
Cox, D. J. (2002). Psychological differences between children with and without chronic encopresis. *Journal of Pediatric Psychology*, *27*(7), 585–591. http://doi.org/10.1093/jpepsy/27.7.585.
Davis, S. F., & Buskist, W. (2008). *21st century psychology: A reference handbook*. Los Angeles, CA: Sage.
De Leon, G., & Mandell, W. (1966). A comparison of conditioning and psychotherapy in the treatment of functional enuresis. *Journal of Clinical Psychology*, *22*(3), 326–330.
de Seze, M., Ruffion, A., Denys, P., Joseph, P.-A., Perrouin-Verbe, B., & International Francophone Neuro-Urological expert study group (GENULF). (2007). The neurogenic bladder in multiple sclerosis: Review of the literature and proposal of management guidelines. *Multiple Sclerosis Journal*, *13*(7), 915–928. http://doi.org/10.1177/1352458506075651.

De Wachter, S., Vermandel, A., De Moerloose, K., & Wyndaele, J. J. (2002). Value of increase in bladder capacity in treatment of refractory monosymptomatic nocturnal enuresis in children. *Urology, 60*(6), 1090–1094.

Doleys, D. M. (1977). Behavioral treatments for nocturnal enuresis in children: A review of the recent literature. *Psychological Bulletin, 84*(1), 30–54.

Dorsher, P. T., & McIntosh, P. M. (2012). Neurogenic bladder. *Advances in Urology, 2012*, 1–16. http://doi.org/10.1155/2012/816274.

dos Santos Junior, A. C. S., de Miranda, D. M., & Simões e Silva, A. C. (2014). Congenital anomalies of the kidney and urinary tract: An embryogenetic review. *Birth Defects Research Part C: Embryo Today: Reviews, 102*(4), 374–381. http://doi.org/10.1002/bdrc.21084.

Drysdale, B., Lee, C. Y. Q., Anderson, A., & Moore, D. W. (2015). Using video modeling incorporating animation to teach toileting to two children with autism spectrum disorder. *Journal of Developmental and Physical Disabilities, 27*(2), 149–165. http://doi.org/10.1007/s10882-014-9405-1.

Duby, J. J., Campbell, R. K., Setter, S. M., & Rasmussen, K. A. (2004). Diabetic neuropathy: An intensive review. *American Journal of Health-System Pharmacy, 61*(2), 160–173.

Edgar, C. L., Kohler, H. F., & Hardman, S. (1975). A new method for toilet training developmentally disabled children. *Perceptual and Motor Skills, 41*(1), 63–69. http://doi.org/10.2466/pms.1975.41.1.63.

Eikeseth, S., Smith, T., Jahr, E., & Eldevik, S. (2002). Intensive behavioral treatment at school for 4- to 7-year-old children with autism. A 1-year comparison controlled study. *Behavior Modification, 26*(1), 49–68.

Equit, M., Klein, A.-M., Braun-Bither, K., Gräber, S., & von Gontard, A. (2013). Elimination disorders and anxious-depressed symptoms in preschool children: A population-based study. *European Child & Adolescent Psychiatry, 23*(6), 417–423. http://doi.org/10.1007/s00787-013-0468-9.

Faaborg, P. M., Christensen, P., Kvitsau, B., Buntzen, S., Laurberg, S., & Krogh, K. (2009). Long-term outcome and safety of transanal colonic irrigation for neurogenic bowel dysfunction. *Spinal Cord, 47*(7), 545–549. http://doi.org/10.1038/sc.2008.159.

Feeney, D. J. (2005). Elimination disorders: Enuresis and encopresis. In *Clinical child psychiatry* (2nd ed.pp. 327–341). Chichester: Wiley. doi:10.1002/0470022116.ch18

Fernald, P. S., & Fernald, L. D. (1999). Shaping behavior through operant conditioning. *Activities Handbook for the Teaching of Psychology, 4*, 176–180.

Fernberger, S. W. (1943). Edwin Burket Twitmyer: 1873–1943. *Psychological Review, 50*(3), 345–349. http://doi.org/10.1037/h0063068.

Fischer, N., Church, P., Lyons, J., & McPherson, A. C. (2015). A qualitative exploration of the experiences of children with spina bifida and their parents around incontinence and social participation: Incontinence in children with spina bifida. *Child: Care, Health and Development, 41*(6), 954–962. http://doi.org/10.1111/cch.12257.

Florin, I., & Tunner, W. (1970). Principles of operant conditioning in the treatment of severely retarded children. *Praxis der Kinderpsychologie und Kinderpsychiatrie, 19*(7), 253–259.

Fontaine, W. (2008). 21st century psychology: A reference handbook. *CHOICE: Current Reviews for Academic Libraries, 3*, 488.

Friman, P. C., & Jones, K. M. (2005). Behavioral treatment for nocturnal enuresis. *Journal of Early and Intensive Behavior Intervention, 2*(4), 259–267. http://doi.org/10.1037/h0100319.

Galiano, M., Guillot-Tantay, C., Sivaraman, A., Slaoui, H., Barret, E., Rozet, F., …, & Cathelineau, X. (2016). Superficial implantation of the I-Stop TOMS transobturator sling in the treatment of postprostatectomy urinary incontinence: Description of a novel technique and 1-year outcomes. *Urology, 90*, 195–199. http://doi.org/10.1016/j.urology.2015.10.040.

Gelber, D. A., Good, D. C., Laven, L. J., & Verhulst, S. J. (1993). Causes of urinary incontinence after acute hemispheric stroke. *Stroke, 24*(3), 378–382. http://doi.org/10.1161/01.STR.24.3.378.

Gomez, R. G., Ceballos, L., Coburn, M., Corriere, J. N., Dixon, C. M., Lobel, B., & McAninch, J. (2004). Consensus statement on bladder injuries. *BJU International*, *94*(1), 27–32. http://doi.org/10.1111/j.1464-410X.2004.04896.x.

Gor, R. A., Katorski, J. R., & Elliott, S. P. (2016). Medical and surgical management of neurogenic bowel. *Current Opinion in Urology*, *26*(4), 369–375. http://doi.org/10.1097/MOU.0000000000000299.

Hamano, S., Yamanishi, T., Igarashi, T., Ito, H., & Murakami, S. (2000). Functional bladder capacity as predictor of response to desmopressin and retention control training in monosymptomatic nocturnal enuresis. *European Urology*, *37*(6), 718–722. http://doi.org/10.1159/000020224.

Hanneman, M. J. G., Sprangers, M. A. G., De Mik, E. L., van Heurn, E. L. W., De Langen, Z. J., Looyaard, N., …, & Aronson, D. C. (2001). Quality of life in patients with anorectal malformation or hirschsprung's disease: Development of a disease-specific questionnaire. *Diseases of the Colon & Rectum, 44*(11), 1650–1660. http://doi.org/10.1007/BF02234386.

Havenga, K., Maas, C. P., DeRuiter, M. C., Welvaart, K., & Trimbos, J. B. (2000). Avoiding long-term disturbance to bladder and sexual function in pelvic surgery, particularly with rectal cancer. *Seminars in Surgical Oncology*, *18*(3), 235–243. http://doi.org/10.1002/(SICI)1098-2388(200004/05)18:3<235::AID-SSU7>3.0.CO;2-7.

Hindley, G. B., Filliozat, A. M., Klackenberg, G., Nicolet-Meister, D., & Sand, E. A. (1965). Some differences in infant feeding and elimination disorders: Enuresis training in five european longitudinal samples. *Journal of Child Psychology and Psychiatry*, *6*(3–4), 179–201. http://doi.org/10.1111/j.1469-7610.1965.tb02158.x.

Hinds, J. P., Eidelman, B. H., & Wald, A. (1990). Prevalence of bowel dysfunction in multiple sclerosis. *Gastroenterology*, *98*(6), 1538–1542.

Hoebeke, P., De waard, W., Raes, A., Dehoorne, J., Johan, V. w., & Van laecke, E. (2009). Extended experience with the use of botulinum toxin a in children with overactive bladder (OAB). *Journal of Pediatric Urology*, *5*, S72. http://doi.org/10.1016/j.jpurol.2009.02.124.

Holschneider, A., Hutson, J., Peña, A., Beket, E., Chatterjee, S., Coran, A., …, & Kunst, M. (2005). Preliminary report on the international conference for the development of standards for the treatment of anorectal malformations. *Journal of Pediatric Surgery, 40*(10), 1521–1526. http://doi.org/10.1016/j.jpedsurg.2005.08.002.

Hundziak, M., Maurer, R. A., & Watson, L. S. (1965). Operant conditioning in toilet training of severely mentally retarded boys. *American Journal of Mental Deficiency*, *70*(1), 120–124.

Hyams, G., McCoull, K., Smith, P. S., & Tyrer, S. P. (2008). Behavioural continence training in mental handicap: A 10-year follow-up study. *Journal of Intellectual Disability Research*, *36*(6), 551–558. http://doi.org/10.1111/j.1365-2788.1992.tb00573.x.

Ikeda, K., Koga, A., & Minami, S. (2006). Evaluation of a cure process during alarm treatment for nocturnal enuresis. *Journal of Clinical Psychology*, *62*(10), 1245–1257. http://doi.org/10.1002/jclp.20301.

Joinson, C., Heron, J., Butler, U., von Gontard, A., & Avon Longitudinal Study of Parents and Children Study Team. (2006). Psychological differences between children with and without soiling problems. *Pediatrics*, *117*(5), 1575–1584. http://doi.org/10.1542/peds.2005-1773.

Joinson, C., Heron, J., Emond, A., & Butler, R. (2007). Psychological problems in children with bedwetting and combined (day and night) wetting: A UK population-based study. *Journal of Pediatric Psychology*, *32*(5), 605–616.

Joinson, C., Heron, J., von Gontard, A., & the ALSPAC Study Team. (2006). Psychological problems in children with daytime wetting. *Pediatrics*, *118*(5), 1985–1993. http://doi.org/10.1542/peds.2006-0894.

Jorge, M. J. N., & Wexner, S. D. (1993). Etiology and management of fecal incontinence. *Diseases of the Colon & Rectum*, *36*(1), 77–97. http://doi.org/10.1007/BF02050307.

Kaerts, N. (2013). Studies on toilet training in healthy children. In *Including when to start, the use of readinees signs, current toilet training practices in day care and the relation between day care and parents*. Antwerpen, Belgium: Universiteit.

Kay, S., Tolley, K., Colayco, D., Khalaf, K., Anderson, P., & Globe, D. (2013). Mapping EQ-5D utility scores from the Incontinence Quality of Life Questionnaire among patients with neurogenic and idiopathic overactive bladder. *Value in Health, 16*(2), 394–402. http://doi.org/10.1016/j.jval.2012.12.005.

Kimble, G. A. (1967). *Foundations of conditioning and learning*. New York, NY: Appleton-Century-Crofts. Retrieved from http://libezp.lib.lsu.edu/login?url=http://search.ebscohost.com/login.aspx?direct=true&db=cat00252a&AN=lalu.679399&site=eds-live&scope=site&profile=eds-main.

Kocaoglu, M., & Frush, D. P. (2006). Pediatric presacral masses. *Radiographics: A Review Publication of the Radiological Society of North America, Inc, 26*(3), 833–857. http://doi.org/10.1148/rg.263055102.

Kohen, D. P., Olness, K. N., Colwell, S. O., & Heimel, A. (1984). The use of relaxation-mental imagery (self-hypnosis) in the management of 505 pediatric behavioral encounters. *Journal of Developmental & Behavioral Pediatrics, 5*(1), 21–25.

Konorski, J. (1948). *Conditioned reflexes and neuron organization*. Cambridge, UK: Cambridge University Press.

Koraitim, M. M., Marzouk, M. E., Atta, M. A., & Orabi, S. S. (1996). Risk factors and mechanism of urethral injury in pelvic fractures. *British Journal of Urology International, 77*(6), 876–880. http://doi.org/10.1046/j.1464-410X.1996.01119.x.

Krogh, K., & Christensen, P. (2009). Neurogenic colorectal and pelvic floor dysfunction. *Best Practice & Research Clinical Gastroenterology, 23*(4), 531–543. http://doi.org/10.1016/j.bpg.2009.04.012.

Krogh, K., Christensen, P., Sabroe, S., & Laurberg, S. (2006). Neurogenic bowel dysfunction score. *Spinal Cord, 44*(10), 625–631. http://doi.org/10.1038/sj.sc.3101887.

Krogh, K., Ostergaard, K., Sabroe, S., & Laurberg, S. (2007). Clinical aspects of bowel symptoms in Parkinson's disease. *Acta Neurologica Scandinavica, 117*(1), 60–64. http://doi.org/10.1111/j.1600-0404.2007.00900.x.

Lancioni, G. E., Singh, N. N., O'Reilly, M. F., Sigafoos, J., Bosco, A., Zonno, N., & Badagliacca, F. (2011). Persons with mild or moderate Alzheimer's disease learn to use urine alarms and prompts to avoid large urinary accidents. *Research in Developmental Disabilities, 32*(5), 1998–2004. http://doi.org/10.1016/j.ridd.2011.04.011.

Landman, B. W. M., Van capelle, J. W., Kollen, B. J., & Steffens, M. G. (2009). Intravesical botox injections in children with a therapy resistant idiopathic overactve bladder. *Journal of Pediatric Urology, 5*, S72. http://doi.org/10.1016/j.jpurol.2009.02.125.

LeBlanc, L. A., Carr, J. E., Crossett, S. E., Bennett, C. M., & Detweiler, D. D. (2005). Intensive outpatient behavioral treatment of primary urinary incontinence of children with autism. *Focus on Autism and Other Developmental Disabilities, 20*(2), 98–105. http://doi.org/10.1177/10883576050200020601.

Lie, H. R., Lagergren, J., Rasmussen, F., Lagerkvist, B., Hagelsteen, J., Börjeson, M.-C., … Taudorf, K. (2008). Bowel and bladder control of children with myelomeningocele: A Nordic study. *Developmental Medicine & Child Neurology, 33*(12), 1053–1061. http://doi.org/10.1111/j.1469-8749.1991.tb14827.x.

Longstaffe, S., Moffatt, M. E., & Whalen, J. C. (2000). Behavioral and self-concept changes after six months of enuresis treatment: A randomized, controlled trial. *Pediatrics, 105*(4 Pt 2), 935–940.

Lottmann, H. B., & Alova, I. (2007). Primary monosymptomatic nocturnal enuresis in children and adolescents. *International Journal of Clinical Practice, 61*(155), 8–16. http://doi.org/10.1111/j.1742-1241.2007.01464.x.

Lovibond, S. H. (1964). *Conditioning and enuresis*. Elmsford, NY: Microforms International Marketing Corp.

Lukac, M., Sindjic-Antunovic, S., Vujovic, D., Petronic, I., Nikolic, D., Radlovic, V., … Krstic, Z. (2016). Effectiveness of various surgical methods in treatment of Hirschsprung's disease in children. *Vojnosanitetski Pregled, 73*(3), 246–250. http://doi.org/10.2298/VSP140516002L.

Luxem, M., & Christophersen, E. (1994). Behavioral toilet training in early childhood: Research, practice, and implications. *Journal of Developmental and Behavioral Pediatrics, 15*(5), 370–378.

Macias, M. M., Roberts, K. M., Saylor, C. F., & Fussell, J. J. (2006). Toileting concerns, parenting stress, and behavior problems in children with special health care needs. *Clinical Pediatrics, 45*(5), 415–422. http://doi.org/10.1177/0009922806289616.

Madersbacher, H. (1990). The various types of neurogenic bladder dysfunction: An update of current therapeutic concepts. *Paraplegia, 28*(4), 217–229. http://doi.org/10.1038/sc.1990.28.

Mark, S. D., & Frank, J. D. (1995). Nocturnal enuresis. *British Journal of Urology, 75*(4), 427–434. http://doi.org/10.1111/j.1464-410X.1995.tb07259.x.

Marquis, D. G., & Porter, J. M., Jr. (1939). Differential characteristics of conditioned eyelid responses established by reflex and voluntary reinforcement. *Journal of Experimental Psychology, 24*(4), 347–365. http://doi.org/10.1037/h0061007.

Masel, B. E. (2004). Rehabilitation and hypopituitarism after traumatic brain injury. *Growth Hormone & IGF Research, 14*, 108–113. http://doi.org/10.1016/j.ghir.2004.03.024.

Mash, E. J., & Barkley, R. A. (2006). *Treatment of childhood disorders*. New York, NY: Guilford press.

McCartney, J. R., & Holden, J. C. (1981). Toilet training for the mentally retarded. In J. L. Matson & J. R. McCartney (Eds.), *Handbook of behavior modification with the mentally retarded* (pp. 29–60). Boston, MA: Springer US. Retrieved from http://link.springer.com/10.1007/978-1-4615-7130-8_2.

Mellon, M. W. (2000). Empirically supported treatments in pediatric psychology: Nocturnal enuresis. *Journal of Pediatric Psychology, 25*(4), 193–214. http://doi.org/10.1093/jpepsy/25.4.193.

Mellon, M. W., Natchev, B. E., Katusic, S. K., Colligan, R. C., Weaver, A. L., Voigt, R. G., & Barbaresi, W. J. (2013). Incidence of enuresis and encopresis among children with attention-deficit/hyperactivity disorder in a population-based birth cohort. *Academic Pediatrics, 13*(4), 322–327. http://doi.org/10.1016/j.acap.2013.02.008.

Moffatt, M. E., Kato, C., & Pless, I. B. (1987). Improvements in self-concept after treatment of nocturnal enuresis: Randomized controlled trial. *The Journal of Pediatrics, 110*(4), 647–652.

Moore, E. E., Jackson, S. L., Boyko, E. J., Scholes, D., & Fihn, S. D. (2008). Urinary incontinence and urinary tract infection: Temporal relationships in postmenopausal women. *Obstetrics & Gynecology, 111*(2, Part 1), 317–323. http://doi.org/10.1097/AOG.0b013e318160d64a.

Mowrer, O. H., & Mowrer, W. M. (1938). Enuresis—A method for its study and treatment. *American Journal of Orthopsychiatry, 8*(3), 436–459. http://doi.org/10.1111/j.1939-0025.1938.tb06395.x.

Murphy, E. S., & Lupfer, G. J. (2014). Basic principles of operant conditioning. In F. K. McSweeney & E. S. Murphy (Eds.), *The Wiley Blackwell handbook of operant and classical conditioning* (pp. 165–194). Oxford, UK: John Wiley & Sons, Ltd.. Retrieved from http://doi.wiley.com/10.1002/9781118468135.ch8.

Murphy, K. P., Boutin, S. A., & Ide, K. R. (2012). Cerebral palsy, neurogenic bladder, and outcomes of lifetime care. *Developmental Medicine and Child Neurology, 54*(10), 945–950. http://doi.org/10.1111/j.1469-8749.2012.04360.x.

Nakai, H., Asanuma, H., Shishido, S., Kitahara, S., & Yasuda, K. (2003). Changing concepts in urological management of the congenital anomalies of kidney and urinary tract, CAKUT. *Pediatrics International, 45*(5), 634–641. http://doi.org/10.1046/j.1442-200X.2003.01782.x.

Nevéus, T., von Gontard, A., Hoebeke, P., Hjälmås, K., Bauer, S., Bower, W., … Djurhuus, J. C. (2006). The standardization of terminology of lower urinary tract function in children and adolescents: Report from the standardisation committee of the International Children's Continence Society. *The Journal of Urology, 176*(1), 314–324. http://doi.org/10.1016/S0022-5347(06)00305-3.

Norton, P. A., Zinner, N. R., Yalcin, I., & Bump, R. C. (2002). Duloxetine versus placebo in the treatment of stress urinary incontinence. *American Journal of Obstetrics and Gynecology, 187*(1), 40–48. http://doi.org/10.1067/mob.2002.124840.

Olness, K. (1975). The use of self-hypnosis in the treatment of childhood nocturnal enuresis. A report on forty patients. *Clinical Pediatrics*, *14*(3), 273–275, 278–279.

Önol, F. F., Guzel, R., Tahra, A., Kaya, C., & Boylu, U. (2015). Comparison of long-term efficacy of desmopressin lyophilisate and enuretic alarm for monosymptomatic enuresis and assessment of predictive factors for success: A randomized prospective trial. *The Journal of Urology*, *193*(2), 655–661. http://doi.org/10.1016/j.juro.2014.08.088.

Peña, A. (1995). Anorectal malformations. In *Seminars in pediatric surgery* (vol. 4, pp. 35–47). Philadelphia, PA: WB Saunders Co.

Pierce, W. D., & Cheney, C. D. (2004). *Behavior analysis and learning* (3rd ed.). Mahwah, NJ: Lawrence Erlbaum Associates.

Plant, K. M., & Sanders, M. R. (2007). Predictors of care-giver stress in families of preschool-aged children with developmental disabilities. *Journal of Intellectual Disability Research*, *51*(2), 109–124. http://doi.org/10.1111/j.1365-2788.2006.00829.x.

Pomeranz, A., Abu-Kheat, G., Korzets, Z., & Wolach, B. (2000). Night-time polyuria and urine hypo-osmolality in enuretics identified by nocturnal sequential urine sampling: Do they represent a subset of relative adh-deficient subjects? *Scandinavian Journal of Urology and Nephrology*, *34*(3), 199–202. http://doi.org/10.1080/003655900750016599.

Poussaint, A. F., & Ditman, K. S. (1965). A controlled study of imipramine (Tofranil) in the treatment of childhood enuresis. *The Journal of Pediatrics*, *67*(2), 283–290. http://doi.org/10.1016/S0022-3476(65)80252-9.

Rabadi, M. H., & Aston, C. (2014). Complications and urologic risks of neurogenic bladder in veterans with traumatic spinal cord injury. *Spinal Cord*, *53*, 200–203. http://doi.org/10.1038/sc.2014.205.

Radomski, S. B. (2014). Update on medical therapy for male LUTS. *Canadian Urological Association Journal*, *8*(7–8 Suppl 5), S148.

Radvanska, E., Kovács, L., & Rittig, S. (2006). The role of bladder capacity in antidiuretic and anticholinergic treatment for nocturnal enuresis. *The Journal of Urology*, *176*(2), 764–769. http://doi.org/10.1016/S0022-5347(06)00595-7.

Rasquin, A., Di Lorenzo, C., Forbes, D., Guiraldes, E., Hyams, J. S., Staiano, A., & Walker, L. S. (2006). Childhood functional gastrointestinal disorders: Child/adolescent. *Gastroenterology*, *130*(5), 1527–1537. http://doi.org/10.1053/j.gastro.2005.08.063.

Redsell, S. A., & Collier, J. (2001). Bedwetting, behaviour and self-esteem: A review of the literature. *Child: Care, Health and Development*, *27*(2), 149–162.

Robertson, G. L. (2016). Diabetes insipidus: Differential diagnosis and management. *Best Practice & Research Clinical Endocrinology & Metabolism*, *30*(2), 205–218. http://doi.org/10.1016/j.beem.2016.02.007.

Robson, W. L., Jackson, H. P., Blackhurst, D., & Leung, A. K. (1997). Enuresis in children with attention-deficit hyperactivity disorder. *Southern Medical Journal*, *90*(5), 503–505.

Romeo, G., Ronchetto, P., Luo, Y., Barone, V., Seri, M., Ceccherini, I., … Martucciello, G. (1994). Point mutations affecting the tyrosine kinase domain of the RET proto-oncogene in Hirschsprung's disease. *Nature*, *367*(6461), 377–378. http://doi.org/10.1038/367377a0.

Schulze, P. A. (2000). The cultural structuring of universal developmental tasks (Doctoral dissertation). Retrieved from http://digitalcommons.uconn.edu/dissertations/AAI9982001.

Schulze, P. A., Harwood, R. L., Schoelmerich, A., & Leyendecker, B. (2002). The cultural structuring of parenting and universal developmental tasks. *Parenting*, *2*(2), 151–178. http://doi.org/10.1207/S15327922PAR0202_04.

Sharma, S. (2015). Sacral agenesis with neurogenic bladder dysfunction— A case report and review of the literature. *Journal of Clinical and Diagnostic Research.*, *9*(6), RD08–RD09. http://doi.org/10.7860/JCDR/2015/13694.6113.

Shrestha, A., Anderson, A., & Moore, D. W. (2013). Using point-of-view video modeling and forward chaining to teach a functional self-help skill to a child with autism. *Journal of Behavioral Education*, *22*(2), 157–167. http://doi.org/10.1007/s10864-012-9165-x.

Skinner, B. F. (1937). Two types of conditioned reflex: A reply to Konorski and Miller. *The Journal of General Psychology*, *16*(1), 272–279. http://doi.org/10.1080/00221309.1937.9917951.
Skinner, B. F. (1953). *Science and human behavior*. New York, NY: Simon and Schuster.
Skinner, B. F. (1990). *The behavior of organisms: An experimental analysis*. Cambridge, MA: B. F. Skinner Foundation.
Sloane, E. (1994). *Anatomy and physiology: An easy learner*. Boston ; London: Jones & Bartlett Learning.
Stanhewicz, A. E., & Larry Kenney, W. (2015). Determinants of water and sodium intake and output. *Nutrition Reviews*, *73*(suppl 2), 73–82. http://doi.org/10.1093/nutrit/nuv033.
Stenberg, A., & Lackgren, G. (1994). Desmopressin tablets in the treatment of severe nocturnal enuresis in adolescents. *Pediatrics*, *94*(6), 841.
Stephany, H. A., Clayton, D. B., Tanaka, S. T., Thomas, J. C., Pope, J. C., Brock, J. W., & Adams, M. C. (2014). Development of upper tract stones in patients with congenital neurogenic bladder. *Journal of Pediatric Urology*, *10*(1), 112–117. http://doi.org/10.1016/j.jpurol.2013.07.005.
Stout, N. R., Kenny, R. A., & Baylis, P. H. (1999). A review of water balance in ageing in health and disease. *Gerontology*, *45*(2), 61–66. http://doi.org/10.1159/000022063.
Stover, A. C., Dunlap, G., & Neff, B. (2008). The effects of a contingency contracting program on the nocturnal enuresis of three children. *Research on Social Work Practice*, *18*(5), 421–428. http://doi.org/10.1177/1049731507314007.
Stover, S. L., Lloyd, L. K., Waites, K. B., & Jackson, A. B. (1991). Neurogenic urinary tract infection. *Neurologic Clinics*, *9*(3), 741–755.
Thompson, I. M., & Lauvetz, R. (1976). Oxybutynin in bladder spasm, neurogenic bladder, and enuresis. *Urology*, *8*(5), 452–454. http://doi.org/10.1016/0090-4295(76)90273-9.
Thorndike, E. L. (1965). *Animal intelligence: Experimental studies*. New Brunswick, NJ: Transaction Publishers.
Tomasi, P. A., Siracusano, S., Monni, A. M., Mela, G., & Delitala, G. (2001). Decreased nocturnal urinary antidiuretic hormone excretion in enuresis is increased by imipramine. *BJU International*, *88*(9), 932–937.
Twitmyer, E. B. (1905). Knee-jerks without stimulation of the patellar tendon. *Psychological Bulletin*, *2*, 43–44.
Van Hoecke, E., Baeyens, D., Vande Walle, J., Hoebeke, P., & Roeyers, H. (2003). Socioeconomic status as a common factor underlying the association between enuresis and psychopathology. *Journal of Developmental and Behavioral Pediatrics: JDBP*, *24*(2), 109–114.
Van Hoecke, E., Hoebeke, P., Braet, C., & Walle, J. (2004). An assessment of internalizing problems in children with enuresis. *The Journal of Urology*, *171*(6), 2580–2583. http://doi.org/10.1097/01.ju.0000110521.20103.14.
van Londen, A., van Londen-Barentsen, M. W., van Son, M. J., & Mulder, G. A. (1995). Relapse rate and subsequent parental reaction after successful treatment of children suffering from nocturnal enuresis: A 2 1/2 year follow-up of bibliotherapy. *Behaviour Research and Therapy*, *33*(3), 309–311.
van Nunen, K., Kaerts, N., Wyndaele, J.-J., Vermandel, A., & Hal, G. V. (2015). Parents' views on toilet training (TT): A quantitative study to identify the beliefs and attitudes of parents concerning TT. *Journal of Child Health Care*, *19*(2), 265–274. http://doi.org/10.1177/1367493513508232.
von Gontard, A. (2013). The impact of DSM-5 and guidelines for assessment and treatment of elimination disorders. *European Child & Adolescent Psychiatry*, *22*(S1), 61–67. http://doi.org/10.1007/s00787-012-0363-9.
von Gontard, A., Baeyens, D., Van Hoecke, E., Warzak, W. J., & Bachmann, C. (2011). Psychological and psychiatric issues in urinary and fecal incontinence. *The Journal of Urology*, *185*(4), 1432–1437. http://doi.org/10.1016/j.juro.2010.11.051
von Gontard, A., Mauer-Mucke, K., Plück, J., Berner, W., & Lehmkuhl, G. (1999). Clinical behavioral problems in day-and night-wetting children. *Pediatric Nephrology*, *13*(8), 662–667.
von Gontard, A., Moritz, A. M., Thome-Granz, S., & Freitag, C. (2011). Association of attention deficit and elimination disorders at school entry: A population based study. *The Journal of Urology, 186*(5), 2027–2032. http://doi.org/10.1016/j.juro.2011.07.030.

Walker, C. E., Kenning, M., & Faust-Capanille, J. (1989). Enuresis and encopresis. In E. J. Mash, R. A. Barkley, & E. J. Mash (Eds.), *Treatment of childhood disorders* (pp. 423–448). New York, NY: Guilford Press. Retrieved from http://libezp.lib.lsu.edu/login?url=http://search.ebscohost.com/login.aspx?direct=true&db=psyh&AN=1989-97947-012&site=ehost-live&scope=site.

Wallner, C., Lange, M. M., Bonsing, B. A., Maas, C. P., Wallace, C. N., Dabhoiwala, N. F., … van de Velde, C. J. H. (2008). Causes of fecal and urinary incontinence after total mesorectal excision for rectal cancer based on cadaveric surgery: A study from the cooperative clinical investigators of the dutch total mesorectal excision trial. *Journal of Clinical Oncology*, *26*(27), 4466–4472. http://doi.org/10.1200/JCO.2008.17.3062.

Wassom, M. C., & Christophersen, E. R. (2014). A clinical application of evidence-based treatments in pediatric functional constipation and incontinence. *Clinical Practice in Pediatric Psychology*, *2*(3), 294–311. http://doi.org/10.1037/cpp0000069.

Waye, M. F., & Melnyr, W. T. (1973). Toilet training of a blind retarded boy by operant conditioning. *Journal of Behavior Therapy and Experimental Psychiatry*, *4*(3), 267–268. http://doi.org/10.1016/0005-7916(73)90085-2.

Welk, B., Al-Hothi, H., Winick-Ng, J., Chou, Q., MacMillan, B., & Lawendy, A.-R. (2015). The effect of pelvic factures on future stress incontinence and pelvic organ prolapse surgery. *International Urogynecology Journal*, *26*(6), 805–811. http://doi.org/10.1007/s00192-014-2624-2.

Werry, J. S., & Cohrssen, J. (1965). Enuresis – An etiologic and therapeutic study. *The Journal of Pediatrics*, *67*, 423–431.

Wille, S. (1994). Primary nocturnal enuresis in children. Background and treatment. *Scandinavian Journal of Urology and Nephrology. Supplementum*, *156*, 1–48.

Yang, T.-K., Guo, Y.-J., Chang, H.-C., Yang, H.-J., & Huang, K.-H. (2015). Attention deficit-hyperactivity disorder symptoms and daytime voiding symptoms in children with primary enuresis: An observational study to evaluate the effectiveness of desmopressin treatment. *The Scientific World Journal*, *2015*, 1–6. http://doi.org/10.1155/2015/356121.

Problems Associated with Toilet Training

David A. Wilder and Ansley C. Hodges

Incontinence can impose residential, educational, and vocational limits on individuals. For example, children who are incontinent may be barred from day care settings, camps, and some school settings. Adolescents and adults with intellectual and other disabilities who are incontinent may have difficulty securing day placement programs, jobs, and some living arrangements. In addition, incontinence can create social and health problems. Incontinent individuals are often socially ostracized, and may be at increased risk of infection from contact with fecal matter. Appropriate toileting enables a level of independence that is often not otherwise achieved and is one of the most important skills an individual learns in his or her lifetime (Cicero & Pfadt, 2002; Kroeger & Sorensen-Burnworth, 2009; Lott & Kroeger, 2004).

Typically developing children are trained to use the toilet between 20 and 36 months of age, although there may be a trend toward earlier toilet training in recent decades (Luxem & Christophersen, 1994; Tarhan et al., 2015). Individuals with intellectual disabilities are often trained to use the toilet later in life. In some cases, toilet training may even occur well into adulthood (Averink, Melein, & Duker, 2005; Wilder, Higbee, Williams, & Nachtwey, 1997). Not surprisingly, research suggests that individuals with disabilities who have fewer skills are less likely to master toilet training (Lohmann, Eyman, & Lask, 1967).

Surprisingly, there is a dearth of empirical literature on toilet training typically developing children (Vermandel, Van Kampen, Van Gorp, & Wyndaele, 2008; Warzak, Forcino, Sanberg, & Gross, 2016). The existing studies are largely based off the pioneering toilet training procedures described by Foxx and Azrin (1973), in

D.A. Wilder (✉)
Florida Institute of Technology, School of Behavior Analysis,
150 West University Blvd, Melbourne, FL 32901, USA
e-mail: dawilder@fit.edu

A.C. Hodges
Florida Institute of Technology, Melbourne, FL, USA

J.L. Matson (ed.), *Clinical Guide to Toilet Training Children*, Autism and Child Psychopathology Series, DOI 10.1007/978-3-319-62725-0_6

which the authors successfully trained 34 children between the ages of 20 and 36 months to use the toilet. Training took less than 4 h on average, and a 4-month follow-up showed that participants were nearly accident-free. The Foxx and Azrin procedure consisted of a number of components, including fluid loading (i.e., increased liquid consumption), frequent practice trials in which participants sit on the toilet, immediate delivery of high-preference items contingent upon urination in the toilet, overcorrection contingent upon accidents, and fading of prompts and reinforcers. Since Foxx and Azrin, subsequent studies have used some of these components in refined toilet training procedures. For example, Simon and Thompson (2006) and Halligan and Luyben (2009) reported using fluid loading, reinforcement for urinating in the toilet, and prompted practice trials, but not overcorrection, to train typically developing children.

Toilet training individuals with disabilities was pioneered by Ellis (1963), who used a fairly simple approach, highlighting the delivery of positive reinforcement for appropriate urination. Some years later, Azrin and Foxx (1971) developed a comprehensive toilet training protocol for individuals with disabilities, called the "rapid toilet training" method. Many features of this method were subsequently incorporated into the Foxx and Azrin (1973) procedure for training typically developing children described above. The rapid toilet training method consists of fluid loading, scheduled practice trials, delivery of social and edible reinforcement for urination in the toilet, a urine alarm (attaches to participant underwear) which produces sound when wet, graduated guidance (a prompting hierarchy for dressing and undressing), and a 1-h time-out from reinforcement procedure contingent upon accidents. Azrin and Foxx trained 9 individuals with intellectual disabilities to use the toilet with very few accidents after training. The procedure took about 4 days per participant.

Since Azrin and Foxx (1971), a number of related procedures have been developed to toilet train individuals with disabilities. Nearly all of these procedures are at least partially based on the rapid toilet training method. For example, Cicero and Pfadt (2002) made use of fluid loading, graduated guidance, positive reinforcement, and a punishment procedure. Averink et al. (2005) used similar features, and added a response restriction component, in which participants were prevented from engaging in responses incompatible with appropriate toileting.

Regardless of the details of the procedure used, toilet training both typically developing children and individuals with disabilities is not without complications. In some cases, individuals have behavioral problems that may interfere with the acquisition of toileting skills (Lohmann et al., 1967). These behavioral problems include aggression, self-injury, and noncompliance with the toileting procedure. In addition, because it is parents who often train their children to use the toilet appropriately, problems involving parents sometimes arise. These include resource barriers and problems with parent implementation of specific techniques.

Behavioral Problems and Toilet Training

Behavioral problems such as aggression, self-injury, and noncompliance can make toilet training difficult. Although not common among young children, aggression and self-injury are relatively common among individuals with intellectual disabilities (Lundqvist, 2013). Noncompliance, the most common behavioral problem, is often a concern among young children as well as individuals with disabilities (McMahon & Forehand, 2003). In this section, we review these behavioral problems and provide some suggestions for managing them during the toilet training process.

A few empirical studies have illustrated the assessment and treatment of behavioral problems occurring in the context of toilet training. Hagopian, Fisher, Piazza, and Wierzbicki (1993) used a water prompting procedure to toilet train a 9 year-old boy with an intellectual disability who engaged in severe self-injurious behavior (SIB): body slamming, head banging, and knee biting during toileting. Other procedures, such as reinforcement for appropriate voids, reinforcement plus overcorrection, and reinforcement plus a differential reinforcement of other behavior (DRO) schedule for the absence of SIB, were ineffective. The water prompting procedure consisted of the therapist pouring lukewarm water over the participant's genitals when he was sitting on the toilet and was implemented with a DRO schedule. This procedure resulted in an increase in urinations on the toilet and a decrease in SIB. The authors speculate that the DRO procedure, in which access to preferred music was delivered contingent upon the absence of SIB, was essential to decreasing the self-injury.

More recently, Brown and Peace (2011) used Azrin and Foxx's (1971) rapid toilet training method to train a 13 year-old boy with a disability who exhibited aggression when prompted to urinate on the toilet at school. The authors posited that aggression occurred to avoid or escape the instructions delivered during the toilet training procedure. Through the use of escape extinction (continuing to deliver instructions despite aggression), the authors reported that continence was achieved within 2 weeks and maintained during a 24-month follow-up. After success at school, the program was successfully implemented at home.

Luiselli (1977) described a 15 year-old boy with an intellectual disability who exhibited a phobia of toileting, which resulted in avoidance of the toilet and vocal protests when prompted to use the toilet. The child was noncompliant with most toileting instructions. The author used social and token reinforcement for appropriate urination and time-out from positive reinforcement contingent upon accidents. This reduced accidents and resulted in an increase in appropriate urinations even after discontinuation of the program.

As these studies illustrate, behavioral problems such as self-injury and aggression may occur during the context of toilet training. Clinicians should conduct a functional assessment of these behavioral problems prior to initiating toilet training. The purpose of a functional assessment is to identify the environmental variables maintaining the behavioral problems. Possible functions of these behaviors include social positive reinforcement (access to attention, access to preferred items or activities), social negative reinforcement (escape from demands), or automatic reinforcement (access to non-socially mediated sources of reinforcement).

The results of the functional assessment can be thought of as a description of the "purpose" of the behavioral problems. If the results of the functional assessment suggest that the behavioral problems function to access attention or a preferred item, a few intervention options exist. The first is to provide attention or access to items independent of toileting instructions. The second is to refrain from providing attention or access to items contingent upon behavioral problems. The third intervention option is to provide attention or access to items contingent upon an appropriate request for attention or an item / activity.

In some cases, these behavioral problems may function to escape toilet training. If this is the case, different intervention options exist. The first is to provide frequent, short breaks independent of the problematic behavior (i.e., regardless of when it occurs). The second is to continue to deliver toileting instructions and, if necessary, physically guide compliance with these instructions. The third is to provide short breaks from toileting instructions contingent upon an appropriate request for a break.

If results of the functional assessment suggest that the behavioral problems function to produce access to automatic reinforcement, other intervention options exist. The first is to provide free access to items or activities that provide stimulation similar to the type of stimulation produced by the problematic behavior. For example, if an individual hits himself in the eye to produce visual stimulation, providing free access to visually stimulating items (e.g., toys, digital games, lighting conditions) during toilet training may decrease self-injury. Another intervention option is to block the occurrence of the behavioral problem and proceed with training. For a more detailed description of intervention options for behavioral problems maintained by various environmental events, see Wacker, Berg, Harding, and Cooper-Brown (2011). If these interventions are ineffective, medications may be available to assist.

Although self-injury, aggression, and toileting phobias can be severe, the most common type of behavioral problem associated with toilet training is noncompliance. Many individuals may not comply with one or more toilet training procedures. When confronted with noncompliance, parents, teachers, and therapists may postpone or even abandon training.

Boelens, Van den Broek, and Beieshuizen (2003) described four typically developing children (ages 4–10) who were noncompliant with toilet training procedures. A urine alarm was part of the toileting procedure, and three of the four children were noncompliant with wearing the alarm or with wearing the alarm correctly. Although the authors tried a number of techniques to manage participant noncompliance, including a token system in which the children could earn special time with a parent and a trip to an amusement park, these methods were ultimately ineffective for 3 of the 4 children. Only 1 participant was successfully trained to urinate in the toilet.

Luxem, Christophersen, Purvis, and Baer (1997) describe 11 participants who were noncompliant with toilet training. They used 3 treatments, each consisting of a combination of medical and behavioral procedures, to decrease toileting refusal. The procedures included bowel cleansing, diet modifications, reinforcement of urination in the toilet, and time-out from positive reinforcement for accidents. The procedures took between 16 and 87 days to produce an effect, but were eventually effective for all participants. Measures of parent satisfaction showed that parents were satisfied with the outcome.

As the study described above illustrates, noncompliance with toilet training might be addressed in a variety of ways. Two broad classes of interventions have been developed to increase compliance. Antecedent-based interventions involve some manipulation of the stimulus or events that precede the opportunity to comply (e.g., changing the way the instruction is delivered). Consequence-based interventions involve manipulation of events that come after the opportunity to comply (e.g., changing how someone responds to the noncompliance).

Antecedent-based interventions to increase compliance include making eye contact when delivering instructions (Hanley, Heal, Tiger, & Ingvarsson, 2007), and phrasing instructions in "do" form as opposed to "don't" form (Neef, Shafer, Egel, Cataldo, and Parrish, 1983). Both of these interventions have been shown to be effective to increase compliance with at least some individuals, and should be used when delivering instructions related to toilet training. Although these techniques have not been specifically applied to toilet training, there is no reason to believe their effects would differ in this context.

Another antecedent-based intervention to increase compliance is the high-probability (high-p) sequence (Mace et al., 1988). The high-p sequence consists of a series of instructions with which an individual is likely to comply immediately followed by a lower-probability, or target, instruction. Reinforcement is delivered for compliance with each instruction. The high-p sequence is based on behavioral momentum, which states that the "momentum" of compliance generated via the high-p instructions might increase the likelihood of compliance to the low-probability instruction. In the context of toileting, this might take the form of a parent or therapist telling a child to "Touch your nose", "Give me five", "Give me a fist bump" and then "Sit on the toilet". Of course, as with all interventions to increase compliance, the individual's noncompliance must be due to a lack of appropriate contingencies (i.e., a motivational problem) as opposed to a skill deficit. If noncompliance is due to a skill deficit, such a procedure is unlikely to be effective.

The high-p sequence has received mixed support in the empirical literature. Although some studies have found it to be effective (Mace et al., 1988), others have not (Rortvedt & Miltenberger, 1994). It has not been specifically applied to increase compliance with toilet training, but there is no reason to believe its effects would be any different in this context.

Consequence-based interventions to increase compliance include guided compliance, or three-step prompting (Horner & Keilitz, 1975). Guided compliance incorporates three progressively intrusive prompts to increase compliance. Noncompliance with any of the prompts results in the parent or therapist moving to the next prompt. For example, a parent first provides the instruction (i.e., "sit on the toilet"). If the individual complies, the parent delivers praise. Contingent upon the absence of compliance, the parent reissues the vocal prompt while simultaneously modeling the task. If the individual complies, the parent delivers praise. Contingent upon the absence of compliance, the parent reissues the vocal prompt while simultaneously guiding the individual to comply.

Guided compliance procedures have been shown to be effective in many, but not all, applications (Wilder & Atwell, 2006). As with the high-p sequence, guided compliance procedures have not been specifically applied to increase compliance with toileting. However, there is no reason to believe their effects would be any different in this context.

Another commonly-used consequence-based intervention to increase compliance is differential reinforcement (i.e., delivering reinforcement for compliance and withholding reinforcement for noncompliance) or providing contingent access to preferred items or activities. This procedure has been used to increase compliance in a variety of contexts (Russo, Cataldo & Cushing, 1981). It is also a component of many toilet training protocols, including Azrin and Foxx (1971) and Foxx and Azrin (1973). When using differential reinforcement, one of the most important components is to deliver items or activities that are highly preferred by the individual. For that reason, a stimulus preference assessment (Fisher et al., 1992) might be conducted with the individual being trained to identify high preference items.

In summation, trainee behavioral problems such as aggression, self-injury, and noncompliance may occur in the context of toilet training. These behaviors may impede successful training and should be addressed as early as possible in the toilet training process to increase the likelihood of a successful outcome. Table 1 provides a description of behavioral problems commonly observed in the context of toilet training and a summary of interventions to address these problems.

Problems Involving Parent Implementation of Toilet Training Procedures

In addition to behavioral problems exhibited by individuals undergoing training, in some cases the trainers themselves experience barriers or exhibit performance problems that may impede successful training of the individuals under their care. This section describes research on training parents to implement toilet training procedures, as well as some limitations and problems that have been reported. Some brief suggestions to address these problems are also provided.

Research has identified several barriers that may impede a parent's ability to effectively and efficiently toilet train their child. According to the American Academy of Pediatrics (2003), parents might push their child too early to be toilet trained and ignore the developmental level of their child. Thus, teaching parents about developmental milestones and readiness, rather than emphasizing readiness based solely on chronological age, might help mitigate these issues.

Table 1 Suggestions to address behavioral problems during toilet training

Behavioral problem	Suggestion	Specific suggestions
Self-injury	Conduct functional assessment (see specific suggestions for behavior maintained by social positive reinforcement, social negative reinforcement, or automatic reinforcement)	If behavior is maintained by *social positive reinforcement*- use free access to attention or items, withhold attention or items after behavioral problem If behavior is maintained by *social negative reinforcement*- use breaks independent of problematic behavior or provide breaks for appropriate behavior. If maintained by *automatic reinforcement*- provide free access to similar stimulation or use blocking
Aggression	See self-injury suggestions	See self-injury specific suggestions
Noncompliance	Provide direct eye contact when delivering instruction Use "Do" instead of "Don't" phrasing High-P sequence Guided compliance Differential reinforcement	

A study by Van Nunen, Kaerts, Wyndaele, Vermandel, and Van Hal (2015) highlights this concern. The authors used questionnaires to examine parental beliefs and attitudes concerning toilet training. Specifically, 2000 questionnaires were distributed across 50 schools to parents of children between the ages of 30–36 months. Approximately 58% of questionnaires were returned. Results showed 61% of the parents reported that children should be toilet trained before 30 months. When training occurred later than 30 months, most parents reported that late training was due to parental time constraints (39%), use of disposable diapers (36.4%), or that toilet training was not as important as other demands (19.7%).

Another potential barrier associated with toileting is parental stress. Macias, Roberts, Saylor and Fussell (2006) examined the correlation between parental stress, toilet training concerns, and behavioral problems exhibited by children with special needs. Multiple questionnaires were completed by 170 parents of children with or without toileting concerns. One was the Child Behavior Checklist (CBCL), the results of which indicated significantly more personal distress for parents of incontinent children versus parents of continent children. Moreover, parents of children with an IQ of 70 or below reported more stress associated with incontinence than did parents with children whose IQ was above 70. Overall, this study suggests that parental stress is increased when a child is incontinent. The authors recommended using a parental stress index prior to implementing toilet training procedures, and then perhaps selecting the most appropriate procedures for parents given their stress level.

Ritblatt, Obegi, Hammons, Ganger, and Ganger (2003) compared how parents and childcare professionals implement toilet training, and what resources each group consults during the process. In this study, 89 parents and 97 child care professionals served as participants; the latter were predominately teachers, but also included teachers' aides. Parent questionnaires consisted of 23 questions, and childcare professional questionnaires comprised 16 questions; most questions required only a "yes" or "no" response. This study examined four essential toilet training topics: age of initiation, readiness, practices, and response to accidents. The authors also examined toilet training resources in their questionnaires.

Over 84% of childcare professionals sought advice from books or magazines. Conversely, parents who reported soliciting toilet training advice said they would be more likely to ask friends and family members. The authors reported that less than 50% of parents solicited advice on toilet training; if they did ask for recommendations, they approached other family members (48%) or friends (24%). Only 15–21% of parents reported that they consulted with medical professionals or childcare providers. Finally, although both parents and professionals agreed that children should not be punished for accidents, the Ritblatt et al. (2003) study did suggest differences in the approach to toilet training taken by parents and childcare professionals. Parents were somewhat more likely to use a punishment-based procedure. Overall, this study suggests that when parents, childcare providers, or teachers do not collaborate on toilet training procedures, the process may become more challenging for the child, delay implementation, and create more stress for the family as a whole (Kaerts et al., 2014).

Lack of time, stress, and potential disagreement with teachers and aides at school regarding when and how to toilet train can impede parental implementation of toilet training programs. However, other problems, such as the effort involved in training, the number of individuals to train or simply parental noncompliance with procedures, are also concerns. The studies described below illustrate these problems.

Mahoney, Van Wagenen, and Meyerson (1971) investigated five males diagnosed with an intellectual disability and three children without a known disability. The authors conducted sessions in a school setting. Baseline data were collected on appropriate toileting skills. Then, the experimenters trained a sequence of toileting skills including walking to the toilet, lowering pants, sitting on (or standing in front of) the toilet, voiding, and pulling up pants. Results of this phase of the experiment showed that seven of the eight participants acquired toileting skills at the school.

After initial training was completed, the experimenters conducted three sessions that focused on maintenance of acquired skills, saying "potty" while going to the toilet, and parent training. In the latter, parents were brought into the training location and instructed in the procedures. After the three sessions, two parents, one of whom had a child diagnosed with a disability and one of whom had a typically developing child, were selected for follow-up in the home. Over a span of 6 months, each parent provided information on their child's toileting skills. For the parent of the child without a disability, interviews suggested that toileting accidents decreased from 4 per week to 1 per week over 6 months. For the parent of the participant diagnosed with a disability, approximately four toileting accidents per week occurred for the entire 6-month follow-up period. The experimenter visited the home and noted that the parent was prompting the child to use the toilet. As a result, toileting accidents tended to occur when the parent was not present. The authors reported that feedback had no effect on the parent's behavior. Thus, this study illustrates that problems with parent adherence might relate to the effort involved in cleaning up after toileting accidents. For some parents, prompting a child to toilet might be easier (even if it results in accidents when the parent is absent) than implementing the many steps involved in correctly implementing a toilet training protocol.

Although parents were not involved, Smith, Britton, Johnson, and Thomas (1975) reported some problems when toilet training a group of adults with intellectual disabilities who resided in an institution. Some of the problems involved noncompliance on the part of the residents being trained, but the authors reported more difficulty with the nurses who were training the residents. They found that the most effective approach was to assign one nurse to each individual resident, instead of having one nurse responsible for training many residents. As this study illustrates, time and number of other responsibilities (i.e., competing contingencies) can impact the integrity of toilet training procedures.

More recently, Kroeger and Sorensen-Burnworth (2010) evaluated the effects of a parent-training program to increase continence. Participants included a 4-year-old boy without a history of toilet training and a 4-year-old boy with a failed history of toilet training; both children were diagnosed with autism. Baseline data were collected on the number of toileting accidents, as well as the number of self-initiations. Parent training consisted of explanations, demonstrations, and feedback to the parents as they implemented the procedures with their child. Written instructions were also provided. After the training was completed, the trainer was available for consultation.

The toileting intervention included five components. In the first component, both participants had increased access to fluids for 3 days prior to the intervention through the first day of treatment. In the second component, participants were scheduled to sit on the toilet. Initially, participants sat on the toilet for 30 min with a 5-min break for successful voids on the toilet. While on the toilet, participants had access to preferred toys. In the next phase, participants sat on the toilet for 25 min with a 10-min break for voids. The last phase consisted of 20 min periods of sitting with a 15-min break for voids. If the required sitting time expired without a void, participants were released from sitting on the toilet for 2 min, but were required to remain in the bathroom until the next sitting period.

In the third component, preferred edibles and activities were delivered for voiding and self-initiation of toileting. In the fourth component, toileting accidents were followed by a statement describing where toileting should occur; then, a toilet sitting session was implemented. If the participant finished voiding in the toilet, preferred items and activities were presented as described above. In the final component, self-initiation was trained. The participants sat in a chair next to the toilet for the scheduled sessions. When a void began, if the participant did not move to the toilet, physical guidance was provided. The chair was moved in increments of 2 ft until it was 20 ft from the toilet. When self-initiation without toileting accidents was achieved, generalization was programmed by requiring participants to toilet in other bathrooms in the home, as well as other bathrooms outside the home.

Results of the intervention showed that the number of toileting accidents substantially decreased, while the number of self-initiations increased. During a return to baseline condition, improvements were maintained. Finally, during a follow up assessment after 2 weeks, 6 months, and 3 years, there were no toileting accidents and participants self-initiated on 100% of occasions. This study showed that parents can successfully implement toilet training in a relatively brief period of time, as the training duration was only 4 days. Finally, a social validity assessment was conducted after follow-up, and the parents reported a high degree of satisfaction with the procedures and their effectiveness. The authors noted two advantages of training the primary caregivers, rather than part-time caregivers, such as teachers' assistants. First, primary caregivers have a strong motivation to teach and maintain continence; second, primary caregivers may be more sensitive to subtle cues and behaviors of the trainee, so training may proceed more rapidly.

Interestingly, the authors reported that both participants' parents contacted the trainer on five occasions. Both parents had questions regarding prompt dependency, how to fade out their prompts, and how to fade out the protocol. Similar prompting issues were reported in Mahoney et al. (1971). Parents in these studies struggled with how and when to stop prompting their child to use the toilet and may not always understand that the goal is that the sensation of needing to urinate or defecate comes to "control" going to and sitting on the toilet, not a parental prompt. Thus, prompts should be initially paired with that sensation (or evidence or reports of it) and then faded, both in frequency and topography or magnitude (e.g., begin with vocal and physical prompt, fade to vocal only, and then fade to partial vocal prompt, if necessary). Future research should examine this topic.

LeBlanc, Carr, Crossett, Bennett, and Detweiler (2005) also evaluated the effects of a toilet training procedure. Their study included three children diagnosed with autism ranging in age from 4 years 1 month to 4 years 11 months, all of whom had been previously unsuccessful with toilet training. The participants' parents included two single mothers and a mother and father. This study was initially conducted in an outpatient clinic (Day 1) and then transferred to the home environment on subsequent days (Day 2 and 3) with a follow-up training in the preschool classroom (Day 4). The toilet training protocol included six components: a sitting schedule, rewards for successful voids on the toilet and self-initiations, increased fluid intake, communication training, a urine alarm, and positive practice for accidents. However, some elements of the Azrin and Foxx (1971) procedure were omitted. Accidents were followed with positive practice, but not restitutional overcorrection as in the Azrin and Foxx (1971) study. In the positive practice procedure, voids outside of the toilet resulted in a brief reprimand and then a 1 min toilet sit. Then, participants were required to practice the appropriate steps four consecutive times. Scheduled sittings were programmed across 12 different levels. Participants progressed through one level per hour on day 1, one level per half day on days 2 and 3, and then one level every 2 days until the schedule was completely faded.

Much like the sitting schedule, fluid delivery was also programmed. On the first day, participants were prompted to drink fluids every 5 min for the first hour, every 10 min during the second hour, every 15 min during the third hour, and every 30 min throughout the remainder of day 1. The authors estimated that participants consumed between 2 and 4 ounces of fluid per hour.

The initial training was conducted in an outpatient clinic from 9:00 AM to 4:00 PM. Additionally, parents observed the training during the first 2 h and then began to conduct the training with feedback and support from the researchers. At the end of Day 1, all participants achieved at least level six of scheduled sitting, allowing the participants to be off the toilet for 45 min. When training commenced in the parents' home on days two and three, the researchers were available via phone consultation. On the fourth day, the participants returned to their preschool environments for level eight of the scheduled sitting. At the preschool, the researchers trained the teachers and remained in the classroom throughout the duration of the morning to ensure proper carryover and accurate toileting protocol implementation.

All participants decreased the number of accidents from baseline. Self-initiation data were less consistent and compelling. Self-initiations were at 80% for one participant, but at lower levels for the other two. LeBlanc et al. (2005) suggested that problems with self-initiations might have occurred because the parents often prompted the children to use the restroom. Moreover, the authors suggested that the parents fade out the prompts, but the parents did not follow this recommendation, which was also reported by Mahoney et al. (1971), and Kroeger and Sorensen-Burnworth (2010). Again, it is possible that parents were unsure as to how and when to fade the prompts.

Taylor, Cipani, and Clardy (1994) investigated the effects of a toilet training procedure based on modifications of Azrin and Foxx (1971). Procedures were implemented by the father of a 10-year-old boy; this child was diagnosed with autism and had a developmental age of 2 years and 1 month. Initial attempts with the standard procedure (Azrin & Foxx, 1971) were unsuccessful. The authors hypothesized that the sensation of wearing undergarments had acquired stimulus control over urination; thus, urination occurred only when the undergarments were on and frequently occurred just after putting on the undergarments. Therefore, the procedural modification involved removal of the undergarments for periods of time during training, and then gradually increasing the duration of undergarment use. Results showed a substantial decrease in toileting accidents and an increase in appropriate urination. At a 10-month follow up, toileting accidents were eliminated. Parent evaluation of the procedure was positive.

This study is an example of hypothesis-driven intervention, as the authors identified a potential stimulus control problem that was addressed by their procedural modification. One concern with the procedure was the time spent without wearing any undergarments. Although the parent reported that the total time was not appreciably different from the time without undergarments when frequently changing diapers throughout the day, this procedure may not be feasible for parents whose children are enrolled in a childcare or educational setting.

Coehlo (2011) examined encopresis, which is defined as defecation anywhere other than the toilet, either involuntary or intentionally, at least once a month. The prevalence of encopresis is over 4% among 5–6 year-old children (Van Der Wal, Benninga, & Hirasing, 2005), but Coehlo suggested that it may be underreported. Indeed, the failure to report encopresis could be attributed to parents' feelings of guilt, as some report that encopresis may be linked to sexual abuse, poor diet, or low physical activity. Moreover, treatment for encopresis is demanding, as it involves some or all of the following: dietary changes, bowel training (e.g., taking child to the toilet 10 min after meals and remaining on the toilet for 20 min), use of behavior management techniques (e.g., schedules, pictures, rewards), and possibly medications (e.g., oral stool softeners, bran). To illustrate their points, the authors presented a case study of an 8-year-old boy, Joel, who exhibited encopresis and nightly bed-wetting. Joel was a typically developing 8-year-old with some fine and gross motor delays. Treatment required his parents to administer a quarter teaspoon of bran once a day, and increase this by an additional quarter teaspoon every third day until bowel movements were soft and occurring daily. Joel consumed 64 oz. of water daily, and had a variety of dietary restrictions and exercise requirements. He was prompted to attempt bowel movements 20 min after each meal. A reward system for having a dry bed each night was also used. The authors reported success during the school year, but parents could not adhere to the stringent and demanding schedule when they traveled for summer vacation; as a result, a medication was ultimately required. Thus, this study shows that adherence to toileting protocols can be a challenge, especially over extended periods of time. Practitioners should consider informing parents of the time and resources toilet training might require before beginning training, and obtain a commitment to stick with the procedure at that time.

Rinald and Mirenda (2012) evaluated the effects of parent training workshops on toileting skills. The experimenters presented a 4–5 h workshop that involved written descriptions, video demonstrations, role playing with a doll, and quizzes. Feedback was provided on quiz performance. The workshops focused on toileting procedures similar to those reported by Azrin and Foxx (1971), and included periodic toilet sitting, increased fluids to provide more toileting opportunities, and reinforcement for appropriate toileting. Toileting accidents were followed by changing clothes without specifically commenting on the accident. Scheduled delivery of reinforcement was thinned to either one at the end of an accident-free day, or after every 10 successful voids in the toilet.

After the workshop, a PowerPoint™ presentation and other materials were given to the parents for reference at home. Then, the parents began the toilet training process for approximately 8 h per day over 5–8 days. A researcher was available by phone for consultation. Included in the toilet training procedure was data collection on toileting accidents, child-initiated toileting, and adult-initiated toileting. After the initial training, there was a follow-up conducted after 2 weeks, and again after 1 month. For all participants, toileting accidents decreased, and urination in the toilet increased. However, the proportion of child-initiated versus adult-initiated sittings varied across participants and time. Only one participant showed exclusive child-initiated toileting.

Thus, the study showed positive results, as accidents decreased, but child-initiation data were less compelling. Interestingly, the researchers reported between 2 and 11 parent requests for assistance over the 8 days. Moreover, a social validity rating scale suggested that the parents were very pleased with the results, but several reported the toilet training as quite difficult and time consuming. In fact, one parent reported it was the most arduous task she had ever done. These reports are not surprising, given the time required over the course of 5–8 days. A cost analysis suggested their procedure was more economical than training implemented by a behavior analyst or other professional. Nevertheless, although the cost of their procedure may be more economical than some alternatives, the procedure could still be cost prohibitive for families with limited financial means; a 4–5 h workshop and 5–8 days of training at home can be expensive. Moreover, the time required to implement this procedure could limit some parents' ability to effectively and consistently adhere to the demanding procedural requirements. In addition to obtaining a parental commitment, practitioners might solicit assistance from outside of the home to help parents train, particularly in cases in which the trainee exhibits behavioral problems or has been unsuccessful in the past.

Ardiç and Cavkaytar (2014) evaluated a modified rapid toilet training method to train three children with autism. The procedural modifications included: (a) a reduction in the training procedure from 8 to 6 h; (b) elimination of the urination detection device; and (c) elimination of overcorrection for toileting accidents. The latter was included because Chung (2007) reported that overcorrection did not increase the number of voids in the toilet. In addition, this study only required children to sit on the toilet for 10 min and conduct dry pants checks every 30 min. The authors also reported that the parents were satisfied with the modified protocol. Two of the three participants successfully voided in the toilet, and parent training was effective for two of the three participants. One of the parents did not implement the procedures at home. The authors did not explicitly report why this occurred, although it is possible that the effort involved (i.e., 6 h per day over as many as 6 days) could have been a factor.

In addition to obtaining a commitment and soliciting assistance for difficult cases, practitioners might consider reducing the number of components of the toilet training procedure so that only those that are essential are used. Indeed, researchers have examined the effects of protocols with fewer, less time-consuming procedures and have had some success (Ardiç & Cavkaytar 2014). These procedural modifications are particularly important given the fact that toileting children, particularly those with special needs, is associated with a high degree of stress and a lot of time (Macias et al. 2006). Thus, future research might continue to refine toilet training protocols to decrease the time and effort involved in their implementation and ultimately increase parental compliance.

In summation, the parent training research on toileting skills has focused on different training methods such as direct training of skills with a parent (e.g., Kroeger & Sorensen-Burnworth, 2010; Leblanc et al., 2005), workshops (Rinald & Mirenda, 2012), consultations (e.g., Kroeger & Sorensen-Burnworth, 2010; Rinald & Mirenda, 2012; LeBlanc et al., 2005), and written materials (Rinald & Mirenda, 2012). One commonly reported problem is parental adherence to the toilet training protocols

Table 2 Suggestions to address parental barriers and performance problems during toilet training

Parental barrier/performance problem	Suggestions
Time/stress	Provide advanced notice of time and effort involved Obtain a commitment to finish the protocol Solicit assistance from others outside the home
Noncompliance with implementation	Use only essential toilet training protocol components

(e.g., Leblanc et al., 2005). The time and effort involved is an important factor in the success of the training. Table 2 provides a summary of common implementation barriers and potential solutions.

Conclusion

Toileting is an important life skill to master for young children and individuals with disabilities. A number of problems may occur in the context of training, including trainee behavioral problems such as aggression, self-injury, and noncompliance. In addition, trainer implementation barriers, such as the time and cost of training, may also impede progress. Relatively few studies have focused on behavioral problems occurring in the context of toileting; implementation barriers have also received little empirical attention. Clinicians should evaluate and address these problems as soon as they are detected to increase the likelihood of successful toilet training.

References

Ardiç, A., & Cavkaytar, A. (2014). Effectiveness of the modified intensive toilet training method on teaching toilet skills to children with autism. *Education and Training in Autism and Developmental Disabilities*, *49*(2), 263–276.

Averink, M., Melein, L., & Duker, P. C. (2005). Establishing diurnal bladder control with the response restriction method: Extended study on its effectiveness. *Research in Developmental Disabilities*, *26*(2), 143–151. doi:10.1016/j.ridd.2004.02.001

Azrin, N. H., & Foxx, R. M. (1971). A rapid method of toilet training the institutionalized retarded. *Journal of Applied Behavior Analysis*, *4*(2), 89–99. doi:10.1901/jaba.1971.4-89

Boelens, H., van den Broek, S., & Beishuizen, J. (2003). Using a pants alarm for the treatment of day wetting: Problems with compliance. *Psychological Reports*, *93*(3 Pt 2), 1073–1076. doi:10.2466/PR0.93.8.1073-1076

Brown, F. J., & Peace, N. (2011). Teaching a child with challenging behaviour to use the toilet: A clinical case study. *British Journal of Learning Disabilities*, *39*(4), 321–326. doi:10.1111/j.1468-3156.2011.00676.x

Chung, K. (2007). Modified version of Azrin and Foxx's rapid toilet training category. *Journal of Developmental and Physical Disabilities*, *19*(5), 449–455. doi:http://dx.doi.org.portal.lib.fit.edu/10.1007/s10882-007-9062-8

Cicero, F. R., & Pfadt, A. (2002). Investigation of reinforcement-based toilet training procedure for children with autism. *Research in Developmental Disabilities*, *23*, 319–331. doi:10.1016/s0891-4222(02)00136

Coehlo, D. P. (2011). Encopresis: A medical and family approach. *Pediatric Nursing*, *37*(3), 107–113.

Ellis, N. R. (1963). Toilet training the severely defective patient: An SR reinforcement analysis. *American Journal of Mental Deficiency*, *68*(98), 98–103.
Fisher, W., Piazza, C. C., Bowman, L. G., Hagopian, L. P., Owens, J. C., & Slevin, I. (1992). A comparison of two approaches for identifying reinforcers for persons with severe and profound disabilities. *Journal of Applied Behavior Analysis*, *25*, 491–498. doi:10.1901/jaba.1992.25-491.
Foxx, R. M., & Azrin, N. H. (1973). Dry pants: A rapid method of toilet training children. *Behavior Research and Therapy*, *11*(4), 435–442. doi:10.1016/0005-7967(73)90102-2
Hagopian, L. P., Fisher, W., Piazza, C. C., & Wierzbicki, J. J. (1993). A water prompting procedure for the treatment of urinary incontinence. *Journal of Applied Behavior Analysis*, *26*(4), 473–474. doi:10.1901/jaba.1993.26-473
Halligan, S. M., & Luyben, P. D. (2009). Prompts, feedback, positive reinforcement, and potty training. *Journal of Prevention & Intervention in the Community*, *37*(3), 177–186. doi:10.1080/10852350902976031
Hanley, G. P., Heal, N. A., Tiger, J. H., & Ingvarsson, E. T. (2007). Evaluation of a classwide teaching program for developing preschool life skills. *Journal of Applied Behavior Analysis*, *40*, 277–300. doi:http://dx.doi.org/10.1901/jaba.2007.57-06.
Horner, R. D., & Keilitz, I. (1975). Training mentally retarded adolescents to brush their teeth. *Journal of Applied Behavior Analysis*, *8*(3), 301–309. doi:10.1901%2Fjaba.1975.8-301.
Kaerts, N., Vermandel, A., Van Hal, G., & Wyndaele, J. (2014). Toilet training in healthy children: Results of a questionnaire study involving parents who make use of day-care at least once a week. *Neurology and Urodynamics*, *33*(3), 316–323. doi:10.1002/nau.22392.
Kroeger, K., & Sorensen-Burnworth, R. (2010). A parent training model for toilet training children with autism. *Journal of Intellectual Disability Research*, *54*(6), 556–567. doi:10.1111/j.1365-2788.2010.01286.x
Kroeger, K. A., & Sorensen-Burnworth, R. (2009). Toilet training individuals with autism and other developmental disabilities: A critical review. *Research in Autism Spectrum Disorders*, *3*(3), 607–618. doi:10.1016/j.rasd.2009.01.005
LeBlanc, L. A., Carr, J. E., Crossett, S. E., Bennett, C. M., & Detweiler, D. D. (2005). Intensive outpatient behavioral treatment of primary urinary incontinence of children with autism. *Focus on Autism and Other Developmental Disabilities*, *20*(2), 98–105. doi:10.1177/10883576050200020601
Lott, J. D., & Kroeger, K. A. (2004). Self-help skills in persons with mental retardation. In J. L. Matson, R. B. Laud, & M. L. Matson (Eds.), *Behavior modification for persons with developmental disabilities: Treatment and supports* (vol. 2). New York, NY: National Association for the Dually Diagnosed.
Lohmann, W., Eyman, R. K., & Lask, E. (1967). Toilet training. *American Journal of Mental Deficiency*, *71*(4), 551–557.
Lundqvist, L. O. (2013). Prevalence and risk markers of behavior problems among adults with intellectual disabilities: A total population study in Örebro County, Sweden. *Research in Developmental Disabilities*, *34*, 1346–1356. doi:10.1016/j.ridd.2013.01.010
Luiselli, J. K. (1977). Case report: An attendant-administered contingency management programme for the treatment of toileting phobia. *Journal of Intellectual Disability Research*, *21*(4), 283–288. doi:10.1111/j.1365-2788.1977.tb01591.x
Luxem, M., & Christophersen, E. (1994). Behavioral toilet training in early childhood: Research, practice, and implications. *Journal of Developmental & Behavioral Pediatrics*, *15*(5), 370-378. doi:10.1097/00004703-199410000-00009
Luxem, M. C., Christophersen, E. R., Purvis, P. C., & Baer, D. M. (1997). Behavioral-medical treatment of pediatric toileting refusal. *Journal of Developmental & Behavioral Pediatrics*, *18*(1), 34–41. doi:10.1097/00004703-199702000-00007
Mace, F. C., Hock, M. L., Lalli, J. S., West, B. J., Belfiore, P., Pinter, E., & Brown, D. K. (1988). Behavioral momentum in the treatment of noncompliance. *Journal of Applied Behavior Analysis*, *21*(2), 123–141. doi:10.1901/jaba.1988.21-123
Macias, M. M., Roberts, K. M., Saylor, C. F., & Fussell, J. J. (2006). Toileting concerns, parenting stress, and behavior problems in children with special health care needs. *Clinical Pediatrics*, *45*(5), 415–422. doi:10.1177/0009922806289616

Mahoney, K., Van Wagenen, R. K., & Meyerson, L. (1971). Toilet training of normal and retarded children. *Journal of Applied Behavior Analysis*, *4*(3), 173–181. doi:10.1901/jaba.1971.4173

McMahon, R. J., & Forehand, R. L. (2003). *Helping the noncompliant child: Family-based treatment for oppositional behavior* (2nd ed.). New York, NY: Guilford Press.

Neef, N. A., Shafer, M. S., Egel, A. L., Cataldo, M. F., & Parrish, J. M. (1983). The class specific effects of compliance training with "do" and "Don't" requests: Analogue analysis and classroom application. *Journal of Applied Behavior Analysis*, *16*, 81–99. doi:10.1901/jaba.1983.16-81

Rinald, K., & Mirenda, P. (2012). Effectiveness of a modified rapid toilet training workshop for parents of children with developmental disabilities. *Research in Developmental Disabilities*, *33*(3), 933–943. doi:10.1016/j.ridd.2012.01.003

Ritblatt, S. N., Obegi, A. D., Hammons, B. S., Ganger, T. A., & Ganger, B. C. (2003). Parents' and child care professionals' toilet training attitudes and practices: A comparative analysis. *Journal of Research in Childhood Education*, *17*(2), 133–146. doi:10.1080/02568540309595005

Rortvedt, A. K., & Miltenberger, R. G. (1994). Analysis of a high-probability instructional sequence and time-out in the treatment of child noncompliance. *Journal of Applied Behavior Analysis*, *27*, 327–330. doi:http://dx.doi.org/10.1901/jaba.1994.27-327.

Russo, D. C., Cataldo, M. F., & Cushing, P. J. (1981). Compliance training and behavioral covariation in the treatment of multiple behavior problems. *Journal of Applied Behavior Analysis*, *14*, 209–222. doi:http://dx.doi.org/10.1901/jaba.1981.14-209.

Simon, J. L., & Thompson, R. H. (2006). The effects of undergarment type on the urinary continence of toddlers. *Journal of Applied Behavior Analysis*, *39*(3), 363–368. doi:10.1901/jaba.2006.124-05

Smith, P. S., Britton, P. G., Johnson, M., & Thomas, D. A. (1975). Problems involved in toilet -training profoundly mentally handicapped adults. *Behaviour Research and Therapy*, *13*(4), 301–307. doi:10.1016/0005-7967(75)90035-2

Tarhan, H., Çakmak, Ö., Akarken, İ., Ekin, R. G., Ün, S., Uzelli, D., & Cun, S. (2015). Toilet training age and influencing factors: A multicenter study. *The Turkish Journal of Pediatrics*, *57*, 172–176.

Taylor, S., Cipani, E., & Clardy, A. (1994). A stimulus control technique for improving the efficacy of an established toilet training program. *Journal of Behavior Therapy and Experimental Psychology*, *25*(2), 155–160. doi:10.1016/0005-7916(94)90010-8

Van Der Wal, M. F., Benninga, M. A., & Hirasing, R. A. (2005). The prevalence of encopresis in a multicultural population. *Journal of Pediatric Gastroenterology and Nutrition*, *40*(3), 345–348. doi:10.1097/01.mpg.0000149964.77418.27

Van Nunen, K., Kaerts, N., Wyndaele, J., Vermandel, A., & Van Hal, G. V. (2015). Parents' views on toilet training (TT): A quantitative study to identify the beliefs and attitudes of parents concerning TT. *Journal of Child Health Care*, *19*(2), 265–274. doi:10.1177/1367493513508232

Vermandel, A., Van Kampen, M., Van Gorp, C., & Wyndaele, J. (2008). How to toilet train healthy children? A review of the literature. *Neurology and Urodynamics*, *27*(3), 162–166. doi:10.1002/nau.20490.

Wacker, D., Berg, W., Harding, J., & Copper-Brown, L. (2011). Functional and structural approaches to behavioral assessment of problem behavior. In W. Fisher, C. Piazza, & H. Roane (Eds.), *Handbook of applied behavior analysis*. London: The Guilford Press.

Warzak, W. J., Forcino, S. S., Sanberg, S. A., & Gross, A. C. (2016). Advancing continence in typically developing children: Adapting the procedures of Foxx and Azrin for primary care. *Journal of Behavioral Pediatrics*, *37*(1), 83–87. doi:10.1097/DBP.0000000000000232

Wilder, D. A., & Atwell, J. (2006). Evaluation of a guided compliance procedure to reduce noncompliance among preschool children. *Behavioral Interventions*, *21*, 265–272. doi:10.1002/bin.222.

Wilder, D. A., Higbee, T. S., Williams, W. L., & Nachtwey, A. (1997). A simplified method of toilet training adults in residential settings. *Journal of Behavior Therapy and Experimental Psychiatry*, *28*(3), 241–246. doi:10.1016/S0005-7916(97)00022-0

Wolraich, M. L., & Tippins, S. (2003). *American academy of pediatrics guide to toilet training*. New York, NY: Bantam Dell.

Monitoring Progress in Toilet Training

William J. Warzak, Abigail E. Kennedy, and Kayzandra Bond

Toilet training research is far more recent than toilet training itself, yet the practical challenges of training children to become continent have remained the same whether they take place in a research setting or in the home. While toilet training is a universal experience, cultural, familial, and historical variables affect the final common procedural pathway to toileting independence. Nevertheless, successful attainment of continence is the rule and a developmental milestone eagerly anticipated by parents.

Many training protocols have been developed to facilitate acquisition of continence skills. These range from structured, parent-directed protocols epitomized by the work of Foxx and Azrin (1973a; hereafter referred to as the *Foxx and Azrin* procedure) to unstructured, child-guided protocols such as those of Brazelton (1962), Schmitt (2004), and Spock (1946; hereafter collectively referred to as the *child-oriented* method). While both procedures have their adherents and history of success, structured protocols are more frequently evaluated in research settings, in part because they lend themselves to precise measurement (e.g., Klassen et al., 2006) and precise progress monitoring. Regardless of the protocol, measuring progress is an important element of any behavior change program, and acquisition of continence skills is no different.

W.J. Warzak, PhD (✉)
Department of Psychology, 985450 Nebraska Medical Center, Omaha, NE 68198-5450, USA

Munroe-Meyer Institute, University of Nebraska Medical Center, Omaha, NE, USA
e-mail: wwarzak@unmc.edu

A.E. Kennedy, MS • K. Bond, PhD
Department of Psychology, 985450 Nebraska Medical Center, Omaha, NE, 68198-5450, USA

J.L. Matson (ed.), *Clinical Guide to Toilet Training Children*, Autism and Child Psychopathology Series, DOI 10.1007/978-3-319-62725-0_7

Focus of this Chapter

This chapter provides a review of methods and measures commonly used to evaluate the acquisition of continence skills in young children. In the larger view, measuring toilet training progress entails more than simply counting voids in the toilet or episodes of wet pants. Measurement also encompasses recording the integrity with which a protocol is implemented (e.g., Gresham, Gansle, & Noell, 1993; Peterson, Homer, & Wonderlich, 1982) as well as the reliability of the dependent measures (e.g., Johnston & Pennypacker, 2009). In turn, this requires an appropriate candidate for toilet training as well as having the necessary materials to initiate the protocol successfully. Therefore, while methods of direct observation and measures of toileting behavior will be a primary focus here, measures related to verifying the fidelity of methods, materials, and procedures necessary for the successful implementation of toilet training with integrity also are presented.

Prerequisite Measures

Before a child is ready to be toilet trained, an assessment of developmental, behavioral, and physical readiness should be obtained to determine if the child is an appropriate candidate. Typically developing children are most commonly toilet trained when they are between 2 and 3 years old (Bloom, Seeley, Ritchey, & McGuire, 1993; Schum et al., 2002), but older children and those with developmental delays also are trainable, as exemplified by Foxx and Azrin (1973b) or, more recently, Cicero (2012; Cicero & Pfadt, 2002). The ideal time to initiate toilet training is by no means agreed upon and there is great variability in training windows depending upon the readiness signs selected by the trainer (Kaerts, Van Hal, Vermandel & Wyndaele, 2012; Schum et al., 2002). Kaerts et al. (2012) provide an example of 21 directly observed readiness signs (e.g., "children understand potty words," "pull clothes up and down," "can sit still on the potty for 5–10 min"), but their individual predictive power relative to successful toilet training has not been evaluated.

Indirect measures of readiness take the form of structured retrospective parent report. For example, the Denver II Developmental Screening test (Frauman & Brandon, 1996) and the Ages and Stages Questionnaire (Squires & Bricker, 2009) are popular screening devices, among many (e.g., Battelle Developmental Inventory in Mota & Barros, 2008; Bayley Scales of Infant Development in Schum et al., 2001) that have been used to assess toileting training readiness within the context of broad assessment of early child development. Both screening measures are recommended by the American Academy of Pediatrics (Bright Futures Steering Committee & Medical Home Initiatives for Children with Special Needs Project Advisory Committee, 2006). Nevertheless, there is no significant research that evaluates the functional relationship between individual readiness skills and successful toilet

Table 1 Child prerequisite abilities

Physiological readiness
Bowel peristalsis
Normal bladder capacity
Voluntarily tightens sphincter muscles
Perceives full bladder
Sits independently
One to two bowel movements per day
Periods of time between voids
Recognizes being wet or soiled
Mobility/ dexterity/ walking
Pull pants down and up
Imitates behavior
Follows directions
Unafraid of toilet or flush
Understands words for elimination
Understands the social expectations that bladder emptying takes place in toilet

Note. Adapted from Frauman, & Brandon (1996), Foxx & Azrin (1973b), and Harris (2004)

training (Blum, Taubman & Nemeth, 2003; Kaerts et al., 2012). A number of commonly agreed upon prerequisite skills are noted in Table 1.

Progress toward achieving readiness criteria can be evaluated over time by using the above components with the caveat that readiness criteria are loosely defined. These measures should not be influenced by developmental or medical status, although attaining these readiness milestones may vary as a function of developmental and medical factors. Measures of prerequisite behaviors may be established as binary events (e.g., recognizes being wet or soiled, pull pants down and up) or occur on a continuum (e.g., child follows what percentage of parental requests, how much time typically elapses between voids).

Of the many readiness skills, following directions is one of the most crucial to toilet training success. Children who are not under effective instructional control are poor candidates for toilet training (Polaha, Warzak, & Ditmer-McMahon, 2002). For these children, successful toilet training may be enhanced by implementing compliance training prior to toilet training. A child's compliance can be evaluated by simply asking parents about the likelihood of a child complying with a number of age appropriate one-step commands, or by providing parents with a formal protocol for assessing compliance, as in Shriver & Allen (1997; see Table 2). Seventy percent compliance to one-step commands in young children is often considered satisfactory prior to teaching trials (Shriver & Allen, 1997). In addition, there are a number of child behavior rating scales, such as the Child Behavior Checklist (Achenbach & Rescorla, 2000) and the Eyberg Child Behavior Inventory (Eyberg, Boggs, & Reynolds, 1980) that assess disruptive and otherwise difficult behaviors in young children that may suggest deferring toilet training until the child comes under instructional control.

Table 2 Evaluating child compliance

Component	Definition, measurement, and mean response
Compliance	The child initiating and completing the parent instructed task Measured as completed or not completed
Initiation latency	The time from the end of the initial command to an initial change in the child's behavior directed toward task completion Measured in seconds Mean time for 2–4 year olds 6.5 s (SD =3.4)
Completion latency	The time from initiation to the completion of the task Measured in seconds Mean time for 2–4 year olds 14.9 s (SD = 9.5)
Compliance rate	The number of commands the child complied with divided by the total number of parent provided commands Measured as a percentage Mean percentage for 2–4 year olds 79.4% (SD = 24.1)

Note. Taken from Shriver & Allen (1997)

Dependent Measures

In- vs. out-of-toilet voids The behaviors most central to progress in toilet training are successful voids in the toilet versus voids occurring outside of the toilet (e.g., Beaudry Bellefeuille, Schaaf & Polo, 2013; Kroeger & Sorensen, 2010). In-toilet voids have been variously referred to as in-toilet urination (Luiselli, 1997; Rinald & Mirenda, 2012), successful urination (Chung, 2007), continent urination (Hagopian, Fisher, Piazza, & Wierzbicki, 1993; Simon & Thompson, 2006), and correct urination (Cocchiola, Martino, Dwyer, & Demezzo, 2012). Out-of-toilet voids have been described as accidents (Cicero & Pfadt, 2002), incontinence (Luiselli, 1997), incontinent urinations (Simon & Thompson, 2006), and urinary incontinency (Smith, 1979). Although accidents may be a misnomer, as the child may intend to void outside of the toilet, the use of the terms *successes* and *accidents* to refer to in- and out-of-toilet voids, respectively, has become commonplace (Hanney, Jostad, LeBlanc, Carr, & Castile, 2012; LeBlanc, Carr, Crossett, Bennett & Detweiler, 2005).

Several toilet training procedures include a provision for interrupting out-of-toilet voids, if possible, to provide children with the opportunity to finish the void appropriately in the toilet (Cicero & Pfadt, 2002; LeBlanc et al., 2005). In these procedures, once voids are detected and interrupted, children are quickly taken to the toilet. Hanney et al. (2012) described this behavior chain as accident/success conversions. Other authors have included this condition within their accident definition (Cicero & Pfadt, 2002), or treated such occurrences as successes (LeBlanc et al., 2005).

Researchers have reported toileting successes, accidents (Cicero & Pfadt, 2002; LeBlanc et al., 2005), or both (Brown & Peace, 2011; Luiselli, 1997). Recording and evaluating both accidents and successes has the advantage of allowing a comprehensive analysis of all voids. However, as voids are largely binary events (with the exception of accident/success conversions), clinicians and authors may allocate effort to recording just one or the other of these behaviors. In addition, researchers may be interested in assessing the level of independent toileting, which authors have measured by the percentage of voids that are self-initiated. Self-initiation occurs when a child requests to use the toilet, or moves to the bathroom, and completes a void in the toilet without the assistance of physical or verbal prompts (Kroeger & Sorensen, 2010; LeBlanc et al., 2005). Self-initiation may be tailored to accommodate the communication abilities of the child. For example, self-initiation may occur with a verbal request for one child, an ASL sign for another, and the exchange of a communication card (e.g., PECS; Bondy & Frost, 1994) for yet another.

The definition of voiding episodes is important to consider before toilet training begins. Few would argue that a large puddle of urine represents an accident. However, small urine stains on underwear may less clearly meet criteria for voids outside of the toilet, as it is possible that such a small amount of urine may contact the underwear when a child pulls up their pants at the end of the toileting routine (Foxx, 1986). Thus, it may be necessary to operationalize accidents. One may physically measure the size of the wet spot, as in Lancioni and Marcus (1999), who scored large accidents when both the child's pants and underwear were wet or the child's underwear had a wet spot larger than 6 cm in diameter, and small accidents for wet spots less than 6 cm in diameter and dry pants. In the case of Foxx (1986), parents measured accidents by placing the lid of an olive jar over the wet spot. If the wet spot exceeded the diameter of the lid, the child was considered to have an accident.

Finally, one must consider *moisture alarms* as a potential means of accurately detecting voids that occur outside of the toilet. Moisture alarms have a long history in the treatment of elimination disorders. Mowrer and Mowrer (1938) pioneered their use as an enuresis intervention and Azrin and Foxx (1971) implemented them in early toilet training efforts, but alarms subsequently fell into disuse. More recently, however, moisture alarms once again have been included in toilet training procedures (Cicero & Pfadt, 2002; Vermandel, Van Kampen, De Wachter, Weyler, & Wyndaele, 2008a; Vermandel, Weyler, De Wachter, & Wyndaele, 2008b). Although the primary function of a urine alarm is to alert the child to the release of urine, it also has the effect of alerting caregivers that a void is occurring. However, alarms may introduce artifact by sounding when no accident has occurred, such as when sweat triggers the alarm, or failing to detect accidents (e.g., due to misplacement of the sensor). Therefore, direct observation of target behaviors and permanent products may be a more reliable measure of continence skills.

Toilet training completion Toilet training is a procedure and a process. The primary procedure addresses mechanics of toilet training, the nuts and bolts of sit schedules, fluid loading, schedules of reinforcement, etc. The process of toilet training accrues over time and trials, as child development and environmental contingencies shape and maintain successful toilet training trials, eventually culminating in control of bowel and bladder and independent use of the toilet for elimination.

It is unclear which components of toileting a child must accomplish independently, such as undressing and dressing, flushing the toilet, or washing hands, to be considered toilet trained. Whether or not a child must be completely hygiene independent or not is a function of cultural norms and the goals of caregivers. Typically, children must initiate toileting to be considered toilet trained, but it is unlikely that a 3-year-old who self-initiates toileting also is hygiene independent and unfailingly continent throughout the day and night. It is not uncommon for children to be dry during the day, but still wet the bed at night (Foxx, 1986; Schum et al., 2002; von Gontard, Heron, & Joinson, 2011).

Furthermore, there is no agreed upon percentage of voiding episodes that must occur in the toilet to have achieved mastery. One could argue that 100% of elimination events must occur in the toilet to be considered toilet trained, but there are innumerable young children who intermittently wet their pants let alone the numerous examples of adults who void under conditions where toilets are not available (e.g., camping, swimming). So, the standard for "toilet trained" is clearly less than 100%, but how much less than 100% is a function of culture, community, and family norms and may reflect the presence of behavioral or developmental handicaps.

A number of additional dimensions may affect the definition of "toilet trained." For example, Blum et al. (2003) defined toilet training completion as when the child wore underwear during the day and had fewer than four urine accidents per week and less than two fecal accidents per month. LeBlanc et al. (2005) completed training when participants achieved 80% success for two consecutive days after scheduled sits were discontinued. Kroeger and Sorensen (2010) completed training when the sit schedule had been thinned to 30 min break/5 min sits, with self-initiations occurring 50% of the time or more. Finally, one study included not only dryness criteria but also a latency criterion wherein voids needed to occur within 10 min of sitting on the toilet (Didden, Sikkema, Bosman, Duker, & Curfs, 2001).

Task analyses enable documentation of each discrete task over time as a function of intervention (Donlau, Mattsson & Glad-Mattsson, 2013). Change in the number of steps completed over time represents progress, and can be reported as a percentage of steps completed, with and without prompting. In addition, the level of assistance, or prompt (i.e., physical, gestural, verbal) required at each step of the protocol can be recorded to monitor progress toward successful toileting. For example, Azrin and Foxx (1971) ranked levels of prompting from most invasive and detailed to least starting with physical guidance, then direct verbal guidance, to a touch, a hand motion, a head or finger motion, and finally no prompt. Donlau, Mattsson, and Glad-Mattsson (2013) labeled independence in toileting skills into five categories: does not perform, performs with physical and verbal support, performs with physical support, performs with verbal support, and performs independently.

Problem behaviors Resistance to toilet training was reported by several early researchers of the Azrin and Foxx procedure (Butler, 1976; Foxx & Azrin, 1973a; Matson & Ollendick, 1977). Butler (1976) noted severe emotional reactions to the positive practice component of toilet training. Matson and Ollendick (1977) stated that all mothers reported emotional side effects, specifically tantrums and avoidance behavior, primarily during the positive practice and graduated guidance components. Foxx and Azrin (1973a) reported that most children responded to toilet training as a pleasurable experience, but a few children engaged in tantrums at the start of training. Problem behavior has not been as commonly reported during more recent evaluations of toileting training (Klassen et al., 2006), yet problem behaviors such as tantrums, aggression, noncompliance, and negative vocalizations are likely in children with a history of challenging behavior in response to instructions and physical guidance (Cicero & Pfadt, 2002). Problem behavior during toilet training also may be an indication of distress in response to specific toilet training components (e.g., positive practice; Matson & Ollendick, 1977). It would be beneficial to record ongoing problem behaviors during toilet training given its occurrence, its potential effect on the caregiver's response effort, and as an indication of the child's distress.

Measurement Procedures

Achieving continence is a developmental milestone that typically occurs outside of clinical intervention and experimental arrangements (Choby & George, 2008). As such, monitoring toilet training progress presents unique challenges. Measurement allows determination if intervention is warranted and if so, if it is effective. Methods of data collection have to be selected for their feasibility in children's homes, schools, and day care settings and for use by parents, teachers, and day care providers. It should be noted that the more effort required by data collectors to obtain information the less likely it will be collected (Friman & Poling, 1995). The effectiveness of toilet training can be directly measured and recorded in a number of ways using time sampling, permanent product, and event recording measures.

Time sampling Toileting events occur intermittently throughout the day. They are brief, discrete, unpredictable, yet certain. As such, time-sampling is relevant, especially during baseline, when no schedule (i.e., structured/scheduled sits) is applied to a child's voids, and continuous observation for toileting occurrences may not be feasible. Time-sampling involves the division of an interval of time into smaller, equal intervals and recording the presence or absence of a behavior during that interval. There are several types of time-sampling methods, including whole-interval, partial-interval, and momentary time sampling. Partial-interval recording, which is used to assess whether a behavior occurred at any point in an interval, may be the most relevant procedure for recording voiding events.

For example, Simon and Thompson (2006) conducted pants checks to assess wetness every 15 min. Pants checks identify the occurrence of voids even if they are otherwise not easily noticeable. As a urine stain only reveals the occurrence of an accident, rather than its precise occurrence in time, pants checks during regular, short intervals may be the most accurate means of detecting the number of voids and their approximate distribution in time, in lieu of moisture alarms, which allow timely detection but are subject to artifact.

Time sampling also is relevant to recording problem behavior during toilet training. As noted above, problem behavior has the potential to interfere with toilet training, yet is rarely reported in research. Problem behaviors, such as yelling and hitting, occur with varying frequency and duration. As such, a partial-interval data collection procedure may be most appropriate. However, time sampling is more complex than other data collection procedures because it requires a response during each interval, and therefore, may be most feasible in research settings. At the most basic level, a data collection system could include recording the presence or absence of problem behavior at any point in the chain of behavior involved in each toilet training trial, although this would reflect the limits of any large interval recording procedure and would underestimate occurrences of problem behavior (Cooper, Heron & Heward, 2007).

Permanent product recording Permanent product measurement occurs after a behavior takes place by detecting the effect of the target behavior on the environment, rather than by observing the behavior itself (Cooper et al., 2007). As urination occurs quietly, detection often occurs after the fact. Permanent product of out of-toilet voids are detected by feeling or seeing wetness on the child's clothes or nearby items after the behavior occurred (Simon & Thompson, 2006). For example, there are diaper products that change colors as a function of urination and these can be used in combination with time sampling procedures to record the presence or absence of wetting during standard intervals of time.

Event recording Event recording captures the occurrence of a target behavior (e.g., a child's voids) reported as the frequency (i.e., absolute number) or rate (i.e., the frequency of voids over unit of time), such as per day (LeBlanc et al., 2005) or school day (Cicero & Pfadt, 2002). Event recording is relevant to toilet training because in- and out-of-toilet voids are discrete events with a clear beginning and end, and are relatively brief. Event recording also is feasible from a resources point of view as voids are relatively infrequent and successes and accidents, as well as self-initiations, are easily detectable and easily recorded. Event recording holds advantages over time sampling in that recording only needs to occur in response to voids, and therefore, requires less response effort than time sampling methods. However, event recording assumes a reliable observational procedure that captures all relevant occurrences of the target behavior as they occur in real time, which is not always possible.

Procedural Integrity

Procedural integrity is important to successful implementation of either the child-oriented method or the Foxx and Azrin procedure. The latter procedure is the most commonly researched (Warzak, Forcino, Sanberg, & Gross, 2016) and requires the more structured protocol of the two. The Foxx and Azrin procedure is a

Table 3 Suggested materials used for toilet training

Cotton briefs with moisture detecting snaps inserted in the crotch area
Potty chair or toilet with foot stool and ring.
Urine alerts
Pants alarms
Small table
Variety of fluids
Available reinforcers (reinforcement menu of tangible rewards, special activities, friends who care, etc.)
Individually marked drinking glasses
Kitchen timer or pocket timer
Cloths
Toilet training procedure protocol
Progress record forms or chart

Note. Adapted from Azrin and Foxx (1974), Foxx and Azrin (1973b), and Schaefer (1979)

multi-component procedure, but over time, many of the components have fallen into disuse and are not commonly found in research with typically developing children (Warzak et al., 2016). A small number of components comprise the majority of commonly reported procedures used with typically developing children. A checklist of these components–that is, fluid loading, differential response to dry/wet pants upon pants checks, prompted practice trials, fading prompts, and thinning the schedule of reinforcement for dry pants and voids in the toilet–would provide a measure of procedural integrity. Combining this with measures of readiness skills (Table 1), instructional control (Table 2) and basic materials (Table 3) provides monitoring of procedural integrity that affects the success or failure of the training procedure.

Inter-Observer Agreement

Reliability refers to the consistency with which an event was measured (Cooper et al., 2007) and is often assessed with inter-observer agreement (IOA) procedures. These procedures require that at least two individuals independently observe and record a portion of the events (e.g., 33% of sessions) under study. To determine the level of observer agreement, data from two observers are compared, and the level of agreement between them is expressed as a percentage. Although IOA does not provide information regarding how accurately the measures reflect the true value of the event under study, it has the potential to increase the believability of the measures by indicating how often two independent observers recorded the same outcome when observing the same event.

Interobserver-agreement procedures are standard throughout much of behavioral research, but occasionally absent from toilet training research. Cicero and Pfadt (2002) stated that they did not conduct reliability checks because accidents and self-initiations were clearly defined and easily observed. Another reason that IOA may occasionally not be collected is because a second observer may not be available, given the unpredictable timing and relatively low frequency of toileting events. This issue may be accommodated in schools, when a second staff member may serve as a reliability observer, but appears as a particular obstacle relevant to toilet training in home settings. For example, in-home training programs frequently use a parent as the primary data collector, but it may be intrusive and unrealistic to have a second experimental observer in the home to obtain sufficient amounts of IOA data. This issue may be resolved by having a second parent record IOA data when possible (e.g., nights and weekends). It is also possible that the frequency of toilet training research in children's natural environments may increase if it was acceptable to conduct IOA on a lower proportion of the data that is commonly done in behavioral research, or to include indirect measures of IOA (e.g., phone calls) as supplements to direct measures.

Summary and Future Directions

Most toilet training procedures occur without benefit of measurement, data collection, or experimental design. Training is conducted by parents without professional assistance and it is not uncommon for children to practically train themselves. Nevertheless, there are children who require professional assistance, as well as researchers who pursue the most effective and efficient training procedures. For these individuals, measurement is essential. We have highlighted the most commonly implemented data collection procedures and dependent measures in pursuit of these goals.

Comprehensive progress monitoring entails measures of child readiness and procedural integrity as well as measures of toileting itself. Data collection and dependent measures must conform to children's natural environments and caregivers' ability to observe and record. Confusing the situation is the lack of a consensus definition of what comprises successful toilet training. Just how much of the routine must be completed independently and what percentage of the time remain open questions.

We would note that compliance issues are among the least referenced in the toilet training literature, yet we believe these are among the most important prerequisite skills in toilet training. Training a child who is not under instructional control of parent or staff can become a major challenge emphasizing the importance of compliance assessment and careful measurement of behavioral disturbance as a function of different training procedures.

There are a number of unresolved questions pertaining to the importance of particular readiness skills and which toilet training procedures are most efficient and effective. One practical obstacle to answering these questions is the fact that continence is the norm and the number of individuals who experience difficulty acquiring continence skills is very small relative to the overall population, limiting research funds to support related projects. Perhaps the larger issues raised here could be enfolded within large longitudinal population based studies which investigate demographics and public health outcomes. In this way, the relationship between toileting readiness, for example, and toileting independence could be economically evaluated over time. Regardless, inroads in toilet training, whether they be through large population-based efforts or the result of small-*n* studies, as featured here, require precise measurement and progress monitoring.

References

Achenbach, T. M., & Rescorla, L. A. (2000). *Manual for the ASEBA preschool forms & profiles: An integrated system of multi-informant assessment; child behavior checklist for ages 1 1/2–5; language development survey; caregiver-teacher report form*. Burlington, VT: University of Vermont.

Azrin, N. H., & Foxx, R. M. (1971). A rapid method of toilet training the institutionalized retarded. *Journal of Applied Behavior Analysis, 4*, 89–99.

Azrin, N. H., & Foxx, R. M. (1974). *Toilet training in less than a day*. New York, NY: Simon and Schuster.

Beaudry Bellefeuille, I., Schaaf, R. C., & Polo, E. R. (2013). Occupational therapy based on Ayres sensory integration in the treatment of retentive fecal incontinence in a 3-year-old boy. *American Journal of Occupational Therapy, 67*(5), 601–606.

Bloom, D. A., Seeley, W. W., Ritchey, M. L., & McGuire, E. J. (1993). Toilet habits and continence in children: An opportunity sampling in search of normal parameters. *The Journal of Urology, 149*(5), 1087–1090.

Blum, N. J., Taubman, B., & Nemeth, N. (2003). Relationship between age at initiation of toilet training and duration of training: A prospective study. *Pediatrics, 111*, 810–814.

Bondy, A. S., & Frost, L. A. (1994). The picture exchange communication system. *Focus on Autistic Behavior, 9*, 1–19.

Brazelton, T. B. (1962). A child-oriented approach to toilet training. *Pediatrics, 29*(1), 121–128.

Bright Futures Steering Committee & Medical Home Initiatives for Children with Special Needs Project Advisory Committee. (2006). Identifying infants and young children with developmental disorders in the medical home: An algorithm for developmental surveillance and screening. *Pediatrics, 118*(1), 405–420.

Brown, F. J., & Peace, N. (2011). Teaching a child with challenging behaviour to use the toilet: A clinical case study. *British Journal of Learning Disabilities, 39*(4), 321–326.

Butler, J. F. (1976). The toilet training success of parents after reading toilet training in less than a day. *Behavior Therapy, 7*(2), 185–191.

Choby, B. A., & George, S. (2008). Toilet training. *American Family Physician, 78*(9), 1059–1064.

Chung, K. (2007). Modified version of Azrin and Foxx's rapid toilet training. *Journal of Developmental Physical Disabilities, 19*, 449–455.

Cicero, F. (2012). *Toilet training success: A guide for teaching individuals with developmental disabilities*. New York, NY: DRL Books.

Cicero, F. R., & Pfadt, A. (2002). Investigation of a reinforcement-based toilet training procedure for children with autism. *Research in Developmental Disabilities, 23*, 319–331.

Cocchiola, M. A., Martino, G. M., Dwyer, L. J., & Demezzo, K. (2012). Toilet training children with autism and developmental delays: An effective program for school settings. *Behavior Analysis in Practice, 5*, 60–64.

Cooper, J. O., Heron, T. E., & Heward, W. L. (2007). *Applied behavior analysis* (2nd ed.). Upper Saddle River, N.J: Pearson Prentice Hall.

Didden, R., Sikkema, S. P., Bosman, I., Duker, P. C., & Curfs, L. M. (2001). Use of a modified Azrin–Foxx toilet training procedure with individuals with Angelman syndrome. *Journal of Applied Research in Intellectual Disabilities*, *14*(1), 64–70.

Donlau, M., Mattsson, S., & Glad-Mattsson, G. (2013). Children with myelomeningocele and independence in the toilet activity: A pilot study. *Scandinavian Journal of Occupational Therapy*, *20*(1), 64–70.

Eyberg, S., Boggs, S. R., & Reynolds, L. A. (1980). *Eyberg child behavior inventory*. Portland, OR: University of Oregon Health Sciences Center.

Foxx, R. M., & Azrin, N. H. (1973a). Dry pants: A rapid method of toilet training children. *Behaviour Research and Therapy*, *11*(4), 435–442.

Foxx, R. M., & Azrin, N. H. (1973b). *Toilet training the retarded: A rapid program for day and nighttime independent toileting*. Champaign, IL: Research Press.

Foxx, R. M. (1986). The successful treatment of diurnal and nocturnal enuresis and encopresis. *Child & Family Behavior Therapy*, *7*, 39–48.

Frauman, A. C., & Brandon, D. H. (1996). Toilet training for the child with chronic illness. *Pediatric Nursing*, *22*(6), 469–493.

Friman, P., & Poling, A. (1995). Making life easier with effort: Basic findings and applied research on response effort. *Journal of Applied Behavior Analysis*, *28*, 583–590.

Gresham, F. M., Gansle, K. A., & Noell, G. H. (1993). Treatment integrity in applied behavior analysis with children. *Journal of Applied Behavior Analysis*, *26*(2), 257–263.

Harris, A. (2004). Toilet training children with learning difficulties: What the literature tells us. *British Journal of Nursing*, *13*(13), 773–777.

Hagopian, L. P., Fisher, W., Piazza, C. C., & Wierzbicki, J. J. (1993). A water-prompting procedure for the treatment of urinary incontinence. *Journal of Applied Behavior Analysis*, *26*, 473–474.

Hanney, N. M., Jostad, C. M., LeBlanc, L. A., Carr, J. E., & Castile, A. J. (2012). Intensive behavioral treatment of urinary incontinence of children with autism spectrum disorders: An archival analysis of procedures and outcomes from an outpatient clinic. *Focus on Autism and Other Developmental Disabilities*, *28*, 26–31.

Johnston, J. M., & Pennypacker, H. S. (2009). *Strategies and tactics for human behavioral research. New York*. New York, NY: Routledge.

Kaerts, N., Van Hal, G., Vermandel, A., & Wyndaele, J. J. (2012). Readiness signs used to define the proper moment to start toilet training: A review of the literature. *Neurourology and Urodynamics*, *31*(4), 437–440.

Klassen, T. P., Kiddoo, D., Lang, M. E., Friesen, C., Russell, K., Spooner, C., & Vandermeer, B. (2006). The effectiveness of different methods of toilet training for bowel and bladder control. *Evidence Report/Technology Assessment (Full Report)*, *147*, 1–57.

Kroeger, K., & Sorensen, R. (2010). A parent training model for toilet training children with autism. *Journal of Intellectual Disability Research*, *54*, 556–567.

Lancioni, G. E., & Markus, S. (1999). Urine-triggered alarm signals and prompts to promote daytime urinary continence in a boy with severe intellectual disability. *Behavioural and Cognitive Psychotherapy*, *27*, 261–265.

LeBlanc, L. A., Carr, J. E., Crossett, S. E., Bennett, C. M., & Detweiler, D. D. (2005). Intensive outpatient behavioral treatment of primary urinary incontinence of children with autism. *Focus on Autism and Other Developmental Disabilities*, *20*, 98–105.

Luiselli, J. K. (1997). Teaching toilet skills in a public school setting to a child with pervasive developmental disorder. *Journal of Behavior Therapy and Experimental Psychiatry*, *28*, 163–168.

Matson, J. L., & Ollendick, T. H. (1977). Issues in toilet training normal children. *Behavior Therapy*, *8*(4), 549–553.

Mota, D. M., & Barros, A. J. (2008). Toilet training: Situation at 2 years of age in a birth cohort. *Jornal de Pediatria*, *84*(5), 455–462.

Mowrer, O. H., & Mowrer, W. M. (1938). Enuresis—A method for its study and treatment. *American Journal of Orthopsychiatry*, *8*(3), 436–459.

Peterson, L., Homer, A. L., & Wonderlich, S. A. (1982). The integrity of independent variables in behavior analysis. *Journal of Applied Behavior Analysis, 15*(4), 477–492.

Polaha, J., Warzak, W. J., & Dittmer-McMahon, K. (2002). Toilet training in primary care: Current practice and recommendations from behavioral pediatrics. *Journal of Developmental & Behavioral Pediatrics, 23*(6), 424–429.

Rinald, K., & Mirenda, P. (2012). Effectiveness of a modified rapid toilet training workshop for parents of children with developmental disabilities. *Research in Developmental Disabilities, 33*, 933–943.

Schaefer, C. E. (1979). *Childhood encopresis and enuresis: Causes and therapy*. New York, NY: Van Nostrand Reinhold.

Schmitt, B. D. (2004). Toilet training: Getting it right the first time. *Contemporary Pediatrics, 21*(3), 105–116.

Schum, T. R., McAuliffe, T. L., Simms, M. D., Walter, J. A., Lewis, M., & Pupp, R. (2001). Factors associated with toilet training in the 1990s. *Ambulatory Pediatrics, 1*(2), 79–86.

Schum, T. R., Kolb, T. M., McAuliffe, T. L., Simms, M. D., Underhill, R. L., & Lewis, M. (2002). Sequential acquisition of toilet-training skills: A descriptive study of gender and age differences in normal children. *Pediatrics, 109*(3), 48.

Shriver, M. D., & Allen, K. D. (1997). Defining child noncompliance: An examination of temporal parameters. *Journal of Applied Behavior Analysis, 30*(1), 173–176.

Simon, J. L., & Thompson, R. T. (2006). The effects of undergarment type of on the urinary continence of toddlers. *Journal of Applied Behavior Analysis, 39*, 363–368.

Smith, P. S. (1979). A comparison of different methods of toilet training the mentally handicapped. *Behavior Research & Therapy, 17*, 33–43.

Spock, B. (1946). *The common sense book of baby and child care*. New York: Duell, Sloan and Pearce.

Squires, J., & Bricker, D. (2009). *Ages and stages questionnaires* (3rd ed.) (ASQ-3). Baltimore, MD: Paul H. Brookes Publishers.

Vermandel, A., Van Kampen, M., De Wachter, S., Weyler, J., & Wyndaele, J. (2008a). The efficacy of a wetting alarm diaper for toilet training of young healthy children in a day-care center: A randomized control trial. *Neurourology and Urodynamics, 28*, 305–308.

Vermandel, A., Weyler, J., de Wachter, S., & Wyndaele, J. (2008b). Toilet training of healthy young toddlers: A randomized trial between a daytime wetting alarm and timed potty training. *Journal of Developmental & Behavioral Pediatrics, 29*, 191–196.

von Gontard, A., Heron, J., & Joinson, C. (2011). Family history of nocturnal enuresis and urinary incontinence: Results from a large epidemiological study. *The Journal of Urology, 185*(6), 2303–2307.

Warzak, W. J., Forcino, S. S., Sanberg, S. A., & Gross, A. C. (2016). Advancing continence in typically developing children: Adapting the procedures of Foxx and Azrin for primary care. *Journal of Developmental & Behavioral Pediatrics, 37*(1), 83–87.

Applications of Operant-Based Behavioral Principles to Toilet Training

Hollie V. Wingate, Terry S. Falcomata, and Raechal Ferguson

Introduction

In this chapter, we describe the application of principles and mechanisms derived from basic experimental analysis of behavior (EAB) and applied behavior analysis (ABA) to toilet training methods and procedures. Going back to the seminal studies published Azrin and Foxx (1971) and Foxx and Azrin (1973), ABA has an effective and extensive record of success in terms of the application of operant-based behavioral principles and mechanisms in the area of toilet training. Specifically, reinforcement, punishment, and stimulus control-based procedures have served, historically, as the operant-based foundations for effective toilet training procedures. Within this chapter, we define operant-based behavioral principles and describe ABA-based procedures and examples of the application of various behavioral principles to toilet training. In this chapter we provide a brief review of the relationship between EAB and ABA, a review of the application of behavioral principles (i.e., reinforcement, punishment, stimulus control) within toilet training procedures, and we discuss additional toilet training behavioral techniques (i.e., prompting strategies, scheduled sitting procedures, increased fluid intake, urinary alarm systems). Each of the subsections pertaining to the application of operant-based behavioral principles begins with a definition of the principle followed by the description of several empirical-based studies illustrating their application within toilet training procedures.

H.V. Wingate • R. Ferguson
University of Texas at Austin, Austin, TX, USA

T.S. Falcomata (✉)
Department of Special Education, University of Texas at Austin,
1 University Station/D5300, Austin, TX 78712, USA
e-mail: falcomata@mail.utexas.edu

J.L. Matson (ed.), *Clinical Guide to Toilet Training Children*, Autism and Child Psychopathology Series, DOI 10.1007/978-3-319-62725-0_8

ABA and the Application of Principles of Behavior

ABA is a field that has existed for more than 50 years. Baer, Wolf, and Risley (1968) asserted that "Applied Behavior Analysis is the process of systematically applying interventions based upon the principles of learning theory to improve socially significant behaviors to a meaningful degree, and to demonstrate that the interventions employed are responsible for the improvement in behavior." ABA is one of three branches of the discipline of behavior analysis, with the other two being behaviorism (i.e., the philosophical focus behavior analysis; e.g., Radical Behaviorism) and EAB. The primary focus of the field of ABA is the direct assessment of functional relations between socially relevant behaviors and environment-based variables (Roane & Betz, 2012). The field of ABA was a direct result of the research developed in the area of EAB. The experimental analysis of behavior began with B.F. Skinner and his research that demonstrated that behavior could be overt, recorded, and studied. Skinner manipulated environmental variables, including the consequences that immediately followed behavior, and how those consequences affected behavior. Through the early works of Skinner and the subsequent works of other researchers conducting work in the area of EAB and ABA, principles and mechanisms of behavior were identified and established and continue to be studied today.

The principles and behavioral mechanisms discovered in EAB are the same principles that underlie ABA and serve as the foundations from which effective practices have been derived, developed, and applied by ABA clinicians. The application of these basic, underlying behavioral principles and mechanisms has enabled ABA to stand as an evidence-based practice across settings including in-home, clinic, and school settings, across populations including individuals with developmental and intellectual disabilities, autism spectrum disorders (ASD), and other disabilities and across myriad target behaviors and child-based clinical issues including toileting issues.

ABA-based procedures, based on behavioral principles, have been applied as behavior change tools across many domains including academic interventions, self-help skills, challenging behavior, functional communication training, and many other socially significant behaviors. One domain with a large body of research in terms of the application of ABA practices is toilet training. Felce and Perry (1995), along with the World Health Organization Quality of Life (WHOQL 1995), established parameters in regard to incontinence that could be considered quality of life impairments including poor hygiene, physical discomfort, restricted access to some environments, stigmatism, and self-esteem issues. For individuals without this critical skill, quality of life may be significantly diminished (Cicero & Pfadt, 2002).

Individuals with developmental disabilities often are more difficult to train with toileting skills due to various deficits and often require more support and more intensive intervention (e.g., Azrin & Foxx, 1971; Ellis, 1963; Foxx & Azrin, 1973; Lancioni, 1980; Luiselli, 1994). Ellis (1963) published the first toilet training study that used a simple paradigm where cues were presented and positive reinforcement was provided contingent on toileting successes. Following several replication studies that utilized procedures involving positive reinforcement (e.g., Hundziak, Maurer, & Watson, 1965; Van Wagenen, Meyerson, Kerr, & Mahoney, 1969), Azrin and Foxx (1971) published the most cited and comprehensive toilet training protocol (Kroeger & Sorenson-Burnworth, 2009). The Rapid Toilet Training (RTT; Azrin & Foxx, 1971) method quickly became a preferred toilet training protocol. RTT incorporated several procedures that involved the application of behavioral principles including reinforcement, punishment, and stimulus control-based procedures. The RTT components will be discussed at various points in this chapter as we discuss the application of these various behavioral principles during toilet training procedures.

Reinforcement

Reinforcement is a basic component of operant conditionings (Skinner, 1953) and is often regarded as the most important principle of behavior specifically as it pertains to applied behavioral programming (Cooper et al. 2007; Roane & Betz, 2012). Three components dictate the presence of reinforcement including (a) the presence of immediate consequences following a behavior, (b) an increase in the likelihood of the behavior occurring in the future, and (c) an increase in the behavior is functionally related to the immediate consequences and not due to other variables. Positive reinforcement and negative reinforcement are the two types (or processes) of reinforcement, and they are distinct in terms of their inherent processes.

If a stimulus is presented, or provided, following a behavior and this produces an increase in the likelihood that the behavior will occur in the future, positive reinforcement has occurred (Skinner, 1953). In other words, positive reinforcement is defined as a process in which the presentation of a stimulus, or reinforcer, following the occurrence of a behavior, increases the likelihood that the behavior will occur again in the future. The stimulus that is presented following the target behavior is referred to as a positive reinforcer, or simply a reinforcer. For example, if a child asks for a cookie and the child's mother immediately gives the child a cookie following the request, the likelihood that the child will ask for a cookie in the future will increase; thus positive reinforcement has occurred. In other words, the future probability of any particular behavior is increased by the consequence in the form of delivery of reinforcers. Positive reinforcers with children can include preferred edibles, such as snacks, candy, or sips of preferred drink items; sensory reinforcers such as tactile stimulation, vibration, or flashing lights; tangible reinforcers such as preferred toys, stickers, or other preferred items; activity reinforcers, such as playing a preferred game or going on a highly desired outing; or social reinforcers in the form of physical contact (i.e., hugs, high fives) and social praise or recognition.

If a stimulus is removed following a behavior and this produces an increase in the likelihood that the behavior will occur in the future, negative reinforcement has occurred (Skinner, 1953). In other words, negative reinforcement is defined as a process in which the removal of a stimulus following the occurrence of a behavior increases the likelihood that the behavior will occur again in the future. The stimulus that is removed following the target behavior may be referred to as an aversive stimulus (Skinner, 1953), in which the removal or avoidance of that stimulus is reinforcing. For example, if a child asks for a break from homework and the child's mother immediately responds by allowing the child to take a break, the likelihood that the child will ask for a break from homework in the future will increase; thus negative reinforcement has occurred. In other words, the future probability of any particular behavior is increased by the consequence in the form of the termination of aversive events. Negative reinforcers with children can include breaks from non-preferred activities such as academic or vocational work; the avoidance of aversive consequences such as error correction, positive practice, or other non-preferred consequences; or the delay of aversive events.

Although the process of reinforcement is a naturally occurring phenomenon that affects the behavior of all organisms on an ongoing basis (Skinner, 1953), applied behavior analysts have utilized knowledge of the principle of reinforcement to bring about socially important behavior changes. Specifically, the behavioral principles of positive and negative reinforcement have been applied effectively across a wide variety of target behaviors and skills, populations, and settings. Likewise, positive and negative reinforcement have played an integral role in effective toilet training programs and methods.

Positive Reinforcement and Toilet Training

Azrin and Foxx (1971) pioneered the seminal study with regard to the application of behavioral principles to toilet training, and their procedures involved a particular focus on the application of positive reinforcement. Azrin and Foxx asserted that toilet training is a social process that relies on operant conditioning, including a primary focus on positive reinforcement. In the study, the authors evaluated toilet training methods with nine adults with severe intellectual disabilities in a residential institutional setting. Specifically, the authors implemented a group design in which the participants were randomly assigned to either a treatment or control condition. Prior to the study, the participants had been exposed to a toileting schedule routine intervention; however, incontinence had continued to be a primary concern. The general procedure implemented by Azrin and Foxx involved, among other components (to be discussed in other sections of this chapter), the provision of reinforcers contingent on appropriate toileting behavior (e.g., demonstration by the participants of correct toilet behaviors, dry pants) based on the behavioral principle of positive reinforcement that suggested that future appropriate toileting behavior would increase as a result of the process. The incorporation of positive reinforcement, within a broader treatment package that included the application of other behavioral principles, was demonstrated to be effective at increasing toileting skills in the participants in the treatment condition.

A large number of subsequent studies following the conceptualization provided by Azrin and Foxx (1971) pertaining to toilet training have demonstrated the positive effects of the application of positive reinforcement. For example, Halligan and Luyben (2009) applied positive reinforcement within a toilet training program with two typically developing individuals. Prior to the study, attempts by their parents to toilet train had been unsuccessful with two sisters (aged 2.5 and 3.5), one of whom was "perfectly content to wear a diaper" (p. 179; Halligan & Luyben, 2009) and the other of whom occasionally requested use of the toilet but wore a diaper the majority of the time. Pretreatment naturalistic and anecdotal observations suggested that both girls preferred social attention and approval, highly preferred foods, and any or all items that involved princesses. The authors utilized a multiple baseline single-subject experimental design to evaluate the effects of positive reinforcement while tracking occurrences of wet diaper as well as engagement in appropriate toilet use. During baseline, salty snacks and juice were provided to the two girls to increase their fluid intake, and no prompts were provided to use the toilet. During the subsequent treatment condition, the authors continued to provide salty foods and juice, and in addition, they (a) conducted diaper checks on a 30-min schedule, (b) prompted the girls to use the toilet (i.e., "do you need to use the potty?"; "would you like to be a big girl and try to use the potty?"; Halligan & Luyben, 2009), and (c) and provided praise and approval contingent on compliance in the form of use of the toilet. Over time, the authors faded their use of vocal prompts in favor the use of the positive reinforcers alone. The authors subsequently introduced an additional procedural variation in which following the girls' demonstration of 90% compliance and initiations, they earned access to princess underwear. The overall results demonstrated that the positive reinforcement procedure effectively decreased the rate of wet diapers and significantly increased the girls' appropriate use of the toilet and their acquisition of toileting skills; and the introduction of princess underwear eliminated accidents completely.

Post and Kirkpatrick (2004) provided another example of the application of positive reinforcement during toilet training. In the study, the authors implemented toilet training with a 3.5-year-old boy diagnosed with pervasive developmental disorder (PDD). Prior to the study, several potential positive reinforcers were identified based on their effectiveness during daily living skill programming and educational activities; reinforcers included praise, attention, and preferred videos. The authors implemented toilet training sessions in the home. Initially, during pre-study assessment, the child wore only training pants during the course of the study, and routines and fluid intake were not changed from what was considered a typical day. The authors collected baseline data on natural occurrences of untrained urination to determine the times in which urinations were most likely to occur. Following the pre-study assessment, Phase I was implemented during which the authors reintroduced the diaper and the participant was taken to the toilet every 30 min for 5-min sittings; he was checked for wet or dryness every 15 min. During Phase I, the 30-min trip schedule was implemented for the entire 8–10 h per day of training. The authors employed a strategy in which the participant spent 20 min on the toilet during each 30-min interval (see also Azrin and Foxx, 1971). The authors provided positive reinforcement in the form of praise for compliant toilet sitting and access to a preferred video for on-toilet urination. When the participant was not on the toilet, the authors conducted checks every 5 min. If the participant was wet, the authors stated "you're wet" in a neutral tone and changed the participant. The authors provided positive reinforcement in the form of enthusiastic praise when the participant was dry. The authors progressively decreased the sitting schedule as the participant demonstrated increased occurrences of urination on the toilet and decreasing accidents off the toilet (i.e., he met an 80% criteria for on-toilet urination across the day). Overall, the results showed that the participant increased urination in the toilet through the use of positive reinforcement in the form of access to social praise and videos. Also, of particular note, Post and Kirkpatrick demonstrated the effectiveness of praise and nonconsumable reinforcers in lieu of edibles.

Luiselli (1997) provided another demonstration of the effectiveness of the application of positive reinforcement during toilet training with an 8-year-old boy with PDD. The participant was recruited for the study because he did not engage in toileting behaviors in the school setting. Although he occasionally engaged in independent toileting in the home setting, while at school he did not urinate while on the toilet even though he independently entered the bathroom and complied with requests to sit on the toilet. As a result, the participant wore a diaper at home and in his school setting. The authors focused on two target behaviors including in-toilet urination and incontinence (i.e., urination in the diaper or underwear). Following a baseline condition in which the author instituted two bathroom visits per day with no other intervention components,

Phase I of intervention was implemented in which the author conducted one scheduled bathroom visit per day. Phase I also included a positive reinforcement component in which the author provided a reinforcer (i.e., drinking water from a preferred bottle) contingent on successful urination in the toilet. In addition, instances of accidents during Phase I resulted in changing into dry underwear or a diaper. During Phase II, the author kept all conditions from Phase I constant with the exception of the addition of a second scheduled daily bathroom visit. Further, the participant was required to successfully urinate in the toilet during both visits to earn access to the reinforcer (i.e., the water bottle). Thus, the author implemented an increasing criterion for reinforcement representing an example of reinforcement thinning. During Phase III, the author implemented further reinforcement thinning with the water bottle by slowly increasing the requirements for reinforcement (i.e., reinforcement was provided every second, then third, then fourth successful urination in the toilet) until the reinforcer was successfully eliminated from the procedure in favor of praise alone. The purpose of the reinforcement-thinning component was to maintain toileting skills within naturalistic conditions and everyday occurrences. The overall results showed that the use of positive reinforcement effectively produced independent toileting behavior.

Negative Reinforcement and Toilet Training

Rolider and Van Houten (1985) utilized a negative reinforcement strategy to address encopresis during toilet training with a typically developing 12-year-old girl. The authors reported that prior to the study, the participant's parents had attempted several unsuccessful strategies over the 5-year period in which she had been exhibiting the toileting issues; these included Rogerian family therapy, reprimands, punishment in the form of keeping her at home contingent on accidents, and planned ignoring. The authors employed a reversal single-subject experimental design to evaluate the effectiveness of negative reinforcement procedures relative to baseline, a differential reinforcement of other behavior (DRO) procedure, and a DRO with overcorrection procedure. It should be noted that the authors attempted positive reinforcement-based procedures (unsuccessfully) prior to their employment of negative reinforcement procedures. The DRO procedure consisted of the provision of chocolate candy and a coupon contingent on clean underwear during hourly checks; the coupons were exchangeable for additional reinforcers. The DRO procedure was unsuccessful, and thus, the authors integrated an overcorrection procedure with DRO that consisted of requiring the participant to hand-wash her dirty underwear; the combination of DRO and overcorrection was not effective. The negative reinforcement procedure the authors implemented subsequently consisted of requiring the participant to sit on the toilet each morning after waking up for a 20-min period or until she defecated. She was not required to sit on the toilet again that day if she defecated during the initial 20-min period in the morning. If she did not defecate during the allotted 20-min period in the morning, she was required to sit on the toilet for a longer period of time (i.e., 40 min) during another scheduled bathroom trip. If she defecated during this time, she was not required again to sit on the toilet during that day; however, if she did not have a bowel movement during this time, the time was automatically increased to 90 min on the toilet during a third scheduled bathroom trip. The results of Rolider and Van Houten demonstrated that the negative reinforcement procedure effectively decreased soiling and increased successful bowel movements in the toilet. Of particular note was the fact that the negative reinforcement procedure was effective in a situation in which positive reinforcement had been tried and shown to be ineffective.

Luiselli (2007) provided an additional example of the use of negative reinforcement during toilet training. Luiselli's procedures were similar to those described by Rolidar and Van Houten (1985) in that the participant was not responsive to positive reinforcement procedures prior to the implementation of negative reinforcement procedures. The participant was a 6-year-old boy with multiple disabilities including deafness, mild vision impairment, and developmental disabilities. He also had deficits in language, and his communication skills included signs and gestures. Prior to the study, the participant had never successfully urinated in the toilet. The authors employed a sequential condition (ABCDC) clinical case study design to evaluate the effects of the negative reinforcement procedure. During the initial baseline condition (and during all subsequent conditions), the participant wore disposable diapers and engaged in nine scheduled bathroom visits throughout the day; each visit entailed 3-min sits on the toilet. During baseline, the staff prompted the participant to urinate in the toilet and provided praise contingent on successful urinations in the toilet. During the first treatment condition (Intervention I), positive reinforcement was provided in the form of a preferred candy contingent on successful urinationss in the toilet; the initial treatment approach was unsuccessful, and thus, the authors implemented a subsequent modified treatment condition. The second treatment condition (Intervention II) was identical to the initial treatment condition except that the participant also received access to play for 10–15 min following successful urinations in the toilet; this treatment approach was also unsuccessful which resulted in additional modifications to the treatment during a subsequent treatment condition. During the third treatment condition (Intervention III), similar to Rolidar and Van Houten, a negative reinforcement component was incorporated in which the participant was required to remain seated on the toilet until he urinated. In addition, the author implemented a component of the Azrin and Foxx (1971) RTT protocol in which the participant was instructed to sit for 20 min each half-hour and on nearby chair during the other 10 min of the 30-min sitting interval. Contingent on successful urination in the toilet, the participant was provided with praise, an edible, and he was allowed to leave the bathroom to play with toys. The results of the study indicated that the use of negative reinforcement was an effective toilet training.

Punishment

Like reinforcement, punishment is a basic component of operant conditioning (Cooper et al., 2007; Skinner, 1953). Punishment can be inferred to have occurred when the likelihood of a behavior occurring in the future is decreased due to a change in the environment immediately following the behavior. Similar to the mechanism of reinforcement described above, two types (or processes) of punishment are positive and negative punishment, and they are distinct in terms of their inherent processes.

If a stimulus is presented, or provided, following a behavior and it produces a decrease in the likelihood that the behavior will occur in the future, positive punishment has occurred (Cooper et al., 2007; Skinner, 1953). In other words, positive punishment is defined as a process in which the presentation of a stimulus, or aversive consequence, following the occurrence of a behavior, decreases the likelihood that the behavior will occur again in the future. For example, if a child is scolded for stealing candy from the candy jar, and the stealing behavior decreases, positive punishment has occurred. In the above example, scolding was the *addition* of an aversive stimulus that resulted in a decrease in the candy-stealing behavior.

If a stimulus is removed following a behavior and this produces a decrease in the likelihood that the behavior will occur in the future, negative reinforcement has occurred (Cooper et al., 2007; Skinner, 1953). In other words, negative punishment is defined as a process in which the removal of a stimulus following the occurrence of a behavior decreases the likelihood that the behavior will occur again in the future. The stimulus that is removed following the target behavior is typically a type of reinforcer, the removal of which is an aversive event for the individual. It should also be noted that a stimulus could be removed from the environment, or access to positive reinforcement could be blocked. An example of a negative punishment is a time-out procedure. During time-out, which is implemented as a result of an individual's engagement in a target problem behavior, the individual's access to reinforcement (e.g., a reinforcing activity) is removed or denied resulting in a decrease in the likelihood that the individual will engage in the problem behavior in the future. Another example is a response cost system in which a child may gain tokens for engaging in appropriate behavior, such as remaining quiet during circle time (i.e., positive reinforcement). However, if the child engages in disruptive behavior, a token is removed (i.e., negative punishment). If the loss of the token decreases the future occurrences of disruptive behavior, negative punishment will have occurred.

Similar to reinforcement, punishment is a naturally occurring phenomenon that affects the behavior of all organisms on an ongoing basis (Skinner, 1953). Also similar to reinforcement, applied behavior analysts have utilized the principle of punishment to decrease undesirable behaviors. Likewise, positive and negative punishment procedures have been utilized frequently as integral roles in effective toilet training programs and methods.

Punishment and Toilet Training

The seminal studies by Azrin and Foxx (1971) and Foxx and Azrin (1973) included positive and negative punishment procedures. Specifically, several procedural components of the treatments implemented by Azrin and Foxx and Foxx and Azrin, among others (i.e., positive reinforcement), entailed either the provision (i.e., positive punishment; e.g., overcorrection, positive practice) or removal (i.e., negative punishment, time-out from reinforcement) of stimuli contingent on accidents and other problematic toileting behaviors. These components were based on the behavioral principle of punishment that suggested that future undesirable toileting behavior would decrease as a result of the application of the negative consequences. The incorporation of punishment procedures, within a broader treatment package that included the application of other behavioral principles (i.e., positive reinforcement) and behavioral-based tactics (i.e., scheduled sits, increased fluid intake, urinary alarm system), was demonstrated to be effective at decreasing problematic toileting behaviors in both Azrin and Foxx and Foxx and Azrin.

As discussed by Kroeger and Sorensen-Burnworth (2009), there appears to be less of an emphasis on punishment-based procedures in recent research pertaining to toilet training. This is likely a result of a general focus and emphasis on reinforcement-based procedures in lieu of, or prior to, the implementation of punishment-based procedures. In ABA, for example, the Behavior Analyst

Certification Board (BACB) code of ethics includes considerations pertaining to the application of punishment procedures including (a) that applied behavior analysts should utilize and recommend reinforcement instead of punishment whenever possible; (b) when punishment procedures are necessary, reinforcement-based procedures should always also be included within the treatment; and (c) prior to the use of punishment-based procedures, reinforcement-based approaches should be evaluated (BACB, 2014). Although recent focus has shifted the emphasis to reinforcement-based approaches with an emphasis on punishment-based procedures, such procedures have a "defined place in toileting history" (Kroeger & Soren-Burnworth, 2009). Further, many recent studies on toilet training procedures include punishment components (e.g., positive practice, vocal reprimands) although they may not be referred to as punishment-based procedures when described within the articles (Kroeger & Soren-Burnworth, 2009). Given the historical use of punishment-based procedures, the success rates of toilet training procedures that include punishment-based procedures, and the fact that many previous and recent studies (e.g., Ardic & Cavkaytar, 2014; Averink, Melein, & Duker, 2005; Didden, Sikkema, Bosman, Duker, & Curfs, 2001; Duker, Averink, & Melein, 2001; Lancioni, 1980; LeBlanc, Carr, Crossett, Bennett, & Detweiler; 2005) have included punishment-based components, any discussion of operant-based behavioral principles and their application to toilet training must include a discussion of punishment-based procedures.

Positive Punishment and Toilet Training

Subsequent studies following the seminal papers by Azrin and Foxx (1971) and Foxx and Azrin (1973) have demonstrated the positive effects of positive punishment during toilet training. For example, Didden et al. (2001) applied positive punishment in the treatment of toileting issues. Specifically, Didden et al. implemented a treatment package similar to the one described by Azrin and Foxx (1971) with six individuals with Angelman syndrome. The authors evaluated the effects of the treatment package using a nonconcurrent multiple baseline across participants of single-subject experimental design. Following a baseline condition in which dry checks were implemented hourly with no consequences for appropriate or problematic toileting behavior, the authors implemented training procedures consisting of both positive reinforcement (i.e., edibles and praise every 5 min contingent on dry pants and correct toileting responses) and positive punishment. The positive punishment procedures consisted of (a) requiring the participant to feel his/her wet pants, (b) a verbal reprimand, (c) requiring the participant to walk to the laundry area to retrieve dry clothes, and (d) requiring the participant to clean the area where the accident occurred. A negative punishment component was also included in the form of the removal of toys from the bathroom area and a 1-h time-out interval from positive reinforcement. When success was achieved with the above procedures (i.e., no accidents for 3 consecutive days), the authors implemented a subsequent treatment condition in which the time-out procedures were discontinued. Over time, the schedule of pants checks was also thinned. The results showed that the treatment package was effective at increasing independent toileting skills and successful urinations and decreasing urination accidents in children with Angelman syndrome.

Averink et al. (2005) provided another example of the effects of positive punishment. Averink et al. conducted toilet training with 40 individuals with a variety of disabilities including Down's syndrome, autism, rhesus antagonism, Noonan syndrome, Williams-Beuren syndrome, and Angelman syndrome. The authors utilized a nonconcurrent multiple baseline across participants of single-subject experimental design to evaluate the effects of the toilet training treatment package on urinary accidents. During baseline, the authors removed the participant's diaper and implemented scheduled toileting visits every 1–2 h. The authors provided praise during baseline contingent on successful urinations in the toilet. During the training phase, a trainer conducted treatment in a bathroom with the participant. The trainer prompted the participant to stand near the toilet and blocked all attempts to sit on the floor, walk away from the toilet, and engage in stereotypy and other behaviors not including lowering their pants and sitting on the toilet. Contingent on successful urinations in the toilet, the trainer delivered positive reinforcement in the form of praise and immediate access to preferred activities. Slowly, over time, the trainer increased the distance the participant was allowed to move away from the toilet. Contingent on all toileting accidents, the trainer immediately implemented a positive punishment procedure in the form of positive practice. The positive practice procedures consisted of requiring the participant to (a) go to the bathroom (the vicinity of distance from the toilet specified by the current trainings step) and (b) approach the toilet, lower his/her pants, and sit on the toilet for 3 s, (c) requiring the participant to raise her/her pants and move to a different part of the bathroom; and (d) the trainer repeated this sequence of steps four times following each accident. The results of the study showed that the treatment package, including the positive practice positive punishment procedure, decreased accidents across the clear majority of the 40 participants.

LeBlanc et al. (2005) provided an additional example of the application of positive punishment within an intensive outpatient behavioral treatment with three children with autism and urinary incontinence. The authors utilized a nonconcurrent multiple baseline across participants of single-subject experimental design to evaluate the effects of their treatment package on accidents and self-initiations. First, LeBlanc et al. conducted a preference assessment (i.e., *Reinforcer Assessment for Individuals with Severe Disabilities*, Fisher, Piazza, Bowman, & Amari 1996) to identify potential positive reinforcers to be incorporated within the treatment procedures. Following a baseline condition in the absence of treatment, the authors implemented a set of intensive training procedures that consisted of, among other components (e.g., sitting schedule, increased fluids), communication training, positive and negative reinforcement contingent on successful urinations and self-initiations (e.g., access to high-preferred toys, foods, and beverages; escape from the toilet), and positive punishment procedures in the form of positive practice. The positive practice procedures consisted of the authors (a) rapidly transitioning the participant to the toilets after providing a vocal verbal prompt ("no wet pants"); (b) requiring the participant to remove his/her pants, sit briefly on the toilet, stand, and replace the wet clothes; and (c) repeating this sequence of steps four times following each accident. The results clearly demonstrated the effectiveness of the training package including the positive punishment procedures.

Negative Punishment and Toilet Training

Azrin and Foxx (1971), in their seminal study, incorporated a negative punishment component within their broader treatment package approach. Specifically, contingent on the occurrence of accidents, the authors implemented 1-h time-out procedures in which they removed the participant's access to edibles and praise that were being provided every 5 min, they removed the participant's access to fluids (every 30 min), and they removed the participant's access to a chair. Thus, the authors removed stimuli contingent on accidents to decrease the likelihood that accidents would occur in the future. Azrin and Foxx combined these negative punishment procedures with positive punishment, reinforcement, and stimulus control procedures. Although it is difficult to determine the relative effects of the different elements of Azrin and Foxx's procedures, that application of negative punishment was a clear component of the treatment package.

Ardic and Cavkaytar (2014) incorporated a negative punishment procedure within a treatment package to decrease occurrences of urination in the pants with three children with autism diagnoses. The authors employed a multiple probe single-subject experimental design to evaluate the effects of their intervention. Following a baseline condition, the authors implemented a treatment consisting of a package of procedures including prompts, scheduled toilet visits, differential reinforcement of sitting (with access to toys provided as long as the participant sat on the toilet), positive reinforcement contingent on urination in the toilet, and negative punishment. With regard to the negative punishment element, specifically, the authors implemented two components that functioned as negative punishment including (a) removal of access to a toy in the case that he urinated in his pants and (b) a time-out from reinforcement for 10 min following urinations in the pants. It should also be noted that if the participant remained dry for the full 10-min time-out period, the authors immediately provided access to reinforcers. The result showed that the treatment package was effective at decreasing urination in the pants and increasing appropriate toileting skills.

Stimulus Control

When a behavior occurs at a higher frequency in the presence of a particular stimulus (i.e., a discriminative stimulus) relative to the absence of the stimulus, the behavior can be considered a discriminated operant that is under stimulus control (Cooper et al., 2007). The process of stimulus control directly involves the behavioral principle of reinforcement in that for a discriminative stimulus to come to reliably occasion a particular behavior, the behavior must be sufficiently reinforced in the presence of the stimulus. Also referred to as the "three-term contingency" (A, antecedent; B, behavior; C, consequence; Cooper et al., 2007), this process entails the reinforcement (C) of a behavior (B) in the presence of a particular antecedent (A). For example, a child's requesting behavior may be considered under stimulus control when a green card signals to the child that a break from work is available contingent on requests for a break if needed; and the child reliably emits requests in the presence of the green card. Further, other stimuli other than the green card (e.g., a red card) reliably signal that requests for breaks will not be reinforced and, thus, requests do not occur in the presence of stimuli other than the green card.

Similar to the behavioral principles of reinforcement and punishment, stimulus control is a naturally occurring phenomenon that affects the behavior of all organisms. In addition, applied behavior analysts often incorporate stimulus control procedures and considerations into their clinical practice with individuals with disabilities in terms of both skill acquisition programming and treatments of challenging behavior. Additionally, stimulus control processes play crucial roles in individuals' demonstration of problematic toileting behaviors, their acquisition of appropriate toileting skills, and their engagement in appropriate toileting skills and behavior over time and across different settings.

Stimulus Control and Toilet Training

Azrin and Foxx (1971) provided an initial example of the application of the behavioral principle of stimulus control in their seminal study. Specifically, Azrin and Foxx sought to establish stimulus control with urination in the toilet. The authors implemented stimulus control procedures by maximizing, to the extent possible, the pairing of urinations with sitting on the toilet. They did this by requiring the participants to sit on the toilet every 30 min for durations of 20 min (or until successful urination occurred) and then immediately providing several reinforcers (e.g., candy bars, drinks, hugs, praise) contingent on the successful urination. In this way, this aspect of the broader RTT method applied the behavioral principle of stimulus control to establish the toilet as a discriminative stimulus for urination (i.e., the discriminated operant). Azrin and Foxx also focused on immediacy of reinforcement, an important component in the establishment of stimulus control, via an apparatus that alerted the authors immediately when urination occurred, either in the toilet or pants. Although the stimulus control aspect of the set of procedures described by Azrin and Foxx was only one component of the treatment package, it is a vital component and has been a facet of successful ABA-based toilet training procedures.

Although stimulus control is considered to be integral to the success of ABA-based toilet training approaches and is often an inherent component of ABA-based treatment packages (i.e., the immediate application of reinforcement in the presence of successful urination in the toilet is intended to establish stimulus control in terms of successful urination and the toilet; e.g., Azrin & Foxx, 1971), several studies have isolated and manipulated treatment components to directly address stimulus control outcomes (e.g., Luiselli, 1996; Post & Kirkpatrick, 2004; Smith, Smith, Lee, & Kwok, 2000; Taylor, Cipani, & Clardy, 1994). For example, Taylor et al. (1994) transferred stimulus control from clothing and undergarments to the toilet to decrease unsuccessful voids and increase successful voids in the toilet exhibited by a 10-year-old male diagnosed with autism and severe intellectual disability. The participant had never been successfully toilet trained through any other method during four previous attempts and was resistant to attempts at toilet training. In addition, prior to the study, the participant had been taken to the toilet four to six times daily (for 8 years previous), but he only voided following his removal from the toilet when he was back in his clothing. Thus, the toilet was not serving as an effective discriminative stimulus for appropriate urination; rather his clothing was serving as the discriminative stimulus (i.e., stimulus control was likely occurring with his clothing; no stimulus control was occurring in terms of the toilet and his voiding behavior). Therefore, the authors sought to transfer stimulus control from his clothing to the toilet. The authors evaluated the effects of the stimulus control transfer procedures using an ABAC single-subject clinical case study design. Baseline consisted of 4-h assessment periods in which the only consequence for voiding outside of the toilet was a change of clothes. During Phase I of treatment, the authors implemented Azrin and Foxx's (1971) RTT procedures for 12 h. The Azrin and Foxx procedures were demonstrated to be ineffective at bringing about correct eliminations and decreasing incorrect eliminations. Thus, the authors implemented a subsequent treatment phase in which they modified the procedures described by Azrin and Foxx by incorporating a stimulus control transfer component. Specifically, they removed the participant's pants 5 min after receiving liquids, and they remained off until the next appropriate void in the toilet. Additionally, the authors increased the time in which the participant wore his clothes by 1-min increments after liquids were given. The participant was prompted to sit on the toilet until voiding or until a 10-min interval had passed. If voiding occurred during the 10-min toileting opportunity, the clothing was replaced, and an additional min of clothing-on time was added; after 15 correct voids, the participant's clothing remained on. The results showed that the procedures successfully transferred stimulus control from the participant's clothing to the toilet, as by the end of the study, he was successfully voiding in the toilet and incorrect urinations ceased completely (even during 4- and 10-month follow-ups). The results of Taylor et al. are particularly noteworthy in that they showed that individuals who are not successful with previous toilet training programs may require additional stimulus control procedural manipulations to supplement basic toilet training approaches. In other words, although the applications of reinforcement and response inhibitory procedures often produce adaptive stimulus control during basic toilet training procedures, there may be occasions in which additional stimulus control-based procedures may be necessary to bring about successful toilet training.

A second example of the effective use of a stimulus control procedure was provided by Luiselli (1996). Luiselli implemented toilet training procedures with a 7-year-old girl with PDD. Prior to the study, standard toilet training procedures (i.e., scheduled toileting trips, positive reinforcement) had been attempted but were not successful; instead, the participant frequently urinated in her diaper. Given the previously unsuccessful toilet training attempts and the participant's tendency to urinate in her diaper, the author implemented procedures aimed at transferring stimulus control, in terms of urination, from the diaper (and wearing the diaper) to the toilet. Luiselli used an AB clinical case study design to assess the effects of the stimulus control transfer procedures. First, during baseline, the staff implemented daily bathroom visits in which the participant was required to sit on the toilet while the staff provided vocal prompts. Following baseline, the staff implemented Phase I of the treatment, which involved the participant arriving at school and being changed from her diaper into training briefs. During each scheduled visit to the bathroom, her briefs were removed and replaced with a diaper, and she was required to sit on the toilet for 3 min. The diaper was only worn while sitting on the toilet and was removed after the 3 min. If the participant voided, staff provided enthusiastic praise, a sticker for her sticker chart, and the training briefs were put back on. Additionally, additional positive reinforcement was delivered in the form of free time or looking at a preferred book. If the participant did not void during the 3-min period, she was neutrally changed into the training briefs and exited the bathroom. The purpose of this phase was to function as the first step in the stimulus control transfer process (i.e., to establish the diaper *while also sitting on the toilet* as the discriminative stimulus for urination rather than the diaper alone). During the second phase of treatment, the author systematically faded out the diaper when urination in the diaper was consistent and reliably occurring while sitting on the toilet. Specifically, Luiselli intended to alter the physical dimensions of the diaper by cutting out progressively larger holes in the diaper; however, before the fading process involving the hole could be implemented, the participant sat on the toilet and independently voided in the absence of the diaper. Thus, the transfer of stimulus control occurred successfully as a result of Phase I pairing, and further fading from the diaper to the toilet was unnecessary. Therefore, the participant transitioned to wearing training briefs during the day and was expected to sit independently on the toilet without a diaper. Staff continued to provide positive reinforcement for successful voids in the toilet. During Phase III, the training briefs were faded during the day, and the participant was able to wear typical clothing and underwear, and in-toilet voiding remained at 100%, while in-pants urinations occurred at 0%. Data collected at a 1-month follow-up indicated 100% in-toilet urinations. Although as systematic fading of the diaper was not necessary, the implications in terms of transfer of stimulus control are important as the participant was conditioned to urinate while wearing a diaper on the toilet which, in turn, transferred to independent urinations on the toilet (i.e., stimulus control was transferred from the diaper to the toilet).

Post and Kirkpatrick (2004) manipulated the parameters of a standard toilet training procedure to address problematic stimulus control with a 3.5-year-old with a PDD diagnosis. The authors implemented a clinical case study design to assess the toilet training procedures. First, the authors implemented a baseline condition in which they documented occurrences of on- and off-toilet urinations while also implementing 5-min toilet sits every 30 min. The authors intended to implement a subsequent treatment condition in which scheduled toilet sits would occur based on the baseline data pertaining to off-toilet urinations (no on-toilet urinations occurred during baseline). However, the authors observed that the participant's training pants appeared to be functioning as a discriminative stimulus for urination (i.e., stimulus control was occurring with the training pants). Thus, the authors modified the toilet-sitting schedule as a tactic for facilitating transfer of stimulus control from the training pants to the toilet. Specifically, by increasing the density of the schedule for visits and the duration of time on the toilet, it was more likely that urination would occur in the toilet allowing for maximization of reinforcement of urination in the presence of the toilet (i.e., the intended discriminative stimulus). Through this process and tactic (in combination with prompting strategies and the application of reinforcement), the authors eventually demonstrated large increases in on-toilet urinations. The authors subsequently increased time off-toilet and decreased the scheduled visits, and on-toilet urinations continued to occur at high levels (with low-to-zero levels of off-toilet urinations). Thus, the authors' manipulation of variables that would increase the likelihood that in-toilet urinationss would contact reinforcement appeared to transfer stimulus control from the participant's training pants to the toilet.

Other Behavior-Based Tactics for Toilet Training

Although not directly derived from basic behavioral principles such as reinforcement, punishment, and stimulus control, there are several tactics that are often used within toilet training procedures that supplement or are applied in conjunction with procedures that entail the direct application of behavioral principles. Such tactics or procedures include prompting, scheduled toilet sits or visits to the bathroom, increased fluid intake procedures, and urinary alarm systems. These tactics are intended to increase the effects of reinforcement and stimulus control procedures by facilitating the occurrence of appropriate toileting behaviors and skills, allowing for the reinforcement (via positive and/or negative reinforcement) and stimulus control-based procedures to exert their effects based on their underlying behavioral principles. Many or most studies on toilet training procedures include these tactics (see Kroeger & Sorensen-Burnworth, 2009).

Prompting Strategies

Prompting strategies are antecedent-based methods used to facilitate correct responses, skills, or behaviors when they are not currently in a person's repertoire, thus requiring assistance to achieve the correct response (Cooper et al., 2007). While prompting is not an explicit behavioral principle, it does facilitate learning of new behavior and supplements the effects of tactics that apply behavioral principles (i.e., reinforcement, stimulus control). Prompting is typically implemented in the presence of a particular target discriminative stimulus and facilitates the occurrence of the behavior so that the behavior contacts positive or negative reinforcement, thus resulting in an increase in the likelihood that the behavior will occur in the future and learning occurs. Prompting is used specifically during the acquisition stage of teaching a new behavior or skill. The overall intent is to facilitate the occurrence of the behavior via prompting, followed by reinforcement of the behavior, and the subsequent transfer of stimulus control from the prompting method to naturally occurring stimuli in the learner's environment. It is this transfer of stimulus control from the prompt to the natural stimuli that indicates the behavior has been learned and added to the individual's repertoire. Prompts take the form of vocal prompts, model prompts, and physical guidance.

Prompting procedures typically play a prominent role within toilet training methods to facilitate engagement in the various behaviors and skills that are necessary for independent toileting (e.g., Adkins & Matthews, 1997; Azrin & Foxx, 1971; Foxx & Azrin, 1973; Halligan & Luyben, 2009; Luiselli, 1997; McLay, Carnett, Van Der Meer, & Lang, 2015; Post & Kirkpatrick, 2004; Taylor et al., 1994). Engagement in those necessary toileting behaviors and skills, through prompting procedures, allows for the direct reinforcement (positive and negative) of the behaviors and skills; this, in turn, increases the likelihood the individual will engage in in those behaviors and skills in the future and learn independent toileting. For example, Adkins and Matthews (1997) were successful in using vocal prompting to increase appropriate voiding for two adults with cognitive impairments. The authors trained care providers to use a verbal prompt to direct the adult participants to use the toilet. The two participants were checked for dryness every hour and praised when they were dry at the time of the check. When dryness was observed, the trainer provided a simple vocal prompt to use the toilet. The prompting procedure resulted in a 22% reduction of urine collected in wet diapers per day across the two participants when the dry checks were increased to 2 h and an additional significant reduction when the dry checks were scheduled 1 h apart and the adults were prompted to use the toilet.

Video modeling has also been used successfully in several studies to toilet train individuals with developmental disabilities. For example, McLay et al. (2015) successfully trained two participants with ASD through the use of video modeling combined with other prompting procedures. The participants were two boys, aged 7 and 8 years old; neither participant was able to urinate or defecate on the toilet, and one participant also engaged in fecal smearing. Both participants had no vocal language skills, and each used a speech-generating device (SGD) to communicate simple one-word requests. Both boys wore diapers throughout the day and night, and previous attempts at toilet training with both participants had been unsuccessful. Both participants were able to engage in motor imitation (a prerequisite skill when employing video modeling) as well as one-step gross motor actions (e.g., knocking on a table), one-step actions with objects (e.g., rolling a ball), facial expressions (e.g., a sad face), and single-word utterances from a video model. Based on the pre-assessment information, the authors chose to break the video model into smaller segments and train each step of the toileting routine individually rather than showing the entire routine in one sitting. Last, a task analysis was developed to identify the key steps in the toileting sequence (e.g., initiation of the toileting procedure, walking to the toilet, removal of clothing, sitting on the toilet, voiding on the toilet, dressing, flushing, and completion with handwashing). During baseline, the authors implemented least-to-most prompting (i.e., vocal, gestural, physical guidance), and reinforcement was withheld. During intervention, the authors first showed the participant a video model demonstrating the first step in the toileting sequence. The video model was shown immediately before the scheduled sit time based on data collected prior to intervention on how often the participants voided (i.e., 5–7 scheduled sits per day across participants). If the child did not respond to the video cue, the authors implemented the least-to-most prompting sequence (i.e., vocal, gestural, physical guidance). Positive reinforcement was delivered in the form of praise after each step of toileting was successfully completed; tangible positive reinforcement was delivered upon successful voids. Results from the study showed that the video-modeling intervention was successful as it increased the number of steps in toileting procedure completed independently when compared with baseline. Overall, the intervention was successful for both participants and their toileting for urination and was successful with one of the children for defecation. In addition, the intervention generalized to the school setting from the home for both participants, and outcomes were maintained at the 4-month follow-up period. McLay et al.'s procedures illustrated how modeling and prompting procedures, antecedent-based behavioral techniques, can facilitate the effects of reinforcement-based procedures that apply the behavioral principle of positive reinforcement. Specifically, the modeling and prompting procedures promoted the occurrence of the individual toileting-related behaviors and skills to facilitate and maximize the contact of those behaviors and skills with positive reinforcement, which, in turn, increased the likelihood that those behaviors would occur in the future in the presence of the toilet and the feeling of needing to use the bathroom. Thus, in addition to facilitating the effects of positive reinforcement, the modeling and prompting procedures facilitated the transfer of stimulus control to the feeling of needing to use the bathroom, as well as the visual cue of seeing a toilet, enabled prompting to be faded and independent toilet use and initiation to increase.

Physical and graduated guidance is another common behavioral tactic used in toilet training procedures for individuals with intellectual disabilities (Kroeger & Sorensen-Burnworth, 2009). Foxx and Azrin (1973) utilized graduated guidance and physical promptings within RTT. Specifically, the authors used graduated guidance to facilitate sitting on the toilet and then progressively lessened the intensity of guidance applied to the participants as they engaged in successful and independent sitting. In addition to several considerations within the procedures (e.g., variety, quality, immediacy, and frequency of reinforcement; detection of correct and incorrect responses accurately), physical guidance was included along with other prompting procedures (i.e., vocal). Specifically, each participant was placed in a non-distracting environment (i.e., restriction to highly preferred activities that could interfere with toileting performance), the authors increased fluid intake to increase the number of potential trials, reinforcement was provided contingent on correct responding, and graduated guidance and vocal prompting procedures were utilized. Graduated guidance was used following any vocal instruction during the toileting routine in which the participant did not respond to the vocal instruction and required manual guidance to complete the step. Graduated guidance involved providing assistance for walking to the bathroom, undressing and dressing, and hand washing. All physical prompts were eventually faded and transfer of stimulus control and independent toileting was achieved.

Scheduled Siting Procedures

Many toileting treatment packages include a scheduled sitting component (e.g., Averink et al., 2005; Azrin & Foxx, 1971; Keen, Brannigan, & Cuskelly, 2007; LeBlanc et al., 2005; Luiselli, 1996, 1997, 2007; Post & Kirkpatrick, 2004; Richmond, 1983). Scheduled sitting procedures entail the establishment of a schedule by which the individual is prompted or moved to the bathroom to sit on or stand in front of the toilet. When combined with increased fluid intake procedures (see below), scheduled sitting procedures are intended to increase the likelihood that successful voiding will occur in the toilet allowing for the application of reinforcement-based procedures. Thus, scheduled sittings can be essential in increasing the effects of reinforcement-based procedures by maximizing the ability of the trainer to apply reinforcement to successful voiding by increasing the chance that the behavior will occur. Schedules that are used for schedule sitting procedures can be predetermined and entail regular intervals (e.g., every 90 min; Luiselli, 2007), or they can be based on pre-training assessment procedures aimed at determining the likeliest times for urination (e.g., LeBlanc et al., 2005; Post & Kirkpatrick, 2004).

As described above in the positive reinforcement section, Post and Kirkpatrick (2004) applied positive reinforcement toilet training procedures with a 3.5-year-old boy with PDD; additionally, the authors incorporated scheduled sitting procedures within a treatment package. Specifically, Post and Kirkpatrick implemented scheduled sittings throughout the day (i.e., every 30 min) in conjunction with the positive reinforcement-based procedures. Initially during treatment, the authors had the child sit on the toilet for 20 min per 30-min intervals, which were implemented every 30 min. The authors based this schedule on data they collected prior treatment on urination times. The authors implemented positive reinforcement-based procedures including praise for compliance with toilet sitting and access to high-preferred items contingent on successful appropriate urinations. By applying the scheduled sitting procedure, the authors maximized the chances for successful urinations in the toilet; thus, they maximized their opportunities to apply positive reinforcement, which, in turn, maximized the effects of the application of the behavioral principle. Further, this also allowed for the establishment of stimulus control in terms of the feeling of the need to go the bathroom occasioning appropriate urinations.

Keen et al. (2007) implemented scheduled sitting procedures in conjunction with a toilet training video prompting procedure with five children with autism diagnoses. The authors employed a multiple baseline across participants of single-subject experimental design to evaluate the treatment package which also included the application of positive reinforcement in addition to scheduled sittings and video-modeling procedures. Specifically, the authors implemented scheduled sittings during which, prior to sitting down on the toilet, they showed 6-min animated videos of successful toileting behaviors. The authors then required the participants to sit on the toilet for 3-min intervals. The authors delivered positive reinforcement contingent on appropriate toileting behaviors. The results showed that the treatment package was successful at increasing in-toilet urinations. The procedures provided an example of the positive effects of scheduled sittings and prompting procedures in facilitating the effects of positive reinforcement. Similar to Post and Kirkpatrick (2004), the combination of procedures also allowed for the establishment of appropriate stimulus control.

Increased Fluid Intake

A standard component of most toileting training treatments involves the increase of fluid intake by the participants (e.g., Ardic & Cavkaytar, 2014; Averink et al., 2005; Azrin & Foxx, 1971; Foxx & Azrin, 1973; Halligan & Luyben, 2009; Keen et al., 2007; LeBlanc et al., 2005; Luiselli, 1997; Taylor et al., 1994). Similar to scheduled sittings and prompting procedures, increasing fluid intake is intended to increase the likelihood that individuals will successfully void in the toilet and thereby allow for the application of positive reinforcement and stimulus control-based procedures. Although increasing fluid during toilet training has been demonstrated to be an effective component of training packages, the potential medical risks of increasing fluid intake should be noted and considered when designing a toilet training protocol (see Kroeger & Sorensen-Burnworth, 2009).

In their seminal study, Azrin and Foxx (1971) utilized fluid intake procedures by providing drinks every 30 min. The increase in fluid intake was intended to supplement and work in conjunction with the reinforcement-based components of the treatment package (i.e., contingent delivery of edible and social reinforcement). The results of the study showed that the treatment package was effective, and it is important to note that the reinforcement-based components' ability to exert their effects on the target behaviors was enhanced by the increase in voiding that resulted from the increase in fluid intake.

Averink et al. (2005) described an additional example of the incorporation of increases in fluid intake within a broader treatment package approach that also included positive reinforcement and positive punishment procedures. Specifically, the authors provided extra liquids at the beginning of each training day. The results showed that the procedures were effective at bringing about decreases in toileting accidents.

Urinary Alarm Systems

Devices that detect moisture in the diaper or underwear and subsequently sound an alarm or provide an indicator sound have been utilized regularly within toilet training procedures (e.g., Azrin & Foxx, 1971; Foxx & Azrin, 1973; Lancioni, 1980; LeBlanc et al., 2005). The inclusion of such devices allow for the instant detection of urinary accidents, which, in turn, allows for the relatively immediate implementation of subsequent procedures (e.g., punishment-based procedures, negative reinforcement-based procedures). For example, Azrin and Foxx utilized an apparatus that sounded an audio signal when the participant urinated or defecated in his/her pants. As discussed above, Azrin and Foxx incorporated positive punishment-based procedures in the form of positive practice and overcorrection and a negative reinforcement-based procedure in the form of time-out from reinforcers. The alarm system facilitated the effects of the punishment- and negative reinforcement-based components by allowing for their relatively immediate implementation by the authors, thereby maximizing their effects in terms of reducing the future occurrence of accidents. Similarly, LeBlanc et al. utilized a urine sensor and alarm within their treatment package that also included a sitting schedule, positive reinforcement-based procedures, increased fluid intake, and positive punishment-based procedures (i.e., positive practice). When the alarm sounded, the authors immediately provided a vocal reprimand (i.e., "no wet pants") and "quickly escorted" the participant to the bathroom and prompted them to sit on the toilet. If successful urination occurred, the positive reinforcement-based procedures were implemented; if the participant did not urinate in the toilet, the authors implemented the positive punishment-based procedures (i.e., positive practice). Thus the urine alarm functioned to increase the impact of both the positive reinforcement-based components and the positive punishment-based components by allowing for the relatively immediate implementation of those procedures following accidents, thereby maximizing their effects.

Summary

In this chapter we described the application of operant-based behavioral principles and mechanisms derived from EAB and ABA within toilet training and procedures. A primary goal of this chapter was to provide the reader with an overview of the strong applicability of behavioral principles and mechanisms across numerous examples of toilet training methods across a wide variety of populations (e.g., ASD, visual and hearing impairments, Angelman syndrome, Down's syndrome, severe intellectual disabilities, PDD, cognitive impairments, typically developing individuals) and age groups (e.g., children, adolescents, adults). The variety of procedures derived from basic behavioral principles and mechanisms that have been utilized within toilet training treatment packages is also diverse, including positive and negative reinforcement-based procedures, positive and negative punishment-based procedures, and stimulus control-based procedures. A wide variety of additional procedures and tactics that function to supplement and increase the effects of procedures based on behavioral principles have also been shown to be successful components including prompting strategies, scheduled toilet sits, increased fluid intake procedures, and urinary alarm systems.

References

Adkins, V. K., & Mathews, R. M. (1997). Prompted voiding to reduce incontinence in community-dwelling older adults. *Journal of Applied Behavior Analysis, 30*, 153–156.

Ardiç, A., & Cavkaytar, A. (2014). Effectiveness of the modified intensive toilet training method on teaching toilet skills to children with autism. *Education and Training in Autism and Developmental Disabilities, 49*, 263.

Averink, M., Melein, L., & Duker, P. C. (2005). Establishing diurnal bladder control with the response restriction method: Extended study on its effectiveness. *Research in Developmental Disabilities, 26*, 143–151.

Azrin, N. H., & Foxx, R. M. (1971). A rapid method of toilet training the institutionalized regarded. *Journal of Applied Behavior Analysis, 4*, 89–99.

Baer, D. M., Wolf, M. M., & Risley, T. R. (1968). Some current dimensions of applied behavior analysis. *Journal of Applied Behavior Analysis, 1*, 91–97.

Board, B. A. C. (2014). Professional and ethical compliance code for behavior analysts.

Cooper, J. O., Heron, T. E., & Heward, W. L. (2007). Applied behavior analysis (2nd ed.). Upper Saddle River, NJ: Prentice Hall.

Cicero, F. R., & Pfadt, A. (2002). Investigation of a reinforcement-based toilet training procedure for children with autism. *Research in Developmental Disabilities, 23*, 319–331.

Didden, R., Sikkema, S. P., Bosman, I., Duker, P. C., & Curfs, L. M. (2001). Use of a modified Azrin–Foxx toilet training procedure with individuals with Angelman syndrome. *Journal of Applied Research in Intellectual Disabilities, 14*, 64–70.

Duker, P. C., Averink, M., & Melein, L. (2001). Response restriction as a method to establish diurnal bladder control. *American Journal on Mental Retardation, 106*, 209–215.

Ellis, N. R. (1963). Toilet training and the severely defective patient: An S-R reinforcement analysis. *American Journal of Mental Deficiency, 68*, 98–103.

Felce, D., & Perry, J. (1995). Quality of life: Its definition and measurement. *Research in Developmental Disabilities, 16*, 51–74.
Fisher, W. W., Piazza, C. C., Bowman, L. G., & Amari, A. (1996). Integrating caregiver report with a systematic choice assessment. *American Journal on Mental Retardation, 101*, 15–25.
Foxx, R. M., & Azrin, N. H. (1973). Dry pants: A rapid method of toilet training children. *Behaviour Research and Therapy, 11*, 435–442.
Halligan, S. M., & Luyben, P. D. (2009). Prompts, feedback, positive reinforcement, and potty training. *Journal of Prevention & Intervention in the Community, 37*, 177–186.
Hundziak, M., Maurer, R. A., & Watson, L. S. (1965). Operant conditioning in toilet training severely mentally retarded boys. *American Journal of Mental Deficiency, 70*, 120–124.
Keen, D., Brannigan, K. L., & Cuskelly, M. (2007). Toilet training for children with autism: The effects of video modeling. *Journal of Developmental and Physical Disabilities, 19*, 291–303.
Kroeger, K. A., & Sorensen-Burnworth, R. (2009). Toilet training individuals with autism and other developmental disabilities: A critical review. *Research in Autism Spectrum Disorders, 3*, 607–618.
Lancioni, G. E. (1980). Teaching independent toileting to profoundly retarded deaf-blind children. *Behavior Therapy, 11*, 234–244.
LeBlanc, L. A., Carr, J. E., Crossett, S. E., Bennett, C. M., & Detweiller, D. D. (2005). Intensive outpatient behavioral treatment of primary urinary incontinence of children with autism. *Focus on Autism and Other Developmental Disabilities, 20*, 98–105.
Luiselli, J. K. (1994). Toilet training children with sensory impairments in a residential school setting. *Behavioral Interventions, 9*, 105–114.
Luiselli, J. K. (1996). A case study evaluation of a transfer-of-stimulus control toilet training procedure for a child with pervasive developmental disorder. *Focus on Autism and Other Developmental Disabilities, 11*, 158–162.
Luiselli, J. K. (1997). Teaching toilet skills in a public school setting to a child with pervasive developmental disorder. *Journal of Behavior Therapy and Experimental Psychiatry, 28*, 163–168.
Luiselli, J. K. (2007). Single-case evaluation of a negative reinforcement toilet training intervention. *Child & family behavior therapy, 29*, 59–69.
McLay, L., Carnett, A., van der Meer, L., & Lang, R. (2015). Using a video Modeling-based intervention package to toilet train two children with autism. *Journal of Developmental and Physical Disabilities, 27*, 431–451.
Post, A. R., & Kirkpatrick, M. A. (2004). Toilet training for a young boy with pervasive developmental disorder. *Behavioral Interventions, 19*, 45–50.
Richmond, G. (1983). Shaping bladder and bowel continence in developmentally retarded preschool children. *Journal of Autism and Developmental Disorders, 13*, 197–204.
Roane, H. S., & Betz, A. M. (2012). Behavior analysis. In V. S. Ramachandran (Ed.), *Encyclopedia of human behavior* (2nd ed.). Elsevier Press: Kidlington, UK.
Rolider, A., & Van Houten, R. (1985). Treatment of constipation-caused encopresis by a negative reinforcement procedure. *Journal of Behavior Therapy and Experimental Psychiatry, 16*(1), 67–70.
Skinner, B. F. (1953). *Science and human behavior*. Simon and Schuster.
Smith, L., Smith, P., Lee, Y., & Kwok, S. (2000). Behavioural treatment of urinary incontinence and encopresis in children with learning disabilities: Transfer of stimulus control. *Developmental Medicine & Child Neurology, 42*, 276–279.
Taylor, S., Cipani, E., & Clardy, A. (1994). A stimulus control technique for improving the efficacy of an established toilet training program. *Journal of Behavior Therapy and Experimental Psychiatry, 25*, 155–160.
Van Wagenen, R. K., Meyerson, L., Kerr, N. J., & Mahoney, K. (1969). Field trials of a new procedure for toilet training. *Journal of Experimental Child Psychology, 8*, 147–159.
WHOQOL Group. (1995). The World Health Organization quality of life assessment (WHOQOL): Position paper from the World Health Organization. *Social Science & Medicine, 41*, 1403–1409.

Toilet Training: Strategies Involving Modeling and Modifications of the Physical Environmental

Laurie McLay and Neville Blampied

Toilet training is a social learning process requiring interactions between young children and their parents and caregivers over extended periods of time, typically in the first 2 to 4 years of life. It is a complex process involving both developmental maturation and learning, and not all children respond sufficiently to the conventional techniques encountered in their specific family and cultural context to achieve excretory continence and culturally appropriate toileting practices (Kaerts, Vermandel, Lierman, van Gestel, & Wyndalele, 2012). Thus, for some, additional strategies are needed in order for continence and toileting to be learned (Kaerts et al., 2012). Such strategies may include motivating and prompting the behavior, manipulation of antecedent stimulus control, and/or facilitative environmental modifications, as well as providing salient consequences for correct performance. In this chapter, selected strategies will be described, guidelines for implementing them provided, and the research base supporting their use evaluated. First, to put these intervention options in context, the chapter begins with a brief biobehavioral analysis of the development of bladder and bowel continence and of the key skills that must be acquired for toileting to be done reliably and independently.

L. McLay (✉)
University of Canterbury, College of Education, Health, and Human Development, Christchurch, New Zealand
e-mail: laurie.mclay@canterbury.ac.nz

N. Blampied
University of Canterbury, College of Science, Psychology Department, Christchurch, New Zealand

J.L. Matson (ed.), *Clinical Guide to Toilet Training Children*, Autism and Child Psychopathology Series, DOI 10.1007/978-3-319-62725-0_9

Toilet Training: A Biobehavioral Analysis

Any behavior analysis of a learned response must begin by considering the nature of the behaviors involved, specifically asking if they are respondent (i.e., reflex based) or operant (i.e., a discriminated operant response determined by a three-term contingency of antecedents, behavior, and consequences) or involving operant-respondent interactions (Cooper, Heron & Heward, 2007). In the case of operant behavior, the role of motivation plus other antecedents (i.e., controlling stimuli), the response and how it might be shaped and facilitated, and the nature of the consequences (i.e., if reinforcing or punishing) need careful attention (Kazdin, 2013).

The achievement of reliable independent toileting by a child requires the coming together in their behavior repertoire of three different domains of skill. First, they must achieve continence, i.e., the ability to withhold the release of urine and feces (voiding) until it is appropriate to do so. This is further broken down into nocturnal fecal continence (NFC), nocturnal urinary continence (NUC), day urinary continence (DUC), and day fecal continence (DFC; Schum, Kolb, McAuliffe, Simms, Underhill, & Lewis, 2002). The natural history of this process is not well documented (Kaerts et al., 2012; Schum et al., 2002), but research suggests that the typical sequence is NFC, then DFC, followed by DUC, and, finally, NUC, with girls typically achieving these milestones before boys (Stein & Susser, 1967). Note that the ages at which these milestones are typically met are not the same across cultures (deVires & deVires, 1977) and have also changed to later ages over recent decades within Western culture (Bakker & Wyndale, 2000).

The second set of skills that must be acquired involve recognizing that the bowel or bladder needs emptying, approaching the potty/toilet and using it appropriately, with correct posture and ultimately with situationally correct behaviors of genital and anal cleaning and flushing the toilet. Finally, some more general skills, such as undressing and dressing and handwashing that are performed in other contexts, must also be used in the toileting context. Fully functional independent toileting requires that all of these skills be chained together in a single fluent performance. This typically requires extensive training and practice over a relatively long period of time (Luxem & Christopherson, 1994).

The Respondent Behavior Substrate

All living organisms must be able to excrete the waste products of metabolism. Humans, in common with other vertebrates, produce urine in the kidneys and feces in the bowel. These wastes are produced all the time but are not discharged continuously because they are stored in specialist organs – the bladder for urine and the rectum for feces – which are kept closed by muscular sphincters. Only when their sphincters are relaxed does tension in the smooth muscles of the bladder and rectal wall expel the contents out of the body. This process can be viewed (at a simplified level) as a reflex initiated by an unconditioned stimulus (US) of bladder or rectal distension at a critical level (which changes with age and experience) and an unconditioned response (UR) of sphincter relaxation. This respondent behavior is present throughout life, from birth to death, and may emerge again even after independent toileting is well established due to emotional distress, illness, intoxication, dementia, and the loss of capacities in old age.

The Operant Behavior Overlay

Continence requires that the child develop the capacity to prevent the reflex release of bowel and bladder contents until they are in a culturally appropriate situation (a toilet of some kind). This is often referred to as learning to "hold on" and involves the voluntary tensing of abdominal and perineal muscles such that the reflex relaxation of the sphincter is inhibited. This is a learned behavior, except perhaps for NFC, which, since it occurs at the earliest age, is first in the sequence and emerges while the child is asleep (Schum et al., 2002), may represent a maturational process.

The other forms of continence require the acquisition of antecedent stimulus control, one component of which is interoceptive (awareness of the sensation of bowel and bladder distension and excretory urgency) and the other exteroceptive (including recognizing the potty/toilet as the correct place for voiding to occur). Both of these are facilitated by the prior learning of excretory and toilet-related words (Schum et al., 2002) and by parents/caregivers discriminating when overt signs of imminent voiding occur and helping the child with the correct toileting behavior (Kaerts et al., 2012; Smeets, Lancioni, Ball, & Oliva, 1985). Parents/caregivers then scaffold the process through which the child makes transitions such as from potty (portable and available in many places) to the toilet (in fixed places) and acquires the skills of undressing, dressing, cleaning, and flushing that constitute the full toileting repertoire (Schum et al., 2002).

Intervention Strategies

As the analysis above shows, many things must be learned for a child to become continent and toilet trained. This chapter focuses on a subset of these involving antecedent control and facilitative environmental modifications that may be deployed to help children who have not become toilet trained by typical family/caregiver training (Halligan & Luyben, 2009). Elementary teaching and learning strategies commonly used in teaching children skills, including toilet training, are noted below. Following Kazdin (2013) these strategies may be differentiated into (1) setting events and establishing operations, (2) prompts and high-probability requests, (3) discriminative stimulus control, and (4) other strategies. In the context of toilet training, setting events and establishing operations involve aspects of the context in which toileting behavior occurs and its motivation, including the emotional tone of parent-child interactions. Prompts are stimuli, such as verbal instructions (e.g., "go sit on the potty"), visual or auditory cues (e.g., a picture of a child sitting on a toilet posted on the toilet door), and gestures (e.g., pointing to the potty); manual guidance (e.g., helping a child undress); and demonstrations (e.g., soaping hands). A special kind of prompt involves the use of high-probability request sequences (e.g., three requests in quick succession that a child is likely to perform) followed immediately by a request that the child has shown little likelihood of complying with (e.g., "go sit on the potty").

The critical feature of prompts is that as skills are acquired the prompts can be faded until they are no longer needed for correct performance. Discriminative stimulus control involves learning that specific features of the environment, which may be interoceptive (internal to the person) or exteroceptive (in the physical or social environment), are associated with correct performances of behavior, for instance, learning that it is the potty or toilet where defecation should occur, not in diapers or clothing. Unlike prompts, discriminative stimuli (SD) cannot be faded – for instance, if we went into a room labeled *Toilet* but could not see a toilet fixture, we would not be able to perform correct toilet behaviors – however, control may be transferred from one SD to another, e.g., a male child who has learned to urinate in a toilet can also learn to use a urinal.

These elementary strategies are often combined in more complex packages that involve modeling procedures (observational learning) and/or some form of environmental or stimulus manipulation. Modeling includes in vivo modeling, video modeling (VM), video self-modeling (VSM), and video point-of-view (POV) modeling. Modeling may function as a prompt – a demonstration of a specific component skill – or provide a demonstration of the full behavior sequence and its consequences. Behavior-facilitating environmental modifications involve provision of prompts, modified discriminative stimuli, and structural supports for achieving competent toileting. The task to be learned also is often broken down into simpler steps, and these are then combined by response chaining. For the purpose of this chapter, reinforcement strategies will be described only to the extent that they are used in combination with key toilet training strategies that are the chapter focus. A combination of Internet webpage and database searching was used to locate research into toilet training strategies that focused on these approaches. First, however, the basic forms of modeling are described.

Varieties of Modeling

The science of social learning reveals that learning may occur when a person who lacks a particular skill observes a model performing an example of that skill. This is commonly referred to as observational learning or modeling (Bandura, 1977a, 1978). Four key conditions are required for observational learning to occur: (1) attention to the behavior being modeled, (2) retention of the observed behavior and the conditions in which the behavior occurred, (3) reproduction of the behavior that was modeled (i.e., imitation), and (4) a sufficient level of motivation to warrant imitation of the observed behavior (Bandura, 1977a). Important additional factors increasing the likelihood that the learner will learn by observation relate to the observation of consequences being experienced by the model and the experience of consequences by the learner in the event that they attempt to imitate the model. These consequences may be rewarding or punishing. Observation and experience of rewarding consequences increases the likelihood of imitation; observation and experience of punishment inhibits imitation (Bandura, 1977a). Other factors that modulate observational learning include the salience of the behavior modeled and the consequences experienced by the observer; the emotional responsiveness of the model during the performance; the perceived social equivalence, attractiveness, and/or status of the model relative to the learner; and the motivational state of the learner (Bandura 1977a; Kazdin, 2013). While observational learning is primarily regarded as providing the learner with information about the topography of the behavior to be learned, it also provides information about salient SDs and about contingent consequences.

The first modeling procedure investigated was in vivo modeling (Bandura, Ross, & Ross, 1961), which involves the use of a live model who demonstrates the target behavior or skills. There is a large body of research demonstrating that in vivo modeling is effective in supporting the learning of typically developing children and children with disabilities (Bandura et al., 1961; Gena, Couloura, & Kymissis, 2005; Hosford, 1980; Meltzoff, 1995; Ollendick & King, 1998).

There are obvious benefits to recording the model's behavior on film or video. The learner can then watch the demonstration repeatedly at any convenient time. Types of VM include adult modeling, in which an adult models the target skills or behavior, and peer modeling, in which an equivalent-aged peer models the target behavior. In VSM the model and the observer are the same individual, while in point-of-view (POV) modeling, the observer experiences the display as if viewed through the eyes of the model. VSM and POV modeling generally require technical means to supply the modeled display. There is considerable evidence supporting the use of each of these types of modeling for the acquisition of many skills (Dowrick, 1999; McCoy & Hermansen, 2007).

When used in clinical practice, VSM can take the form of feedforward or feedback (also known as positive self-review, PSR; Dowrick, 1999, 2012a, 2012b) modeling. In video feedforward, a skill is selected that the individual is unable to perform. The video then provides a successful and errorless demonstration of the target skill or behavior being performed by that individual. To date, video feedforward has been used to teach a variety of skills, including academic skills, language, play, prosocial behavior, and social skills (e.g., Baker, O'Reilly, & Lang, 2009; Dowrick, 2012a; Lang, Shogren, Machalicek, Rispoli, O'Reilly, Regester, & Baker, 2009; Tereshko, MacDonald, & Ahearn 2010).

The process of using video feedback/PSR differs from video feedforward in that it typically involves video recording an individual performing a particular target skill or behavior at some appropriate level of competence and then having the individual review the video in order to review and, perhaps, restore competent performance (Dowrick, 1999, 2012a, 2012b). Much research demonstrates the positive effects of video feedback on educator and practitioner practices (Mead, Dozier, & Bernard, 2014; Pinter, East, and Thrush, 2015; van Vonderen, Duker, & Didden, 2010; van Vonderen, Didden, & Beeking, 2012), parenting practices (Cassibba, Castoro, Costantino, Sette, & Ijzendoorn, 2015; Lam-Cassettari, Wadnerkar-Kamble, & James, 2015; Moss, Tarabylsby, St-Georgesc, Dubois-Comtoisd, Cyr, Bernier, St-Laurentd, Pascuzzo, & Lecompte, 2014), and children's skill acquisition and behavior change (Deitchman, Reeve, Reeve, & Progar, 2010; O'Reilly, O'Halloran, Sigafoos, Lancioni, Green, Edrisinhaa, Cannella, & Olive, 2005; Sibley, Pelham, Mazur, Gnagy, Ross, & Kuriyan, 2012).

Observational Learning, Modeling, and Toilet Training

Several types of modeling can be used in toilet training, including in vivo modeling, VM, VSM, and POV modeling. Each of these processes and the evidence base underpinning these processes are described below.

In Vivo Modeling

When used in toilet training, in vivo modeling would typically involve a parent or sibling demonstrating the toileting sequence, including in-toilet voiding. While this is a commonly reported procedure anecdotally, the authors were unable to identify any research documenting whether this procedure, when used in isolation, is in fact effective in teaching children the steps in the toileting sequence, including in-toilet voiding. Based on the conventions of in vivo modeling, the child should be exposed to the model immediately prior to a toileting opportunity, and the model would demonstrate errorless performance of the toileting sequence (i.e., correct performance of the target behavior performed independently).

In vivo modeling is advantageous as it offers a simple, technology-free option, provided at a teachable moment when the learner's opportunity to imitate is available. It may also be beneficial in that the model is known to the child, that the model and the learner are emotionally attached to each other, and that the emotions demonstrated are authentic. These are all setting events that are likely to promote learning, and there are some suggestions in the literature that using a familiar model (e.g., a peer or family member) may enhance the success of modeling procedures (Dowrick, 1999).

There are also obvious limitations to the use of in vivo modeling, particularly in regard to cultural concerns and ethical issues. While people known to the individual would be able to model some of the steps in the toileting sequence (e.g., flushing the toilet), in many cultures there may be restrictions on who is considered appropriate, other than the child's parent or family caregiver, to model in-toilet voiding. In such cases training is restricted to times when the parent(s) or other family member(s) are present. Further, this means that it is not always possible to provide an in vivo model in settings other than the home environment. While this is not problematic for typically developing children, it may pose problems in situations where clinicians or teachers are supporting the toilet training process (Kaerts et al., 2012; Luxem & Christopherson, 1994), particularly in that there is limited opportunity to promote generalization of the toileting skills to contexts not involving parental supervision and/or the home environment.

Video Modeling and Toilet Training

There are a variety of sources of VM available to support the toilet training process. One is via the purchase of commercially available products; the other is to create individualized video models. Commercially available toileting videos often use generic animated characters (Keen, Brannigan, & Cuskelly, 2007) or people acting as generic models (who are necessarily unfamiliar to the learner) to depict the toileting sequence. Such videos typically demonstrate a person going through the toileting sequence, but do not depict urination or defecation. For example, in the 20-min video "It's Potty Time" (Howard, 1991), various children are demonstrated going through the toileting sequence and shown to be physically and emotionally supported by their parents, though voiding is not demonstrated. Examples of toilet use are occasionally followed by depictions of parental praise. This video includes songs about toilet use and also short interludes of unrelated narrated stories (e.g., Raggedy Ann), a feature common in commercially available toileting videos that is included to motivate watching the video.

Commercial videos have the advantages of being readily available, convenient, and often inexpensive. A caution, however, in purchasing commercially available toilet training videos is that they are not able to be edited or tailored according to each child's unique needs. It is also possible that some children do not relate to the characters demonstrating the procedure or may not be motivated to attend to these characters. If this is the case, individualized videos using familiar models may offer an effective alternative.

Evidence for Video Modeling Including Commercial Toilet Training Products and Toilet Training Research

Only two studies were identified that have examined the effects of commercial VM on the acquisition of toileting skills (Bainbridge & Smith-Myles, 1999; Keen et al., 2007), both using generic models of children or characters. Bainbridge and

Smith-Myles (1999) used commercial VM to teach toilet use to a 3-year-old boy with autism spectrum disorder (ASD) using "It's Potty Time" (Howard, 1991). The child was shown the video three times per day, and immediately afterward, he was told "It's time to go potty" (a prompt). The results were an increase in independently initiated toilet use and a decrease in urination accidents.

Keen et al. (2007) used an animated VM video (6 min in duration) to teach in-toilet urination to five children with ASD between the ages of 4 and 6 years, comparing treatment with a control group in which prompting and reinforcement alone were used. Treatment group children were required to watch the VM immediately prior to the scheduled use of the toilet. The VM depicted the sequence of toileting steps for boys and girls paired with animated characters that provided verbal instructions on the toileting sequence and praise for successful voiding on the toilet. VM was supplemented by a set of pictorial cues that accompanied the video. These cue cards were reportedly used as prompts to redirect children so that they did not urinate in inappropriate areas in the home. Children were also prompted to initiate toilet use using pictures, signs, or language. In this study frequency of in-toilet urination was greater (to an unspecified degree as no effect size was reported) for the three children who watched the animated video, compared to the two children in the control group. Sufficient detail regarding the content and process for using the VM and picture cue card was lacking in this report making it difficult to fully understand all aspects of the procedure.

In summary, while the research examining the use of VM shows promise, the small number of studies and lack of evidence of direct or systematic replication means it is difficult to draw definitive conclusions about the effectiveness of this approach across all children and young people. Surprisingly, no research was identified that investigated the use of personally created VM using models who were familiar to the child. Given the growing popularity of VM and the importance of independent toileting as a life skill (Kaerts et al., 2012), further research examining the effectiveness of VM is required.

Video Self-Modeling and Toilet Training

Feedforward VSM is an alternative to VM and necessarily has to be individually tailored because the model and the learner are the same person. To create the demonstration of the learner performing skills not yet in their repertoire, videos are edited to remove evidence of assistance and errors, and sometimes coaching (not visible on the edited video) is required to achieve a simulation of the required performance. Where culturally/ethically appropriate, the self-model should demonstrate several key steps, beginning with independent approach to the toilet, undressing, flushing of the toilet, redressing, and handwashing. Animations of the child's genital and/or anal area can also be used to depict in-toilet voiding (including urination and defecation, separately or both, depending on what the child needs to learn) and self-cleaning. Animation is used to protect the children's privacy and avoid cultural offense, but also in cases in which in-toilet voiding is unable to be captured on video due to the child being unable to perform this. POV modeling can also be integrated into these videos in order to depict actions as viewed from the perspective of the child. This is used to specifically target fine motor actions that are best demonstrated using a close-up view.

There are many advantages to using VM or VSM over in vivo modeling. The steps in the toileting sequence are modeled consistently each time, can be viewed repeatedly, and be tailored to specifically target the specific needs of each child (e.g., there may only be a few steps in the toileting sequence that the child is yet to learn). VM/VSM typically incorporates examples of the child being rewarded (e.g., by descriptive praise or by some other form of rewarding consequence). This may increase the efficiency of toilet training as children who are going through the toilet training process may not otherwise be aware of the reinforcement contingency between in-toilet voiding and the reward, and this can motivate children to engage in these behaviors during repeated practice. VSM has further advantages over VM in that it is possible that children are better able to relate to the video demonstration of the skill, when the model and the learner are one (Dowrick, 1999, 2012b). Finally, VM/VSM can represent the situation as a fun, positive experience, thus assisting with creating a setting event context that is positively valenced.

Evidence for Video Self-Modeling and Toilet Training

Recent research on VSM in toilet training has focused on children with ASD (Drysdale, Lee, Anderson, & Moore, 2015; Lee, Anderson, & Moore, 2014; McLay, Carnett, van der Meer, & Lang, 2015). No studies were identified that included children who were typically developing or who had developmental disabilities other than ASD. Segments of the child's favorite television show were also sometimes inserted sporadically throughout the video sequence in order to maintain the child's attention (Drysdale et al., 2015; Lee et al., 2014) to the video. Other common features of the research on VSM and the procedures used to implement these techniques in toilet training are noted below.

Errorless Feedforward VSM In each of the studies the child was shown to complete each step in the toileting sequence without prompting or errors, as though they were completing the sequence independently (Drysdale et al., 2015; Lee et al., 2014; McLay et al., 2015), with prompts and coaching edited out. The child also viewed the video immediately prior to each practice opportunity.

Reinforcement Modeled VSM always concluded with a depiction of the child being rewarded with verbal, social, or tangible rewards for successfully voiding in the toilet. Reinforcement for completion of other steps in the sequence was not depicted in the video models; however, two studies also interspersed video of preferred items or television shows (e.g., about railway trains; Drysdale et al., 2015; Lee et al., 2014) in order to maintain children's attention to the video itself and to promote a positively valenced learning context.

Initiation of Toileting VSM always begins with depicting the child making a request to use the toilet using their normal means of communication, such as the child handing a picture cue card to their mother or using a speech-generating device. Initiation is a very important part of establishing independent toilet use, but is an often overlooked component of toilet training intervention. Note that for children who are ultimately able to toilet independently, initiating toileting by requests to a parent/caregiver would eventually be replaced by independently approaching the toilet and executing the toileting sequence. Achievement of this degree of independence may require further training in which prompts are faded and independent performance explicitly rewarded.

Combination of Video Modeling/Video Self-Modeling and POV Modeling Each study also integrated POV modeling within the VSM sequence (Drysdale et al., 2015; Lee et al., 2014; McLay et al., 2015), specifically to depict fine motor actions (e.g., flushing the toilet). This was because it was useful to demonstrate an action from the perspective of the learner where a close-up shot was needed to adequately depict the specific action.

Target Skills It is noteworthy that while all this research used videos demonstrating the steps in the toileting sequence, not all of the research depicted urination (Lee et al., 2014) and only one study depicted defecation (McLay et al., 2015). When included, the voiding process was demonstrated using an animation of the child's genitals and the motion of voiding. This was typically paired with appropriate sound effects (e.g., the sound of urine hitting the water).

Conclusion While further evidence is required, this research suggests that the various components of training noted above may be important inclusions in VSM for toilet training. Note also that in the majority of research to date, VM and VSM have been implemented in the home setting with parents managing the intervention. This seems logical given that this is the natural context for toilet training. Nevertheless, given the growth of out-of-home infant and child care (Bakker & Wyndaele, 2000), the development and evaluation of VM/VSM materials and procedures for use by non-parental caregivers would also be desirable.

Additional Behavioral Strategies Paired with Modeling

None of the research studies reviewed above used VM or VSM in isolation. The procedures were always supplemented with components additional to the video that included physical, gestural, and/or verbal prompting and reinforcement. Some of these supplementary components have been noted above, but they are considered more fully below.

Prompting In many cases, each child was given the opportunity to respond to each step in the sequence. If the child did not respond, responded incorrectly, or was off-task, then they were prompted in order to complete that step (Drysdale et al., 2015; Keen et al., 2007; Lee et al., 2014; McLay et al., 2015). This usually involved a least-to-most prompting procedure (Drysdale et al., 2015; Keen et al., 2007; Lee et al., 2014; McLay et al., 2015) often in the order of verbal, gestural, and then physical prompting. In the case of voiding, if the child did not void while seated on the toilet, a verbal prompt was often provided (e.g., "pee-pee"; Lee et al., 2014; McLay et al., 2015).

Reinforcement In some cases reinforcement was provided for completing each step in the toileting sequence, as well as in-toilet voiding (Drysdale et al.,. 2015; Keen et al., 2007; McLay et al., 2015). Reinforcement was usually provided differentially, so that in-toilet voiding resulted in the highest level of reinforcement, while completing other steps in the sequence, or just remaining seated on the toilet, resulted in verbal praise (McLay et al., 2015) or a moderately preferred tangible reinforcer.

Video Prompting and Response Chaining When a video model demonstrates only a component skill and the learner is shown this only following an error, this can be referred to as video prompting (Le Grice & Blampied, 1995, 1997), and in some of the research reviewed, a behavioral chaining procedure was used in which the video was edited into segments that demonstrated a limited number of steps in the toileting sequence (Drysdale et al., 2015; McLay et al., 2015) making video prompting possible. For example, in the Drysdale et al., (2015) study, the child was shown the video that represented the targeted steps in the sequence. Upon mastery, new steps were introduced, in a sequential order, until all steps were able to be completed; however, the full video prompting procedure does not appear ever to have been implemented in toilet training.

Regularly Scheduled Practice Opportunities In the majority of studies, the children were provided with multiple practice opportunities each day. In order to determine each child's toileting schedule, parents conducted regular diaper checks (e.g., every 30 min), and recorded whether or not the child had urinated or defecated. These checks took place prior to intervention and allowed the parents and researchers to determine the time at which practice opportunities were most likely to result in successful in-toilet voiding (Drysdale et al.,. 2015; Keen et al., 2007; Lee et al., 2014; McLay et al., 2015). Typically, between five and eight practice opportunities were provided each day, during waking hours.

Maintenance of Treatment Effects

It is essential to ensure that any toileting skills that are acquired are maintained long term following the fading of prompting, modeling, and behavior-facilitating environmental modifications. Most research into the effects of VM/VSM gathered follow-up data in order to assess the maintenance (Drysdale et al., 2015; Lee et al., 2014; McLay et al., 2015), at between 5 days (Lee et al., 2014) and 2 months (McLay et al., 2015). Toileting skills were maintained following VSM. In one VM study that reported follow-up data, gains were maintained for three children, but not for those whom practice opportunities ceased post-treatment (Keen et al., 2007). This highlights the importance of providing regular and sustained opportunities for toilet use.

Generalization of Treatment Effects

Stokes and Baer (1977) define generalization as "the occurrence of relevant behavior under different, non-training conditions (i.e., across subjects, settings, people, behaviors, and/or time) without the scheduling of the same events in those conditions as had been scheduled in the training conditions" (p. 350). Generalization (or transfer of training) is said to have occurred when the child responds correctly across a variety of settings, times of day, people, and materials (Cooper et al., 2007). Many individuals, including children with disabilities, may have difficulty generalizing newly acquired skills (Egel, Shafer, & Neef, 1984; Young, Krantz, McLannahan, & Poulson, 1994), meaning that it is very important to program for generalization and transfer. Equally, it is essential that researchers assess whether outcomes have generalized so that the conditions where additional training maybe required are identified (i.e., whether training is acquired across a variety of settings or whether generalization across multiple settings is likely to occur).

When toilet training children using VM/VSM, there are multiple aspects of generalization that need to be considered. For example, if the video model displays the child using a single toilet, will they require additional teaching in order to learn to use toilets in other settings? Or if one family member is responsible for teaching the child to use the toilet, will they maintain toilet use when that parent is not present and another family member is present? These respective processes are referred to as generalization across settings and people.

A number of studies have assessed generalization (Keen et al., 2007; McLay et al., 2015) without actively programing for it (Drysdale et al., 2015; Keen et al., 2007; McLay et al., 2015), i.e., they did not actively teach children to use a variety of toilets or expose children to a variety of teachers. The exception to this was Lee et al. (2014) where the child was prompted using a picture cue and verbal prompt to use the toilet in his school on four occasions (Lee et al., 2014). In most cases training occurred in the home setting, and generalization was assessed at school or similar places (Drysdale et al., 2015; McLay et al., 2015), though in some cases generalization to a community bathroom was assessed (Keen et al., 2007). Generalization was reported to occur when children were taught using VSM (Drysdale et al., 2015; Lee et al., 2014; McLay et al., 2015) though generalization did not occur for all children when VM was used (Keen et al., 2007). Based on these results, it is possible that VSM facilitates generalization, though further research into this possibility is required.

Social Validity of the Treatments

When developing parent-implemented interventions, it is important to measure the social validity of the treatment approach. Social validity refers to clients' (in this case parents') subjective ratings of the acceptability of and satisfaction with the treatment (Wolf, 1978). According to Wolf (1978), there are three key areas to consider: (1) Are the goals socially significant? (2) Are the treatment procedures socially appropriate and acceptable? And (3) are the outcomes satisfactory to the consumer? Given that parents of children with disabilities are most affected by urinary and bowel incontinence and that parents are most often responsible for toilet training their children, it seems pertinent to gauge their perspective on treatment approaches. Where the age and communicative capacity of the children involved in training make it possible, their views on treatment acceptability should also be sought.

Three of the studies described in this chapter assessed the social validity of the treatments provided (Drysdale et al., 2015; Lee et al., 2014; McLay et al., 2015) via parents' ratings of the acceptability of the treatment as well as their understanding of the treatment rationale. This was done using the Treatment Acceptability Rating Form-Revised (TARF-R; Reimers, Wacker, & Cooper, 1991). In some cases treatments using VSM were perceived to be more time consuming (McLay et al., 2015) and disruptive (Drysdale et al., 2015; Lee et al., 2014; McLay et al., 2015) than the parents had anticipated (McLay et al., 2015). Some parents' ratings of the acceptability and effectiveness of the treatment also decreased from pre- to post-intervention (Lee et al., 2014). In the majority of cases, however, VSM was generally perceived to be effective, reasonable, and acceptable (Drysdale et al., 2015; McLay et al., 2015), a finding that should encourage the use of VSM in toilet training.

The most recent example of research to have included VSM is McLay et al. (2015). These researchers used a combination of VSM and POV modeling, plus animation, to teach steps in the toileting sequence, including both in-toilet urination and defecation, to two boys (aged 7 and 8 years) with ASD. Animation was used to represent the processes of urination and defecation to both children by superimposing an animation of genitals and a urination stream to represent urination and by depicting feces being excreted into the toilet. Voiding was paired with sound effects. The video ended with the model being given verbal praise and also a preferred tangible reward for voiding. The boys were shown the video immediately prior to a scheduled practice opportunity and then proceeded to practice the toileting sequence.

In summary, relative to all forms of modeling, VSM appears to be an effective tool to support toilet training in children. Not all children may benefit equally from its use, but it is generally reported to have positive effects on acquisition of toileting sequence steps as well as achievement of in-toilet urination and defecation when paired with additional behavioral strategies (e.g., prompting and reinforcement) and regular practice opportunities. VSM is also likely to result in generalization and maintenance of acquired skills and, importantly, is a strategy that is viewed favorably overall by parents who have used it. VSM also depicts the child in both the role of model and learner and may thereby increase the child's self-efficacy (Bandura, 1977b), and the emotional tone of the learning situation can be depicted as positive, thus providing a setting event context which facilitates learning.

Behavior-Facilitating Modifications of the Environment

The techniques involving modeling reviewed above depict performance via the actions of a model along with salient environmental cues; however, VM and VSM, in particular, expose the learner to a virtual rather than the actual physical environment within which the toileting behavior has to occur in reality. Another set of strategies for promoting learning, therefore, involve modifying the actual environment in ways that guide correct responding and make key behaviors easier to perform, thereby facilitating acquisition of correct performance. These strategies are reviewed next. They can be used independently but, like modeling, are almost always used in treatment combinations.

Many of these strategies involve prompts (e.g., pictorial schedules which outline the toileting sequence), while others are designed to support the correct response topography (e.g., having a stepping stool to enable the child access to the toilet). Kroeger and Sorenson-Burnworth (2009) reviewed research into toilet training for individuals with developmental disabilities, including ASD, which highlighted a number of common procedures involving modification of the toilet environment and/or stimulus conditions to facilitate in-toilet voiding. These approaches are described next.

Manipulation of Environmental Stimuli

Manipulation of stimuli refers to the process of manipulating antecedent variables which function as prompts or SDs in order to facilitate learning and to change the probability of various discriminated operants. Recall that, as outlined above, stimulus prompts are added to the learning context as supplementary stimuli (e.g., verbal instructions or picture cues; Kazdin, 2013) that support acquisition but can be faded as the response becomes established in the behavior repertoire. SDs, however, are essential components of the discriminated operant constituted by the three-term contingency; unlike prompts they cannot be faded from the environment without disrupting performance. Training may, however, fade control from one SD to another, a process typically done by reducing the salience of the initial SD while increasing the salience of the new SD (Cooper et al., 2007). Further, a particular behavior may be established in a new context by moving SDs from one context to another – for instance, if urination is occurring reliably on a potty, placing the potty in the toilet bowl may help transfer stimulus control to the toilet once the potty is removed.

Establishing and manipulating stimulus control (i.e., establishing correct SDs) is usually incorporated with other traditional toilet training techniques, such as reinforcement-based procedures and scheduled toileting visits. Scheduled toileting visits (especially in combination with hydration; see below) provide opportunities for children to practice using the toilet and, if carefully timed, permit whatever natural contingencies may be operating to strengthen the correct behavior. When planning to modify stimulus control, it is essential to first identify the conditions under which the child is likely to urinate or defecate and the signals for these events, i.e., to perform a functional analysis or assessment (Kaerts et al., 2012; Kamiyama & Noro, 2011; Smeets et al., 1985). Where these stimuli can be manipulated, they can be replicated as closely as possible during toilet training, particularly in order to help establish in-toilet voiding.

In the research reviewed below, clear distinctions between stimulus prompting and manipulation of SDs have not consistently been drawn by researchers, and many procedures are a mixture of both processes. In the next sections, we review the use of stimulus prompts, modification of diapers and undergarments, and provision of structural environmental behavioral supports as aids to toilet training.

Visual Prompts

Visual prompts provide children with a pictorial representation of the task or the steps required to complete that task. These visual aids can be presented in the form of photos or generic images. Parents who may be investigating the use of visual aids using online sources will be assailed with a variety of possibilities, including visual picture schedules which depict the toileting sequence; single picture cue cards which the parent uses to indicate to the child that it is time to go to the toilet, or which the child uses to initiate toilet use; and "first-then boards" which depict the contingency of voiding followed by reward. It is thought that visual depiction of this sequence helps children to understand and follow the steps involved in the toileting sequence and any contingencies that have been established relating to toilet training. Visual prompts such as picture schedules can be useful as they can be used independent of third-party involvement (i.e., as a replacement for verbal or physical prompting) and children are not required to retain large amounts of information when learning lengthy and complex behavior chains. As toileting becomes established, they can be withdrawn, but note that even as adults we continue to depend on cues such as signs and gender symbols to select gender-appropriate toilets.

There is some evidence to support the use of visually cued schedules to support children's skill acquisition (Bryan & Gast, 2000; Dettmer, Simpson, Smith-Myles, & Ganz, 2000; MacDuff, Krantz, & McClannahan, 1993). There are also some studies that have used picture cue cards to support toilet training (Drysdale et al., 2015; Keen et al., 2007; Lee et al., 2014), though no studies were identified that used pictorial schedules for this purpose. In instances in which visual prompts have been used, they are always used as part of a multicomponent treatment package, and it is, therefore, difficult to draw any conclusions about their effectiveness as a stand-alone intervention. Nevertheless, visual prompts may be a simple addition to a toilet training package.

Another prompting procedure is the use of high-probability response sequences (Kazdin, 2013; Mace, Hock, Lalli, West, Belifore, Pinter, & Brown, 1988).

This procedure has the trainer/parent who first identifies several requests which a child is highly likely to comply with (e.g., "give me a high five"). In training, a sequence of these requests is made in close succession, with the request to which the child is unlikely to comply (the low-probability request) attached at the end, and this sequence is repeated in appropriate circumstances several times a day during training. This procedure has been shown to increase the likelihood of compliance with previously noncompliant requests (Banda, Neisworth, & Lee, 2003). Humm, Blampied, and Liberty (2005) report a case in which a 6.5-year-old girl with a developmental age of 2.5 years and a diagnosis of cerebral palsy increased her compliance with two parental requests ("Go to the toilet" and "Stay on the toilet") following the high-probability request procedure. Parents were moderately satisfied with this treatment (Humm et al., 2005).

Structural Toileting Aids

In addition to visual aids that may support toilet training, there are a variety of structural supports that may facilitate the toilet training process and may prompt successful toilet use. Structural toileting aids are designed to support children's independent access to the toilet as well as to provide comfort and security for the child while they are seated on the toilet. For example, small step stools have been used for children who have physical limitations or disabilities that may prevent them from accessing the toilet. Small toilet training seats have been developed that are able to be placed on the toilet rim, in order to create a smaller surface area for the child to sit on and to support them to feel comfortable while seated. This feeling of security is particularly important in cases in which children have developed a fear of the toilet. The use of such aids has not been documented in the literature, though, anecdotally, it is something that is viewed very favorably by parents.

The Modification of Diapers and Undergarments

Environmental manipulations also include modification or removal of diapers and removal of undergarments and other clothing. A limited number of research studies have investigated these procedures (Luiselli, 1996a; Taylor, Cipani, & Clardy, 1994). The stated rationale for the modification of diapers or undergarments is that wearing a diaper is one of the SDs that maintains urination. From birth children have a history of urination and defecation while wearing diapers, and the presence of the diaper may come to control voiding so that it is only likely to occur when the diaper SD is being experienced (Taylor et al., 1994). An alternative (but unstated) rationale is that the association of diapers with urination (and defecation) may represent the effect of respondent conditioning via a conditioned stimulus (CS); the CS (diaper) elicits the conditioned response (CR) of urination/defecation. For older children, undergarments may come to serve the same function as CS or SD. The scientific study of the natural history of toileting is insufficiently developed (Schum et al., 2002) for these alternative accounts to be distinguished among. It is clear, however, that whatever the initial role of diapers or undergarments, successful toileting requires key steps in the toileting behavior sequence to come under the control of new stimuli, such as the potty or later the toilet room and the toilet fixture.

An alternative explanation for continued voiding only when undergarments are being worn is that the component skills required to undress have not been established with sufficient fluency to make it easy for the child to undress before voiding, a point addressed by POV modeling described above. Under conditions of urgency, the very act of beginning to undress may control immediate sphincter relaxation (again, possibly an instance of respondent conditioning) leading to an accident. It can take some time for children to learn the correct timing of the components of the toileting sequence as well as learning the skills themselves.

Assuming that diapers function as inappropriate SDs for voiding, this problem has been addressed in several ways. The first one is direct modification of diapers by cutting gradually larger holes in the diaper, placing the child in the diaper (SD for voiding), and then asking them to sit on the toilet. Wearing (modified) diapers while the child is seated on the toilet maintains the SD for urination, and, if the child successfully urinates while on the toilet (via the hole in the diaper), then the opportunity is provided for successful in-toilet urination and its reinforcement. If desired, more and more of the diaper can be cut away so as to facilitate transfer of full stimulus control to the potty or toilet.

In other procedures stimulus control is transferred from the child's undergarments or diapers to the potty or toilet by ensuring that undergarments are completely removed in between scheduled toileting visits and then gradually and systematically reintroduced (Taylor et al., 1994), a procedure used for older children who have not previously been successfully toilet trained (Luiselli, 1996a, 1996b). Each of these approaches is thought to be useful as they can help to establish the transfer of stimulus control for voiding (e.g., from diaper to sitting on the toilet), and if they work, they provide opportunities for the child to be rewarded for successful in-toilet voiding.

Evidence for the Effectiveness of Diaper Modification and the Removal of Clothing

Luiselli (1996b) describes a procedure for toilet training children with developmental disabilities in which stimulus control is systematically transferred from the diaper to the toilet. In summary, a toileting schedule was established so that regular practice opportunities were provided throughout the day. The diapers were removed, and the child was placed in training briefs (similar to underwear but with additional padding to provide some absorbancy). At the scheduled time, the child was placed in a diaper (the assumed voiding SD) and placed on the toilet and was rewarded for successfully urinating in the diaper. If the child failed to urinate, they were told to "try again next time," and the training briefs were replaced until the next scheduled practice opportunity.

Luiselli (1996a, 1996b) intended to use this procedure to toilet train a 7-year-old girl with a diagnosis of atypical pervasive developmental disorder; however, the child initiated sitting on the toilet without the diaper and successfully urinated (an example of spontaneous transfer of stimulus control), and therefore this step was eliminated. Follow-up data 1 month posttreatment indicated that gains were maintained.

Taylor et al. (1994) have conducted the sole investigation into the systematic removal of clothing to manipulate stimulus control. The case was a 10-year-old boy with ASD who had a history of failed toilet training attempts and for whom it was thought that underpants were the SD for urination (i.e., the child would not urinate while seated on the toilet without undergarments, but did so immediately when his undergarments were pulled up). The intervention began with the Azrin and Foxx (1971) procedure for 2 consecutive days. Then a second phase consisted of removing the child's undergarments 5 min after the consumption of liquids and until the child successfully urinated; meanwhile he was prompted to sit on the toilet at 30 min intervals until urination occurred or 10 min had passed. Successful urination let 1 min be added to the period of time that the child could have his clothes on. This continued progressively until 15 successes were achieved, at which point the child's clothes were no longer removed. Improvement in toileting occurred in phase 2, and gains were maintained at a 4-month and 10-month follow-up.

Setting Events/Motivational Strategies

Setting events include features of the learning context that facilitate (or impair) learning (Kazdin, 2013). They include changes in motivation to perform the target responses, the emotional valence of the learning context, and emotions experienced and expressed by the learner in the training situation.

Motivating Voiding: Hydration and Diet Manipulation

Urination and defecation naturally occur only when the bladder or rectum reaches capacity. Natural opportunities to learn continence and toileting skills are, therefore, limited to those occasions when the bladder or rectum is full or nearly so. To increase practice opportunities and promote in-toilet urination during toilet training, hydration procedures are regularly employed, usually by providing the child free access to preferred liquids and encouraging frequent consumption. The equivalent manipulation for defecation is to increase dietary fiber intake and prescribe laxatives (Wassom & Christophersen, 2014). Hydration and dietary fiber manipulations are also ways to make interoceptive discriminative stimuli associated with bladder and bowel functioning more salient and provide opportunities for those stimuli to function as SDs for seeking out and using the toilet. Hydration and dietary fiber/laxative strategies are typically used in conjunction with other strategies, such as scheduled toilet use, prompting, and reinforcement procedures (Wassom & Christophersen, 2014).

Evidence for Hydration Procedures

Since the initial study of toilet training by Azrin and Foxx (1971), increased hydration is commonly reported as a component of toilet training, primarily for encouraging urination, but it is also used when fecal incontinence is the target because it makes defecation more frequent and physically easier, especially for individuals who are constipated (Cicero & Pfadt, 2002; Freeman, Riley, Duke, & Rongwei, 2014; Hagopian, Fisher, Piazza, & Wierzbicki, 1993; Kroeger & Sorensen, 2010; Wassom & Christophersen, 2014; Wilder, Higbee, Williams, & Nachtwey, 1997; Wilson, 1995). Kroeger and Sorenson (2010) used an intensive toileting training procedure (plus rewards) to toilet train two boys with ASD. In preparation for toilet training, the parents were asked to increase their child's access to fluids for 3 days preceding toilet training. Wilder et al. (1997) paired increased daily fluid intake with scheduled toileting visits and the use of an in-toilet alarm that was activated by urination. This successfully taught a 21-year-old intellectually disabled man to urinate in the toilet. The wider use of technologies to support toilet training is described in Chap. 10.

Given that increasing fluid intake is a common component of many toilet training procedures, it is not possible to conclude that increasing fluid intake alone makes a unique contribution to toilet training. However, it is a very simple and nonintrusive procedure with a good rationale, and its use may well be justified. Before it is used, it is important to consult with a health professional in order to avoid overhydration or hyponatremia. In the treatment of fecal incontinence, two recent meta-analytic reviews of the use of dietary manipulations/laxatives combined with behavioral interventions have concluded that the quality of the evidence for the effectiveness of this combined treatment is poor (Brazzelli, Griffiths, Cody, & Tappin, 2011) but that the combined treatment may have some efficacy (Freeman et al., 2014).

Negative Emotions and Toilet Training

It has long been recognized that fear of voiding and the toileting situation may interfere with the achievement of continence and toileting competence by young children (Luiselli, 1977). This is a setting event which represents the interaction of the respondent (fear) and operant (escape/avoidance and resistance) behavior repertoires. The fear may inhibit sphincter release through reflex mechanisms, while fear also motivates escape from, avoidance of, and resistance to toilet training.

Gradual exposure to the toilet setting and to the sensations of voiding while on the toilet, potentiated by the positive affect generated by reinforcement, may be needed to bring about fear extinction/adaptation (Gimpel & Holland, 2003).

Recommendations for Research

To date, little research has been conducted into the effectiveness of modeling and environmental modification strategies as methods to support toilet training. In light of these limitations, there are a number of considerations for future research. Typically, it is necessary to combine treatments in packages, but to further enhance research, it would be helpful to use research designs where components were introduced sequentially, to see if a particular component adds incremental benefits. Alternatively, sequences of dismantling strategy studies need to be done to determine the necessary and sufficient training components; otherwise, randomized controlled trials are necessary.

It is also noteworthy that there are many aspects of VM/VSM that are yet to be established. For example, we still do not have an understanding of optimal viewing schedules for VM/VSM. Furthermore, there are many theoretically related, yet unexplored intervention strategies that may facilitate the toilet training process, e.g., the use of video prompting or social stories. Social stories use a combination of pictures and text to depict a person correctly performing the desired skill or task. While there is evidence that they can have positive effects on children's learning and behavior (Delano & Snell, 2006; Chan & O'Reilly, 2008), there does not appear to be any research into its use in toilet training. Equally, it seems pertinent that the effects of video prompting procedures are investigated for use in toilet training, given the utility of this approach when teaching children a small subset of skills within a task.

To date, the majority of research into toileting difficulties has focused on urinary incontinence rather that fecal incontinence. It is possible that this is a reflection of the epidemiology of the two problems. However, it seems essential that we better understand the strategies that support children to acquire both urinary and fecal continence if they are to achieve independent toileting.

As parents/caregivers are primarily responsible for toilet training their children, it is essential that consumer satisfaction and acceptability ratings are assessed and evaluated. Where possible, this should also include the perspectives of children. Treatments that are socially valid are more likely to be implemented in practice and may be more feasible for parents to implement resulting in greater adherence to treatment procedures and enhanced treatment effectiveness (Finn & Sladeczek, 2001; Kazdin, 1977).

Finally, the synthesis of evidence for supporting evidence-based practice would be greatly enhanced by researchers reporting some kind of effect size (including single-case effect sizes; Parker, Vannest, & Davis, 2011). This would allow us to determine the extent to which particular toilet training tools or strategies were, in fact, effective and provide information to feed into research syntheses such as meta-analyses. Further research in this area would significantly enhance our understanding of the effectiveness of these promising strategies and the conditions under which they are effective.

Overall Conclusions

This chapter has described a variety of modeling, environmental, and stimulus modification strategies currently used to toilet train children and young people. This includes in vivo modeling, VM, VSM, a wide range of prompting strategies, facilitative environmental modification, and modification of setting events/motivation. Accounts of the use of these strategies, mostly in various combinations, are common, but there has been little research investigating their effectiveness. The majority of existing research also focuses on the use of these strategies in people with disabilities who frequently have a history of failed attempts at toilet training. The fact that the identified strategies are always used as a part of a multicomponent treatment package means it is difficult to draw strong conclusions regarding the effectiveness of these approaches if used alone.

Interventions should always be based on a clear rationale, one that is drawn from a comprehensive biobehavioral and functional analysis of toileting and its difficulties. For parents/caregivers, therapists, or teachers planning to modify aspects of the environment or using modeling strategies to support toilet training, it is important to conduct a thorough functional assessment and to then consider additional processes that may enhance the success of any intervention, such as scheduled toileting visits and reinforcement strategies explained in other chapters. It is also important to provide sufficient training to ensure the generalization and maintenance of acquired toileting skills.

References

Azrin, N. H., & Foxx, R. M. (1971). A rapid method of toilet training the institutionalized retarded. *Journal of Applied Behavior Analysis, 4*, 89–99.

Bainbridge, N., & Smith-Myles, B. S. (1999). The use of priming to introduce toilet training to a child with autism. *Focus on Autism & Other Developmental Disabilities, 14*, 106–109.

Baker, S. D., O'Reilly, M., & Lang, R. (2009). Review of video modeling with students with emotional and behavioral disorders. *Education and Treatment of Children, 32*, 403–420.

Bakker, E., & Wyndaele, J. J. (2000). Changes in the toilet training of children during the last 60 years. The cause of an increase in lower urinary tract dysfunction? *BJU International, 86*, 248–252.

Banda, D. R., Neisworth, J. T., & Lee, D. L. (2003). High-probability request sequences and young children: Enhancing compliance. *Child & Family Behavior Therapy, 25*, 17–29.

Bandura, A. (1977a). *Social learning theory*. Englewood Cliffs, NJ: Prentice-Hall.

Bandura, A. (1977b). Self-efficacy: Toward a unifying theory of behavior change. *Psychological Review, 84*, 191–215.
Bandura, A. (1978). Social learning theory of aggression. *Journal of Communication, 28*, 12–29.
Bandura, A., Ross, D., & Ross, S. A. (1961). Transmission of aggression through imitation of aggressive models. *Journal of Abnormal and Social Psychology, 63*, 575–582.
Brazzelli, M., Griffiths, P. V., Cody, J. D., & Tappin, D. (2011). Behavioral and cognitive interventions with or without other treatments for the management of faecal incontinence in children. *Cochrane Database of Systematic Reviews, 2*. doi:10.1002/14651858.CD002240.pub3
Bryan, L. C., & Gast, D. L. (2000). Teachign on-task and on-schedule behaviors to high-functioning children with autism via picture activity schedules. *Journal of Autism and Developmental Disorders, 30*, 553–567. doi:10.1023/A:1005687310346
Cassibba, R., Castoro, G., Costantino, E., Sette, G., & Van Ijzendoorn, M. H. (2015). Enhancing maternal sensitivity and infant attachment security with video feedback: An exploratory study in Italy. *Infant Mental Health Journal, 36*, 53–61.
Chan, J. M., & O'Reilly, M. F. (2008). A social stories intervention package for students with autism in inclusive classroom settings. *Journal of Applied Behavior Analysis, 41*, 405–409.
Cicero, F. R., & Pfadt, A. (2002). Investigation of a reinforcement-based toilet training procedure for children with autism. *Research in Developmental Disabilities, 23*, 319–331.
Cooper, J. O., Heron, T. E., & Heward, W. L. (2007). *Applied behavior analysis* (2nd ed.). Upper Saddle River, NJ: Pearson.
Deitchman, C., Reeve, S. A., Reeve, K. F., & Progar, P. R. (2010). Incorporating video feedback into selfmanagement training to promote generalization of social initiations by children with autism. *Education and Treatment of Children, 33*, 475–488.
Delano, M., & Snell, M. E. (2006). The effects of social stories on the social engagement of children with autism. *Journal of Positive Behavior Interventions, 8*, 29–42.
Dettmer, S., Simpson, R. L., Smith-Myles, B., & Ganz, J. B. (2000). The use of visual supports to facilitate transitions of children with autism. *Focus on Autism and Other Developmental Disabilities, 15*, 163–169.
deVires, M. W., & deVries, M. R. (1977). Cultural relativity of toilet training readiness: A perspective from East Africa. *Pediatrics, 60*, 170–177.
Dowrick, P. W. (1999). A review of self-modeling and related interventions. *Applied and Preventive Psychology, 8*, 23–29. doi:10.1016/S0962-1849(99)80009-2
Dowrick, P. W. (2012a). Self modeling: Expanding the theories of learning. *Psychology in the Schools, 49*, 30–41. doi:10.1002/pits.20613
Dowrick, P. W. (2012b). Self model theory: Learning from the future. WIREs. *Journal of Cognitive Science, 3*, 215–230. doi:10.1002/ wcs.1156
Drysdale, B., Lee, C. Y. Q., Anderson, A., & Moore, D. W. (2015). Using video modeling incorporating animation to teach toileting to two children with autism spectrum disorder. *Journal of Developmental and Physical Disabilities, 27*, 149–165. doi:10.1007/s10882-014-9405-1
Egel, A. L., Shafer, M. S., & Neef, N. A. (1984). Receptive acquisition and generalization of prepositional responding in autistic children: A comparison of two procedures. *Analysis and Intervention in Developmental Disabilities, 4*, 285–298.
Finn, C. A., & Sladeczek, I. E. (2001). Assessing the social validity of behavioral interventions: A review of treatment acceptability measures. *School Psychology Quarterly, 16*, 176–206. doi:10.1521/scpq.16.2.176.18703
Freeman, K. A., Riley, A., Duke, D. C., & Rongwei, F. (2014). Systematic review and meta-analysis of behavioral interventions for fecal incontinence with constipation. *Journal of Pediatric Psychology, 39*, 887–902.
Gena, A., Couloura, S., & Kymissis, E. (2005). Modifying the affective behavior of pre-schoolers with autism using in-vivo or video modeling and reinforcement contingencies. *Journal of Autism and Developmental Disorders, 35*, 545–556. doi:10.1007/s10803-005-0014-9
Gimpel, G. A., & Holland, M. L. (2003). *Emotional and behavioral problems of young children: Effective interventions in the preschool and kindergarten years*. New York, NY: Guliford.

Hagopian, L. P., Fisher, W., Piazza, C. C., & Wierzbicki, J. J. (1993). A water-prompting procedure for the treatment of urinary incontinence. *Journal of Applied Behavior Analysis, 26*, 473–474.

Hosford, R. E. (1980). Self-as-a-model: A cognitive social learning technique. *The Counseling Psychologist, 9*, 45–62.

Howard, B. J. (1991). *It's Potty Time [Video-tape]*. Duke family services: Learning Through Entertainment, Inc..

Humm, S. P., Blampied, N. M., Liberty, & K.A. (2005). Effects of parent-administered, home-based, high-probability sequences on compliance by children with developmental disabilities. *Child & Family Behavior Therapy, 27*, 27–45.

Kamiyama, T., & Noro, F. (2011). Effectiveness of parent-implemented interventions based on functional assessment of toilet skills in young children with autism. *Japanese Journal of Behavior Analysis, 25*, 153–164.

Kaerts, N., Vermandel, A., Lierman, F., vanGestel, A., & Wyndaele, J. J. (2012). Observing signs of toilet readiness: Results of two prospective studies. *Scandinavian Journal of Urology and Neophrology, 46*, 424–430.

Kazdin, A. E. (1977). Assessing the clinical or applied importance of behavior change through social validation. *Behavior Modification, 1*, 427–452.

Kazdin, A. E. (2013). *Behavior modification in applied settings* (7th ed.). Long Grove, IL: Waveland.

Keen, D., Brannigan, K. L., & Cuskelly, M. (2007). Toilet training for children with autism: the effects of video modeling. *Journal of Developmental and Physical Disabilities, 19*, 291–303. doi:10.1007/s10882- 007-9044-x

Kroeger, K. A., & Sorensen-Burnworth, R. (2009). Toilet training individuals with autism and other developmental disabilities: A critical review. *Research in Autism Spectrum Disorders, 3*, 6070618. doi:10.1016/j.rasd.2009.01.005

Kroeger, K. A., & Sorenson, R. (2010). A parent training model for toilet training children with autism. *Journal of Intellectual Disability Research, 54*, 556–567. doi:10.1111/j.1365-2788.2010.01286.x

Lam-Cassettari, C., Wadnerkar-Kamble, M. B., & James, D. M. (2015). Enhancing paren-child communication and parental self-esteem with a video feedback intervention: Outcomes with prelingual deaf and hard-of-hearing children. *Journal of Deaf Studies in Education, 20*, 266–274.

Lang, R., Shogren, K., Machalicek, W., Rispoli, M., O'Reilly, M. F., Regester, A., & Baker, S. (2009). Use of video self-modeling to teach classroom rules to two children with Asperger's syndrome. *Research in Autism Spectrum Disorders, 3*, 483–488. doi:10.1016/j.rasd.2008.10.001

Lee, C. Y. Q., Anderson, A., & Moore, D. W. (2014). Using video modeling to toilet train a child with autism. *Journal of Developmental and Physical Disabilities, 26*, 123–134. doi:10.1007/s10882-013-9348-y

Le Grice, B., & Blampied, N. M. (1995). Using videoprompting to teach video recorder and personal computer operation to pupils with intellectual handicaps. *Education and Training in Mental Retardation and Developmental Disabilities, 29*, 321–330.

Le Grice, B., & Blampied, N. (1997). Learning to use video recorders and personal computers with increasing assistance prompting. *Journal of Developmental & Physical Disabilities, 9*, 17–30.

Luiselli, J. K. (1977). Case report: An attendant-administered contingency management programme for the treatment of a toileting phobia. *Journal of Mental Deficiency Research, 21*, 283–288.

Luiselli, J. K. (1996a). A case study evaluation of a transfer-of-stimulus control toilet training procedure for a child with a pervasive developmental disorder. *Focus on Autism and Other Developmental Disabilities, 11*, 158–162.

Luiselli, J. K. (1996b). A transfer-of-stimulus control prompting procedure applicable to toilet training programs for children with developmental disabilities. *Child and Family Behavior Therapy, 18*, 29–34.

Luxem, M., & Christophersen, E. (1994). Behavioral toilet training in early childhood: Research, practice, and implications. *Developmental and Behavioral Pediatrics, 15*, 370–378.
Mace, F. C., Hock, M. L., Lalli, J. S., West, B. J., Belifore, P., Pinter, E., & Brown, D. K. (1998). Behavioral momentum in the treatment of noncompliance. *Journal of Applied Behavior Analysis, 21*, 123–141.
MacDuff, G. S., Krantz, P. J., & McClannahan, L. E. (1993). Teaching children with autism to use photographic activity schedules: Maintenance and generalization of complex response chains. *Journal of Applied Behavior Analysis, 26*, 89–97.
McCoy, K., & Hermansen, E. (2007). Video modeling for individuals with autism: A review of model types and effects. *Education and Treatment of Children, 30*, 183–213. doi: http://www.jstor.org/stable/42899952.
McLay, L., Carnett, A., van der Meer, L., & Lang, R. (2015). Using a video modelling-based intervention package to toilet train two children with autism. *Journal of Developmental and Physical Disabilities, 27*, 431–451.
Mead, E. B., Dozier, M., & Bernard, K. (2014). Using video feedback as a tool in training parent coaches: Promising results from a single-subject design. *Attachment & Human Development, 16*, 356–370.
Meltzoff, A. N. (1995). Understanding the intentions of others: Reenactment of intended acts by 18-month-old children. *Developmental Psychology, 31*, 838–850. doi:10.1037/0012-1649.31.5.838
Moss, E., Tarabylsby, G. M., St-Georgesc, R., Dubois-Comtoisd, K., Cyr, C., Bernier, A., … Lecompte, V. (2014). Video-feedback intervention with maltreating parents and their children: Program implementation and case study. *Attachment & Human Development, 16*, 329–342.
Ollendick, T. H., & King, N. J. (1998). Empirically supported treatments for children with phobic and anxiety disorders: Current status. *Journal of Clinical Child Psychology, 27*, 156–167. doi:10.1207/s15374424jccp2702_3
O'Reilly, M. F., O'Halloran, M., Sigafoos, J., Lancioni, G. E., Green, V., Edrisinhaa, C., … Olive, M. (2005). Evaluation of a video feedback and self-management to decrease schoolyard aggression and increase pro-social behaviour in two students with behavioural disorders. *Educational Psychology, 25*, 199–206.
Parker, R. I., Vannest, K. J., & Davis, J. L. (2011). Effect size in single-case research: A review of nine nonoverlap techniques. *Behavior Modification, 35*, 303–322. doi:10.1177/014544551139147
Pinter, E. B., East, A., & Thrush, N. (2015). Effects of a video-feedback intervention on teachers' use of praise. *Education and Treatment of Children, 38*, 451–472.
Reimers, T., Wacker, D., & Cooper, L. (1991). Evaluation of the acceptability of treatments for children's behavioral difficulties. *Child and Family Behavior Therapy, 13*, 53–71.
Schum, T. R., Kolb, T. M., McAuliffe, T. L., Simms, M. D., Underhill, R. L., & Lewis, M. (2002). Sequential acquisition of toilet-training skills: A descriptive study of gender and age differences in normal children. *Pediatrics, 109*, 1–7. www.pediatrics.org/cgi/content/full/109/.3/e48.
Sibley, M. H., Pelham, W. E., Mazur, A., Gnagy, E. M., Ross, J. M., & Kuriyan, A. B. (2012). The effect of video feedback on the social behavior of an adolescent with ADHD. *Journal of Attention Disorders, 16*, 579–588.
Smeets, P. M., Lancioni, G. E., Ball, T., & Oliva, D. S. (1985). Shaping self-initiated toileting in infants. *Journal of Applied Behavior Analysis, 18*, 303–308.
Stein, Z. A., & Susser, M. (1967). The social dimensions of a symptom: A socio-medical study of enuresis. *Social Science & Medicine, 1*, 183–201.
Stokes, T. F., & Baer, D. M. (1977). An implicit technology of generalization. *Journal of Applied Behavior Analysis, 10*, 349–367.
Taylor, S., Cipani, E., & Clardy, A. (1994). A stimulus control technique for improving the efficacy of an established toilet training program. *Journal of Behavior Therapy and Experimental Psychiatry, 25*, 155–160.
Tereshko, L., MacDonald, R., & Ahearn, W. H. (2010). Strategies for teaching children with autism to imitate response chains using video modeling. *Research in Autism Spectrum Disorders, 4*, 479–489. doi:10.1016/j.rasd.2009.11.005

Van Vonderen, A., Duker, P., & Didden, R. (2010). Instruction and video feedback to improve staff's trainer behavior and response prompting during one-to-one training with young children with severe intellectual disability. *Research in Developmental Disabilities, 31*, 1481–1490.
van Vonderen, A., Didden, R., & Beeking, F. (2012). Effectiveness of instruction and video feedback on staff's trainer behavior during one-to-one training with children with severe intellectual disability. *Research in Developmental Disabilities, 33*, 283–290.
Wassom, M. C., & Christophersen, E. R. (2014). A clinical application of evidence-based treatments in pediatric functional constipation and incontinence. *Clinical Practice in Pediatric Psychology, 2*, 294–311.
Wilder, D. A., Higbee, T. S., Williams, W. L., & Nachtwey, A. (1997). A simplified method of toilet training adults in residential settings. *Journal of Behavior Therapy and Experimental Psychiatry, 28*, 241–246.
Wilson, M. (1995). Generic habit-training program. *Focus on Autistic Behavior, 10*, 1–8.
Wolf, M. M. (1978). Social validity: The case for subjective measurement or how behaviour analysis is finding its heart. *Journal of Applied Behavior Analysis, 11*, 203–214.
Young, J. M., Krantz, P. J., McClannahan, L. E., & Poulson, C. L. (1994). Generalized imitation and response-class formation in children with autism. *Journal of Applied Behavior Analysis, 27*, 685–697.

Technology Used in Toilet Training

Johnny L. Matson

Technology in the field of toilet training has been an integral part of modern treatment programs since their inception. These methods have been employed for nocturnal and diurnal enuresis as well as encopresis. Obviously, the methods which have been developed have become more complex and varied over time. This chapter reviews research and methods that have used various forms of technology, defined here as the use of any type of equipment or devise. Of course, with the advent of video equipment and computers, these methods have become more sophisticated. Having said that, little research to date has capitalized on these newer devices. In this chapter, a review of studies on these and other technology will be made. An attempt will be made to group procedures based on a chronological format, and the chapter will end with speculation on where new developments will likely occur.

Daytime Treatment

Generally, the initial focus with toilet training involves methods for insuring continence during the daytime. First, there are more problems in general child development that accompanies this problem. For example, many school and preschool programs will only allow children to attend who have obtained daytime continence. Second, because children are eating and drinking during the day, more incidence of voiding occur during waking hours. Third, this problem is compounded by the fact that children are awake for a greater percentage of time than when they sleep. This disparity increases with age. Fourth, intervals between learning attempts (voiding

J.L. Matson (✉)
Department of Psychology, Louisiana State University, Baton Rouge, LA 70803, USA
e-mail: johnmatson@aol.com

J.L. Matson (ed.), *Clinical Guide to Toilet Training Children*, Autism and Child Psychopathology Series, DOI 10.1007/978-3-319-62725-0_10

episodes) are shorter, assisting in attaining continence. Fifth, since caregivers are awake, obviously they can more immediately be involved in treatment. Thus, the procedures and technology differ from nighttime treatment.

Nocturnal Treatment

Nighttime bedwetting is somewhat distinct from daytime toileting and involves methods that differ considerably from both a technology and psychological methods perspective. Also, in most instances bedwetting occurs well beyond the time when daytime training has been successfully accomplished. For example, Stein, Mendelsohn, Obermeyer, Amromin, and Benca (2001) report bedwetting at least once a week by school age children in 5.1% of the population. Thus, often the conceptual and motor skills are considerably more advanced.

Bell and Pad

One of the earliest technological advances in toileting involved nocturnal enuresis. Mowrer and Mowrer (1938) developed an alarm system that is activated when the child wets the bed. The bell is the unconditioned stimulus while a full bladder is viewed as the conditioned stimulus. Over time and conditioning trials, the child learns to wake at a period that is closer and closer to the time when voiding begins. Often the child may still wet the bed nightly for a time, but the diameter of the wet spot becomes smaller and smaller until accidents disappear. Thus, over time the child learns to awake when bladder extension reaches a point where voiding will soon occur.

When used consistently, and very soon after the buzzer sounds, the bell and pad is very effective. In fact, it is considered, even today, to be the most effective of the nocturnal enuresis treatment methods (Kaplan, Breit, Gauthier & Busner, 1989). However, even with this method, relapse can occur in a substantial number of cases (Doleys, 1977). As a result, investigators have attempted to add components to the bell and pad. Azrin, Sneed, and Foxx (1973) added reinforcement and punishment, while Lassen and Fluet (1979) added a token economy and additional practice. Fava, Cracco, and Facco (1981) also included reinforcement procedures with the bell and pad. What all these studies have in common is that the add-on procedures involved operant conditioning. Thus, a more complex intervention, in some cases, may also prove to be more robust.

Some researchers and clinicians have argued that operant methods alone are superior to the bell and pad, even when additional operant procedures are added to the Mowrer and Mowrer method. Kaplan, Breit, Gauthier, and Busner (1989) made such an assertion. In a direct comparison to tangible rewards and fading, they state that the two methods produced similar rates of continence for nocturnal enuresis. They also conclude that the operant conditioning methods resulted in lower rates of relapse compared to the bell and pad plus additional learning-based add-ons. Despite this finding, alarm systems have continued to be commonly studied and more frequently recommended relative to any other treatment method or any other type of technology. Also, this method seems to produce physiological changes. Oredsson and Jorgensen (1998) reported increased nocturnal bladder capacity as a function of bell and pad training. This methodology has been established as the treatment of choice for nighttime bedwetting for normally developing children (Rajigah, 1996). Similarly, this technology has proven useful in the treatment of special needs children's bedwetting problems.

One study of the bell and pad, which compared it to desmopressin alone and a combination of desmopressin and the bell and pad, was reported for a group of children in Saudi Arabia. They randomly assigned 136 kids to the 3 groups ($n = 45$, 45 and 46). They reported the most rapid decrease in accidents for the two groups that employed medication. However, where the drug alone was used relapse was frequent. The bell and pad required more time to achieve effects. The effects were more consistent and long lasting compared to medication. Of note, a no-treatment control group was not included, compromising the confidence in the results.

Other Alarm Methods

Alarm systems have also been reported for a number of daytime toileting problems. Van Wagenen and Murdock (1966) had a sensing electrode grid placed in the underwear of nine children with intellectual disabilities. The auditory signal alerted staff who then used prompts and other training methods to increase continence. Henriksen and Peterson (2013) have also used a urine alarm system for nighttime toileting. In their case study, a 12-year-old child with autism and fetal alcohol syndrome was successfully trained. While the population studied by Azrin and Foxx (1971) involved adults with intellectual disabilities, their methods would also be applicable to children. They devised a wet pants alarm. This principle of training mirrored the bell and pad with added operant methods. When the alarm was activated by urination, a series of consequences were introduced. Components of treatment included time out for soiling, peer modeling, and social reinforcement. Other consequences for accidents included tepid showers, verbal reprimands, and cleaning soiled surfaces. Similar technology and positive reinforcement have also been used to toilet train a 9-year-old boy with intellectual disabilities. The authors of this study, Chang, Lee, Chou, Chen, and Chen (2011), stressed the mobility of this technology and the ability to use it in a school setting.

Azrin, Bugle, and O'Brien (1971) went the pants alarm technology one better by also adding a toilet signal apparatus to the program. (Note: Many commercially available children's portable potties now use an alarm system. In this newer version, the "alarm" consists of a brief recording of cheering or other soundtracks designed to encourage the child.) In the 1971 study, the authors used a commercially available potty chair to teach four children (ages 3, 5, 6, and 6 years) who had profound intellectual disability. Two "male" shapes were affixed to the center of the chair's plastic container. Urination into the potty connected a low-voltage circuit, producing a clicking sound projected from a speaker. The sound from this device differed from the sound produced by the pants alarm sound box. Manual guidance (physical assistance from an adult) and verbal instructions from an adult were used to help then undress prior to setting on the potty and for dressing once they got up. For this study, the primary function of the apparatus was to insure accurate recording of accidents and as a result gauge successful toileting. Also, the authors note the buzzers allowed trainers to attend to other tasks.

Van Wagenen, Meyerson, Kerr, and Mahoney (1969) also describe an alarm system for daytime voiding. They trained nine children with intellectual disability. All the children were seriously impaired and were categorized as profoundly handicapped. One child had echolalic speech, while the remainder of the children had little or no speech. The urine alarm was in a small plastic box affixed to a belt and accompanied by a plastic or rubber urinal. This container allowed for urine to flow through to the stool. An audible sound occurred with continued urine flow. This procedure was accompanied by additional training provided by an adult. When the alarm was activated, the trainer immediately approached the child. The trainer said stop, and then the trainer grasped the child by their arm and escorted them to the stool. When voiding in the stool, the alarm again was activated. The trainer at this point provided lavish verbal praise. This training method resulted in marked improvement in daytime toilet training and generalized to other settings outside the original training environment.

Passman (1975) also used an alarm affixed to the toilet. Edible reinforcers (candy) were provided based on the onset of a tone triggered by voiding into the toilet and contacting moisture-detecting plates which were inside the toilet. The reward was provided very soon after voiding stopped. Once the three adults with profound intellectual handicaps were continent for a little over a month, the alarm and reinforcers were withdrawn. This method was very effective.

Mahoney, Van Wagenen, and Meyerson (1971) also used an alarm system. In their study, the alarm was connected to the participant's pants. A moisture-detecting sensor was connected to the pants and could set off the alarm. However, in a different twist on this training method, the trainer also had the option of activating the alarm with a handheld radio transmitter. The purpose of this latter procedure was to provide a prompt to void. As such, this method was an innovative development. Unfortunately, to date this method has not been developed to the extent its potential deserves. Wright (1975) also used a pants alarm and shaping with children. A second training group used prompts, fading, and graduated guidance, but no alarm. The group which employed the pants alarm in more self-initiations of voiding was the most successful. Others have also set off pants alarm systems manually and have found them to be effective in toilet training (Bettison, 1982; Levanto et al. 2016).

Ease of Application

Another variation of the alarm system is described by Meadow (1977). This study was an uncontrolled case study. The focus was on developing a bedwetting alarm that was very small and easy to service. The author also underscored that the device was less costly than many other methods. Specifically, this system was designed to be a more efficient alternative to the bell and pad. The device was described as a matchbox in size that could be worn on the participant. Thus, this method is similar to the pants alarms described above, although it is designed for nighttime use. The alarm was connected to a moisture sensor which had been put inside a disposable towel. As with the other devices described above, a buzzer is activated by moisture. Also, while the author states that the devices are for nighttime use, it is also suggested that it may prove effective for daytime toileting.

Another study of this type is described by Henriksen and Peterson (2013). They used a nighttime alarm system to eliminate bedwetting in a 12-year-old girl diagnosed with autism and fetal alcohol syndrome. This child's treatment was implemented in her home. The researchers used a urine alarm that was affixed to her pajama top. Also, clipped to her disposable diaper was a moisture sensor. The authors defined bedwetting as visual or tactile indications of wetness in the diaper. When the child's pants wet dry in the morning, she earned preferred edibles and tangible items such as games.

In instances where the alarm went off during the night, a parent would wake their daughter. She was then encouraged to void in the toilet. The child was then asked to put on dry clothes and help change the sheets. Bedwetting was eliminated in 2 weeks, and two bedwetting instances were reported over a 9-month follow-up. Thus, the treatment was both rapid and durable.

Using similar theoretical constructs but more advanced technology, Smith (2014) described where the alarm system technology is headed. An alarm placed in the child's undergarment was connected with wires to a small instrument. Accompanying this device was a wireless iPod which resembled a cell phone. This technology allowed for the incorporation of a considerably greater amount of information. In addition to being able to hear the buzzer go off when soiling occurred, other functions were available such as graphing data. This device also provided reinforcement reminders to staff about whether the participant was able to get to the toilet before voiding stopped. Finally, staff were provided a means to record successful voiding and other relevant clinical data. As such, this device is a far cry from the rudimentary alarm system used in bygone studies. What has not changed, however, are the basic conditioning principles employed along with all of these devices. Basic psychological strategies such as tangible and social reinforcers, graduated guidance, shaping, and efforts to increase the child's psychological awareness as applied to toileting are evident with these programs. Thus, in the future, even more sophisticated alarm systems will likely emerge. However, the basic theories behind the training will remain. The new technology will be smaller, more mobile, and easier to use and will provide more information. As a result, the major advances will be in ease of use, more accurate recording, and staff prompts that can produce more consistent applications of these teaching strategies. In recent years, toileting technology has received minimal research however.

Video Modeling

Lee, Anderson, and Moore (2013) describe toilet training of a 4½-year-old boy in a home-based intervention program. He was diagnosed with autism, and "Andrew" attended a mixture of school programs both special education school and a mainstream program along with an early childhood intervention center. Also, he had 4 h of a home-based intervention per week. Materials for the training program included a flip video camera, pictures of cue cards, a Macintosh computer, a TV with DVDs, and edible rewards. The child watched videos of himself performing the target behaviors which would lead to successful daytime toileting. Segments of favored TV programs were interspersed with toilet training footage. Over time, this procedure along with prompts and in vivo practice of toileting skills resulted in an effective toileting program. This program required less direct intervention in in vivo situations making it easier to implement for parents.

A second study used to teach toileting skills using video modeling is described by Drysdale, Lee, Anderson, and Moore (2014). They taught two children with autism spectrum disorders using real and animated models. Operant methods such as chaining and prompts were also included. The boys improved in their ability to walk to the toilet, undress, sit on the stool and void, and, finally, to pull their pants back up and flush the toilet. This modeling technology was an update from previous studies since an iPad was employed. Using such an approach, of course, adds to the ease and mobility of treatment implementation. Similar strategies were reported by McLay, Carnett, Van der Meer, and Lang (2015). They also taught two boys with autism spectrum disorders. Additionally, they obtained a 3–4-month follow-up where gains were maintained. What is consistent with all these studies is that gains are generally maintained once achieved.

A final study reviewed using video modeling was reported by Lee, Anderson, and Moore (2013). In their study the child with autism who was treated was a 4-year-old boy. The authors used video modeling with picture prompts, a task analysis, and reinforcement methods. The authors used a six-step task analysis which included: (1) going to the toilet, (2) undressing, (3) sitting on the stool, (4) voiding in the stool, (5) dressing, and (6) flushing the toilet. The child learned to go to the toilet and learned many preparatory skills. However, consistent voiding in the stool did not occur. Thus, this study demonstrates that no method is foolproof.

Undergarment Type

This study evaluated the effects of type of undergarment to toilet train normal developing children (Simon & Thompson, 2006). All five participants were normal developing. There were four females and one male aged 21–30 months. Children wore disposable diapers or "pull-ups." The study occurred in a preschool classroom with a spare bathroom with a full-sized toilet. Undergarment checks occurred every 15 min during the 5 h of class. Three treatment conditions were tested. These changes in garments included: (1) a diaper condition using an absorbent material lighter than a diaper affixed by tape or Velcro, (2) a pull-on training pants condition with a pant made of similar material to condition one (however, the pants were pull-ups with a waistband), and (3) the typical 100% cotton underwear without additional padding or waterproof materials. For some children, underwear improved incontinence. However, with this latter condition, cleanup after accidents was part of the procedure. What this study does show nonetheless is that all factors regarding toileting should be evaluated.

Greer, Neibert, and Dozier (2016) provide another example of types of pants worn and the effect on toilet training. Twenty typically developing children with a mean age of 26 months participated. These kids attended a university-based preschool. The children had not responded to low-intensity toilet training prompting to use the toilet by the teacher. This result occurred despite children having adequate readiness skills. (These skills usually consist of recognizing when they are wet, being able to follow instructions, being able to assist with pants being pulled up and down, and being able to sit on the potty.) For training, in addition to frequent prompts to sit on the stool and differential reinforcement, pull-up underwear was used to replace diapers. This procedure proved to be effective for many of the children. With any toileting procedure, there will be some variability in skills, even when readiness skills have been attained. Also, 2–4 months at this age can be a very large gap, and all children do not develop at the same rate. Finally, true independence in toileting is quite different than performing the skill with constant adult physical and verbal prompts. Having said all that, simply using pull-up underwear can be a very useful strategy.

Another study involving diaper wearing and toilet training was conducted by Tarbox, Williams, and Friman (2004). They studied one adult (29-year-old man) with intellectual disabilities. The client had been placed in diapers both at home and in the workplace for an extended period of time. The study was conducted at the participant's workshop. Two experimental conditions were employed. For the diaper condition, he wore this garment for the length of the workshop day. When accidents occurred, the diaper was replaced with a clean one. For the no-diaper condition, the client wore normal underwear during the workshop day. The diaper was replaced just before he went home. Wearing a diaper proved to be a setting event for urinating accidents. Obviously, the person needs to be physiologically ready to be toilet trained. But, when these conditions are in place, normal underwear versus a diaper may facilitate toilet training.

Mobile Phone Application

Another interesting application of technology was described by Kwon et al. (2015). They treated 18 adult males (46–70 years of age) with lower urinary tract symptoms. They used a smartphone to play sound of water and "relaxing melodies" while the participants attempted to void in the toilet. They noted a marked increase in flow rate as a result of their treatment. The failure to use a controlled experimental design does compromise the validity of the author's data. Further study of the topic does seem to be warranted nonetheless.

Toilet Seats

Glass et al. (2013) remind us that when considering issues with technology in the bathroom, it can also involve injuries. They studied injury patterns presented at our emergency room. This data has been compiled in the USA via a National Electronic Injury Surveillance System. The system records injuries that are related to various consumer products. Their data covered the years of 2002–2010. Injuries that occurred at home, school, and other public locations were included in the analysis. During the reporting period, 13,175 participants with toilet-related injuries were identified. The vast majority (over 9000) of the injuries were caused by falling toilet seats. Most injuries were for 2–3-year-olds (7362) followed by 4–7-year-old children (1369). Over 99% of the reported injuries occurred at home and more of the cases were life-threatening. The authors note that the second leading cause of injuries involved slipping on floors. What these data seem to suggest is that young children should be accompanied to the toilet to prevent falls and that the toilet seat, if not lowered already, should be placed down before attempts to void are initiated. The young child should then sit on the toilet seat.

Biofeedback

Satish and Rao (2011) describe a particularly unique approach to technology use for toileting. They describe the goal of their procedure to condition patterns of defecation. These tasks include complete voiding while on the stool and enhancing correct rectal sensation regarding toileting. Various physical tasks were also added to the biofeedback including spreading one's legs, leaning forward, and breathing deeply. Sensors are placed in or near the rectal area and are used to provide visual and auditory feedback regarding muscle movement required for voiding.

Using these biofeedback methods, Chiarioni, Salandini, and Whitehead (2005) describe one such study with 109 participants. These persons were randomly assigned to a five-session EMG biofeedback condition or 14.6 grams/day of polyethylene glycol. The biofeedback conditions were superior, resulting in greater reductions in blocked or incomplete bowel movements. Also, the biofeedback groups had less pain and were able to decrease the use of stool softeners.

In a second study, Rao et al. (2007) compared biofeedback to a placebo biofeedback and to a condition consisting of diet and lifestyle changes. Seventy-seven participants were assigned across these three groups. Biofeedback resulted in better voiding results and produced higher scores on a global bowel satisfaction questionnaire.

The data from these papers were replicated in two additional studies. Heymen et al. (2007) tested 84 participants in one of three conditions: placebo, diazepam, or biofeedback. Biofeedback proved to be superior to both of the other two conditions. Another of these biofeedback studies for constipation was reported by Battaglia et al. (2004). They tested 24 participants, 14 with pelvic floor dyssynergia and 10 with slow transit. This study extended the literature by treating people with slow-transit constipation and long-term follow-up data. Marked positive effects were noted for people suffering from both conditions with biofeedback. At a 1-year follow-up, 50% of people with pelvic floor dyssynergia and 20% with slow-transit constipation maintained their gains. These studies demonstrate effectiveness for constipation. Hopefully, future studies will also expand to other toilet training problems using this technology.

Trends

Most of the efforts involving technology to toilet train children have focused on special populations. Initially these studies highlighted persons in institutions who had intellectual disabilities. Often these people evinced intellectual disabilities. This fact was not surprising at the time. Persons with these disorders had multiple problems in learning (Matson, LeBlanc & Weinheimer, 1999; Matson & Boisjoli, 2007; Matson, Mayville, Kuhn, Land & Cooper, 2005; Matson & Wilkins, 2008). However, as the field has evolved, institutions for the developmentally disabled have been dramatically downsized. The focus has shifted toward a community model. This newer approach implies more training in group homes, family homes, and school settings. In addition to this point, health professionals are focusing more on younger individuals with respect to toilet training. Also, there is an increasing emphasis on including parents in ongoing training (Matson, Mahan & LoVullo, 2009).

Another major trend has been the increased diagnosis of autism. Diagnostic instrument development and more professional focus have gravitated to very young children (Matson, Boisjoli, Hess & Wilkins, 2010). The focus on intensive early intervention has in practice also included daytime toileting programs where applicable. These treatments are not typically discussed in the literature.

Universal preschool programs are now being championed in many countries. This trend will have an effect on daytime toilet training in particular. For example, there will be emphasis on developing toileting and accompanied dressing skills at young ages. Also, there will be multiple situations where teaching staff will need to be versed on toileting skills and the technology that is included in training.

The 1970s and 1980s appear to have been the "golden age" of technology development in the toileting literature. Given the huge technology advances in mobile devices since that time, it is unfortunate that more has not been done to incorporate these devices into toileting methods. As is always the case, more research is needed. This point is particularly important with respect to technology and toilet training. The general lack of research on the many possible devices that could be used to enhance toileting is potentially a field with great possible advancements.

References

Azrin, N. H., Bugle, C., & O'Brien, F. (1971). Behavioral engineering: Two apparatuses for toilet training retarded children. *Journal of Applied Behavior Analysis, 4*, 249–253.

Azrin, N. H., & Foxx, R. M. (1971). A rapid method of toilet training the institutionalized retarded. *Journal of Applied Behavior Analysis, 4*, 89–99.

Azrin, N. H., Sneed, T. J., & Foxx, R. M. (1973). Dry bed: A rapid method of eliminating bedwetting (enuresis) of the retarded. *Behaviour Research and Therapy, 11*, 427–434.

Battaglia, E., Serra, A. M., Buonafede, G., Dughera, L., Chistolini, F., Morelli, A., & Bassotti, E. G. (2004). Long-tern study on the effects of visual biofeedback and muscle training as a therapeutic modality in pelvic floor dyssynergia and slow-transit constipation. *Diseases of the Colon and Rectum, 47*, 90–95.

Bettison, S. (1982). *A comparison of toilet training strategies for the retarded*. University of Adelaide: Unpublished doctoral dissertation.

Chang, Y.-J., Lee, M.-Y., Chou, L.-D., Chen, S. F., & Chen, Y.-C. (2011). A mobile wetness detection system enabling teachers to toilet train children with intellectual disabilities in a public school setting. *Journal of Developmental and Physical Disabilities, 23*, 527–533.

Chiarioni, G., Salandini, L., & Whitehead, W. E. (2005). Biofeedback benefits only patients with outlet dysfunction, not patients with isolated slow transit constipation. *Gastroenterology, 129*, 86–97.

Dolyes, D. M. (1977). Behavioral treatments for nocturnal enuresis in children: A review of the recent literature. *Psychological Bulletin, 84*, 30–54.

Drysdale, B., Lee, C. Y. Q., Anderson, A., & Moore, D. W. (2014). Using video modeling incorporating animation to teach toileting to two children with autism spectrum disorder. *Journal of Developmental and Physical Disabilities, 27*, 149–165.

Fava, G. A., Cracco, L., & Facco, L. (1981). Positive reinforcement and enuresis. *Italian. Journal of Psychology, 8*, 149–152.

Glass, A. S., Bagga, H. S., Tasian, G. E., McGeady, J. B., McCulloch, C. E., Blaschko, S. D., … Breyer, B. N. (2013). No small slam: Increasing incidents of genitourinary injury from toilets and toilet seats. *BJU International, 112*, 398–403.

Greer, B. D., Neider, P. L., & Dozier, C. L. (2016). A component analysis of toilet-training procedures recommended for young children. *Journal of Applied Behavior Analysis, 49*, 69–84.

Henriksen, N., & Peterson, S. (2013). Behavioral treatment of bedwetting in an adolescent with autism. *Journal of Developmental and Physical Disabilities, 25*, 313–323.

Heymen, S., Scarlett, Y., Ringel, J. K., Drossman, D., & Whitehead, W. E. (2007). Randomized controlled trial shows biofeedback to be superior to alternative treatments for patients with pelvic floor dyssynergia-type constipation. *Diseases of the Colon and Rectum, 50*, 428–441.

Kaplan, S. L., Breit, M., Gauthier, B., & Busner, J. (1989). A comparison of three nocturnal enuresis treatment methods. *Journal of the American Academy of Child and Adolescent Psychiatry, 28*, 282–286.
Kwon, W.-A., Kim, S.H., Kim, S., Joung, J.Y., Chung, J., Lee, K.H., ... & Seo, H.K. (2015). Changes in urination according to the sound of running water using a mobile phone application. PLOS ONE.doi:10.1371/journal.pone.0126798
Lassen, M., & Fluet, N. (1979). Multifaceted behavioral treatment for nocturnal enuresis. *Behavior Therapy and Experimental Psychiatry, 10*, 155–156.
Lee, C. Y. Q., Anderson, D. W., & Moore, D. W. (2013). Using video modeling to toilet train a child with autism. *Journal of Developmental and Physical Disabilities, 26*, 123–134.
Levanto, K. E., Aponte, C. A., Wilkins, J., Travis, R., Aiello, R., Zanibbi, K., ... Mruzek, D. W. (2016). Use of urine alarms in toilet training children with intellectual and developmental disabilities: A review. *Research in Developmental Disabilities, 53-54*, 232–241.
Mahoney, K., Van Wagenen, R. K., & Meyerson, L. (1971). Toilet training of normal and retarded children. *Journal of Applied Behavior Analysis, 4*, 173–181.
Matson, J. L., & Boisjoli, J. A. (2007). Multiple versus single maintaining factors of challenging behaviours as assessed by the QABF for adults with intellectual disabilities. *Journal of Intellectual and Developmental Disabilities, 32*, 39–44.
Matson, J. L., Boisjoli, J. A., Hess, J. A., & Wilkins, J. (2010). Factor structure and diagnostic fidelity of the Baby and Infant Screen for children with aUtIsm Traits Part 1 (BISCUIT-Part 1). *Developmental Neurorehabilitation, 13*, 72–79.
Matson, J. L., LeBlanc, L. A., & Weinheimer, B. (1999). Reliability of the Matson Evaluation of Social Skills in Individuals with Severe Retardation (MESSIER). *Behavior Modification, 23*, 647–661.
Matson, J. L., Mahan, S., & LoVullo, S. V. (2009). Parent training: A review of methods for children with developmental disabilities. *Research in Developmental Disabilities, 30*, 961–968.
Matson, J. L., Mayville, S. B., Kuhn, D. E., Laud, R., & Cooper, C. (2005). The behavioral function of feeding problems as assessed by the Questions About Behavioral Function (QABF). *Research in Developmental Disabilities, 26*, 399–408.
Matson, J. L., & Wilkins, J. (2008). Antipsychotic drugs for aggression in intellectual disability. *The Lancet, 371*, 9–10.
McLay, L., Carnett, A., vanderMeer, L., & Lang, R. (2015). Using a video modeling-based intervention package to toilet train two children with autism. *Journal of Developmental and Physical Disabilities, 27*, 431–451.
Meadow, R. (1977). How to use buzzer alarms to cure bed-wetting. *British Medical Journal, ii*, 1073–1075.
Mowrer, O. H., & Mowrer, W. M. (1938). Enuresis: A method for its study and treatment. *American Journal of Orthopsychiatry, 18*, 436–459.
Oredsson, A. F., & Jorgensen, T. M. (1998). Changes in nocturnal bladder capacity during treatment with the bell and pad for monosymptomatic nocturnal enuresis. *The Journal of Urology, 160*, 166–169.
Passman, R. H. (1975). An automatic device for toilet training. *Behaviour Research and Therapy, 13*, 215–220.
Rajigab, L. S. (1996). Treatment of choice for nocturnal enuresis: Review and recommendations. *Journal of Psychological. Practice, 2*, 33–42.
Rao, S. S. C. (2011). Biofeedback therapy for constipation in adults. *Best Practice Research in Clinical Gastroenterology, 25*, 159–166.
Rao, S. S., Seaton, K., Miller, M., Brown, K., Nygaard, I., Stumbo, P., ... Schulze, K. (2007). Randomized controlled trial of biofeedback, sham feedback, and standard therapy for dyssynergic defection. *Clinical Gastroenterology and Hepatology, 5*, 331–338.
Simon, J. L., & Thompson, R. H. (2006). The effects of undergarment type on the urinary continence of toddlers. *Journal of Applied Behavior Analysis, 39*, 363–368.

Smith, T. (2014). Field report: Making toilet training easier-a novel enuresis alarm system. *Behavior Analysis Practice*, *7*, 31–32.
Stein, M.A., Mendelsohn, J., Obermeyer, W.H., Amromin, B.A. & Beuca, R. (2001). Sleep and behavior problems in school-aged children. *Pediatrics*, *1007*(4), e60. Retrieved from http://pediatrics.aappublications.org/content/107/4/e6o.long
Tarbox, R. S. F., Williams, W. L., & Friman, P. C. (2004). Extended diaper wearing: Effects on continence in and out of the diaper. *Journal of Applied Behavior Analysis*, *37*, 97–100.
Van Wagenen, R. K., Meyerson, L., Keer, N. J., & Mahoney, K. (1969). Field trials of a new procedure for toilet training. *Journal of Experimental Child Psychology*, *8*, 147–159.
Van Wagenen, R. K., & Murdock, E. E. (1966). A transistorized signal-package for toilet training of infants. *Journal of Experimental Child Psychology*, *3*, 312–314.
Wright, J.M.C. (1975). Comparison of toilet training techniques with institutionalized retarded children. Unpublished master's thesis. University of Queensland.

Nighttime Toilet Training

Rachel L. Goldin and Delilah Mendes de Gouveia

History of Nocturnal Enuresis

Nocturnal enuresis (NE), commonly known as "bedwetting," is defined as repeated voiding of urine, voluntary or involuntary, into clothing or the bed during sleep, at least twice a week, for 3 consecutive months, in children 5 years of age or older in the absence of a general medical condition (American Psychiatric Association, 2013). Along with NE, daytime wetting is also considered a significant problem but is typically considered separately as it has been suggested that it has an entirely separate etiology. Most cases of daytime wetting are caused by medical conditions (e.g., urinary tract infection; Jarvelin, Huttunen, Seppanen, Seppanen, & Moilanen, 1990).

NE is a common and pathologically benign condition in the pediatric population.

Though benign, the condition has the potential of causing considerable amounts of stress and worry for both the child and parent (Fitzwater & Macknin, 1992). Warzak (1993) found that children who met criteria for NE experienced increased amount of parental disapproval, sibling teasing, and repeated treatment failure, thus increasing the importance of proper treatment. Psychosocial consequences of NE can be problematic when finding the direct cause, possibility of comorbidity, and the best course of treatment (Neveus, 2011). Yeung, Sihoe, Sit, Bower, Sreedhard, and Lau (2004) found that children diagnosed with enuresis experienced an increased level of depressive problems and problems at school and work.

R.L. Goldin, PhD (✉)
Department of Psychiatry, Indiana University School of Medicine, Indianapolis, IN, USA
e-mail: rgoldi3@lsu.edu

D.M. de Gouveia, BCBA
The Emerge Center, Baton Rouge, LA, USA

J.L. Matson (ed.), *Clinical Guide to Toilet Training Children*, Autism and Child Psychopathology Series, DOI 10.1007/978-3-319-62725-0_11

Foxman, Valdez, and Brook (1986) found that only one third of individuals following through age 11 saw a physician about NE. This low percentage could be due to the annual spontaneous cure rate of 14% for 5–9-year-old children (Forsythe & Redmond, 1974). Worried parents of the individual with NE were more likely to seek treatment from a pediatrician (Foxman et al., 1986). Treatments for NE include behavioral, psychological, and pharmacological interventions. Behavioral approaches include scheduled wakenings, reinforcement-based methods, dietary restrictions, overcorrection, retention control, overlearning, and alarm interventions. Psychological approaches include hypnosis and cognitive behavior therapy. Pediatricians frequently prescribe medications for patients with NE (Henriksen & Peterson, 2013). Common medications prescribed to treat NE include desmopressin acetate and tricyclic antidepressants (e.g., imipramine; Glazener, 2008).

Prevalence of NE

Prevalence rates of NE vary because of difficulties reliably defining the condition and the methods of diagnosis (de Jonge, 1973). Fifteen to 20% of 5-year-olds are estimated to meet diagnostic criteria for NE (Axelrod, Tornehl, & Fontanini-Axelrod, 2014). NE in some cases has been found to continue in adolescence with 25% of 6-year-old boys and 15% of 6-year-old girls still wetting the bed (Friman, 2008). In addition, between 1% and 3% continue to meet diagnostic criteria as adolescents (Meltzer, Johnson, Crosette, Ramos, & Mindell, 2010).

Williams, Sears, and Allard (2004) reported that NE occurs at much higher prevalence rates with individuals with autism spectrum disorders (ASD), attention-deficit hyperactivity/disorder (ADHD), and other developmental disabilities (Williams et al., 2004). Boys are more likely to be affected by NE than girls (Neveus, 2011). Oppel, Harper, and Rider (1968) conducted a study in which they compared initial dryness in boys versus girls. They found that girls attained initial dryness at a higher prevalence than did boys.

Etiology

Before considering empirically based behavioral interventions to treat NE, it is important that clinicians and caretakers rule out any medical underlying conditions. Nocturnal polyuria syndrome (NPS), decreased bladder capacity, detrusor overactivity, and sleep arousal disturbances are identified as the most common underlying medical mechanisms that can contribute to NE (DiBianco, Morley, and Al-Omar, 2014; Neveus, 2011).

Nocturnal Polyuria Syndrome (NPS). This syndrome is characterized by an increase in urine output during the night. The antidiuretic hormone (ADH) is responsible for decreasing urine output during sleep. Children diagnosed with NPS commonly lack ADH production resulting in an increase of urine output (Aikawa, Kasahara, & Uchiyama, 1998).

Decreased Bladder Capacity. Yeung, Sit, To, Chiu, Sihoe, Lee, and Wong (2002) reported that children who met diagnostic criteria for NE had significantly decreased bladder capacities compared to healthy children of the same age. Anatomically the bladder is the same size but it tends to contract before it is entirely full (Page & Valentino, 1994).

Detrusor Overactivity. Children with NE may have a lower pressure threshold for detrusor activity as a result of having a significantly decreased bladder capacity during the night (Yeung et al., 2002). A lower pressure threshold can cause children with NE to void in smaller volumes as the overacting detrusor muscle fails to wake them up (Fonseca, Bordallo, Garcia, Munhoz, & Silva, 2009).

Sleep Arousal Disturbances. Researchers have demonstrated that children with NE commonly experience an inability to awaken from sleep when a void sensation occurs. The inability to awaken could be caused by problems between the bladder and brain connection or the child with NE has habituated to the void sensation resulting in failure to arouse from sleep (Watanabe & Azuma, 1989).

Other Diseases. Roche, Menon, Gill, and Hoey (2005) found that NE can also be caused by other diseases including diabetes (mellitus or insipidus) and nonoliguric renal failure. Lastly, urinary tract infection (UTI) and constipation can also produce an increase in the void sensation (Yazbeck, Schick, & O'Regan, 1987).

Family History/Genetics. Fergusson, Hons, Horwood, and Shannon (1986) found that having a family history of enuresis was the strongest predictor of nocturnal bladder control. Children with a family history of enuresis were shown to attain nocturnal bladder control more than 1½ years later versus children with irrelevant family histories.

Developmental Level/Delay in Maturation. The central nervous system (CNS) is hypothesized to play an important role in the etiology of NE. Differences in maturation of the CNS have been suggested in children with NE when compared to typically developing children of the same age. Maturation of the CNS involves bladder stability, recognition of bladder fullness, and the ability to suppress the onset of bladder contractions (Watanabe & Azuma, 1989). Oppel, Harper, and Rider (1968) found that individuals with a low birth weight attained nighttime dryness significantly later than individuals who were born full term.

Typical Age of Bladder Control Attainment

Fergusson et al. (1986) studied a group of children from 4 months of age to 8 years of age. Initial results showed that 96.7% of children 8 years of age had attained nocturnal bladder control. During a follow-up study, authors found that 7.4% of children had relapsed and were experiencing NE. Authors suggested that after 5 years of age, children who were experiencing NE failed to attain primary control and NE was due to secondary or onset enuresis. Oppel et al. (1968) found that 97% of children attained bladder control by 7 and 12 years; however, they also found that one quarter of all children relapsed. These children account for the 25% of 6-year-old boys and 15% of 6-year-old girls still experiencing NE after attaining bladder control (Friman, 2008).

There are different factors that are related to the attainment of nocturnal bladder control including the child's sex, early sleep patterns, and other psychosocial factors. Oppel et al. (1968) found that a higher percentage of girls developed both daytime and nighttime bladder control than boys. They also found that children who were reported to sleep for longer periods of time were slower to attain bladder control versus children who slept for shorter periods. Oppel et al. (1968) identified family social background, presence of stressful life events, consistency of parent figures, and changes of residences as psychosocial factors that could possibly affect bladder control attainment. Taken together, NE is a common childhood disorder that can be the result of and maintained by a multitude of factors. The next section discusses in-depth interventions to treat NE and provides suggestions on best practice.

Interventions

Simple Behavioral Interventions

A common first-line intervention for NE involves using simple behavioral techniques such as star charts and token economies for reducing nighttime bedwetting. Using simple behavioral techniques is less burdensome and stressful for families than frequent night awakenings and alarms. Twelve randomized controlled trials (RCT) assessing the effects of simple behavioral interventions were included in a Cochrane Review. The review suggested that using simple behavioral interventions resulted in significantly less accidents; however, none of the RCTs were good for methodological quality. Additionally, most of the sample sizes were small and the dropout rate was high (Glazener, Evans, & Peto, 2004).

Simple behavioral interventions appear to be beneficial as a first-line treatment (e.g., wakening, reinforcement-based methods, dietary restrictions) or an adjunct treatment (overlearning) to keep the individual motivated throughout treatment and reduce risk of relapse. They are safe and harmless and may be preferred by parents who do not want to use alarms or medication. That being said, one behavioral technique which has been found to be counterproductive and should be avoided is penalties for bedwetting (Glazener, 2008). All behavioral techniques should involve positive reinforcement.

Wakening. The child is woken after going to bed to allow them to urinate. Wakenings can be scheduled or done randomly. As the child experiences dry nights, wakenings are moved progressively earlier in the sleep cycle.

Reinforcement-Based Methods/Reward Systems. The child is provided with rewards for dry nights. As the child achieves more dry nights, the reward system is modified. For example, the child may receive a reward for 2 dry nights in a week; once the child maintains 2 dry nights for another week, the system should be modified so that the child is rewarded only if he or she has 3 dry nights in a week and so on. Rewards should always be given after the preset goal is met. Rewards should involve the child's input and continually be changed so that the child does not lose interest.

Dietary Restriction. Restricting liquids an hour before bed and eliminating caffeinated beverages during the day.

Overcorrection. The child is required to clean up their accident (e.g., placing sheets in the wash) immediately after wetting.

Retention Control. This involves increasing the functional bladder capacity through techniques such as delaying urination for a period of time or drinking increased fluids.

Overlearning. Overlearning is used in conjunction with an alarm intervention. It involves providing the child with extra fluids at bedtime after they have successfully become drying using an alarm. Extra fluids at bed add stress to the detrusor muscles in the bladder. The alarm intervention is then used again until the child has 14 consecutive dry nights.

Standard Alarm Interventions

Urine alarms are one of the most frequently used interventions to treat NE. Urine alarms utilize both classical conditioning and operant conditioning. The classical condition component follows as such:

Unconditioned stimulus (US): awakening stimulus or the alarm sound
Unconditioned response (UR): awakening response and sphincter contraction
Neutral stimulus (NS): feeling produced by bladder distention
Conditioned stimulus (CS): feeling produced by bladder distention
Conditioned response (CR): awakening response and sphincter contraction

The child wets the bed which activates the alarm (US), which prompts awakening and sphincter constriction (UR), therefore stopping urination in the bed and so the child can instead move to the restroom to urinate. After repeated pairing of the alarm (US) and the feeling of having a full bladder (NS), the NS becomes the CS causing the waking response (CR) of waking and going to the restroom to urinate. The operant conditioning component involves the alarm serving as a noxious stimulus, resulting in positive punishment whenever the child wets the bed triggering the alarm. Repeated activation of the alarm elicits an avoidance response; the behavior of not wetting the bed is maintained through negative reinforcement (Lovibond, 1963).

Alarms for NE come in many variations, some are attached to the individual (e.g., clipped on), part of underwear, or placed beneath the individual on the bed. When the individual wets the bed, an electric circuit is activated, which sets off an alarm (e.g., bell, buzzer). As explained above, the noise produced by the alarm causes bladder muscles to reflexively contract, inhibiting further urination. Generally, as part of most alarm interventions, after an alarm goes off, the child must change their clothing and bedding before going back to sleep. Additionally, the child should be encouraged to drink lots of fluids before bed while beginning the intervention to ensure they have accidents.

Alarm interventions are found to be very effective, boasting around a 78% success rate usually occurring within 4 weeks (Mellon & McGrath, 2000); however, they also tend to have a high relapse rate and dropout rate (Fielding, 1985; Kristensen & Jensen, 2003). Rates of relapse have been reported to be as high as 50% and dropout rates as high as 48% (Fielding, 1985; Glazener, 2008). Despite this, many studies have found alarm interventions to be more effective than other treatments such as medications and psychotherapy (Mellon & McGrath, 2000). The best predictor of treatment success is parental motivation (Fielding, 1985). A Cochrane Review of alarm intervention RCTs indicated issues with adherence to this type of intervention, suggesting the undesirability of the intervention (Glazener, Evans, & Peto, 2005). Alarm therapies can be stressful for families and can interfere with normal sleep cycles. Therefore, if the family is not invested in the intervention, they are likely to drop out.

Multicomponent Behavioral Interventions

To deal with the high relapse rate of interventions just involving urine alarms, several interventions have been designed that combine alarms and other behavioral techniques. These multicomponent interventions are found to have around a 79% success rate (Mellon & McGrath, 2000). The combination of alarms with other behavioral techniques reduces the risk of relapse and decreases length of treatment. Common treatment components used in conjunction include retention control training, overlearning, cleanliness training, and positive reinforcement. For example, the relapse rate after successful alarm alone intervention was 49% compared to a 25% relapse rate after successful alarm plus an overlearning intervention (Glazener, 2008). Similarly, alarm interventions with a dry-bed training component have reduced relapse rates from 63% to 27% (Glazener, 2008; Taylor & Turner, 1975).

Dry-bed treatment (DBT) is an example of a complex multicomponent intervention initially proposed and studied by Azrin, Sneed, and Foxx (1974). DBT is designed around the idea that NE is a learning problem, reinforced by a multitude of factors. The urine alarm component of DBT is less about conditioning (Mowrer & Mowrer, 1938) the bladder and rather aimed at creating social and motivational events. DBT pairs a standard urine alarm apparatus with additional features such as training rapid awakening, self-correcting of accidents, increased positive reinforcement of motivation for not having accidents, as well as urine retention practice.

In the original DBT protocol, treatment was done by a trained professional in the child's home. The child's parent then continued the DBT once the child becomes continent. Subsequent studies of DBT have supported its effectiveness and also indicated that parents can be taught to administer the program, making DBT more cost-effective and accessible. Additionally, DBT with the urine alarm component is reported to be more effective than DBT alone or a urine alarm alone, indicating the value of multicomponent interventions (Azrin & Thienes, 1978; Bollard & Nettelbeck, 1981; Nettelbeck & Langeluddecke, 1979). Taken together, multicomponent interventions (including an alarm component) are just as effective as alarms in the short term, but are better at preventing relapse especially when combined with overlearning or using DBT (Glazener, 2008).

Psychological Approaches

Hypnosis is one of the main psychological approaches used to treat NE. Hypnosis for NE involves an induction procedure to place the individual into a trance, deepening the trance, then providing suggestions for urinary continence. Suggestions are specific to enuresis and cover areas such as bladder capacity, reducing fluids before bedtime, holding on as long as possible, and waking up to use the toilet when experiencing a full bladder (Edwards & Spuvy, 1985). Hypnotherapy can be done by a clinician or through teaching children self-hypnosis as a means for self-conditioning to cure their bedwetting (Olness, 1975).

A review by Mellon and McGrath (2000) identified four studies of hypnosis for NE and found an average success rate of 71%. Treatment on average lasted six sessions for about an hour each (Banerjee, Srivastav, & Palan, 1993; Edwards & Spuvy, 1985; Mellon & McGrath, 2000; Olness, 1975). However, only one of the studies reviewed by Mellon and McGrath used quantifiable outcome measures, making it difficult to compare its effectiveness to other treatments.

Cognitive behavioral therapy (CBT) has been proposed as a treatment for NE; however, there is limited research examining its effectiveness as a standalone treatment. CBT for NE has been used in a few different ways including targeting a child's irrational beliefs that cause and maintain bedwetting and teaching self-control skills. Cognitive interventions focusing on self-control suggest that a child must develop both physical and cognitive self-control in order to achieve bladder control. Overtime, a child learns the specific skills required for bladder control such as controlling the sphincter and the urge to go immediately, as well as when and where the appropriate places to void are. Ronen, Wozner, and Rahav (1992) pointed out that poor self-control may be associated with risk for enuresis as boys exhibit higher rates of enuresis and are typically found to have poorer self-control than females and parents with self-control deficits are more likely to have children with enuresis compared to parents with higher self-control levels (Ronen et al., 1992).

Ronen, Wozner, and Rahav compared the effectiveness of a cognitive behavioral intervention to an alarm intervention (i.e., bell and pad) and a token reinforcement intervention. The cognitive behavioral intervention was comprised of five components: modification of misconceptions and irrational beliefs, rational analysis of bedwetting, sensitization to pressure in the bladder, self-control training in different situations, and exercises in self-observation, charting, self-assessment, and self-reinforcement (Ronen et al., 1992). Results indicated that the cognitive behavioral intervention was as effective as the alarm intervention, well accepted by participants and their families, and cost-effective and had a lower but not significantly different dropout rate compared to the alarm group and token reinforcement group. Most noteworthy was that the relapse rate was significantly lower in the cognitive intervention group compared to the other groups (Ronen et al., 1992). Taken together, the evidence for cognitive interventions for the treatment NE is still limited but may be a good option for families that find alarm interventions aversive or in cases which relapse is a persistent issue.

Pharmacological Interventions

Common medications used to treat NE include desmopressin and imipramine due to the antidiuretic effects of the drugs. Medications for NE have been found to be effective while the child is on the medication, but bedwetting tends to return when the medications are discontinued (Glazener, 2008). For example, the long-term effectiveness of imipramine for treating NE ranges from 5% to 40% with a total remission of 10% to 50% (Sukhai, Mol, & Harris, 1989). Wille (1986) studied desmopressin in comparison to an alarm and found that desmopressin reduced the frequency of bedwetting more quickly than the alarm with equal efficacy during the treatment trial; however, in posttreatment there was a significantly higher relapse rate in the desmopressin group compared to the alarm group (Wille, 1994). As such, alarm/conditioning interventions are preferable for the treatment of NE in the long term; however, medication may be useful when other interventions fail or when immediate effects are needed.

Combined Pharmacological/Behavioral Approach

To address the issue of high relapse rates associated with medication use for NE and the undesirability of behavioral intervention, the combined effects of pharmacological and behavioral interventions have been studied in great depth. In terms of overall effectiveness of using a combined approach, most research to date has reported significantly fewer wet nights when alarms and medications are used in combination compared to when they are used alone (Bradbury & Meadow, 1995; Sukhai et al., 1989). Bradford and Meadow (1995) examined the effectiveness of adding the medication desmopressin to an alarm intervention in two groups of children. At baseline, the children in both groups had on average 2.3 dry nights per week. After 6 weeks of treatment, the group with the desmopressin and alarm intervention had 6.3 dry nights per week compared to the alarm-only group, which had 4.8 dry nights per week (Bradbury & Meadow, 1995). Sukhai et al. (1989) reported similar findings but over a 2-week period. Participants were randomly assigned to either the desmopressin and alarm group or placebo and alarm group. After 2 weeks, the desmopressin and alarm group had 5 dry nights a week compared to the placebo and alarm group, which had 4 dry nights per week (Sukhai et al., 1989). These studies illustrate the effectiveness of combining pharmacological and behavioral interventions for treating NE, especially in children who have not improved on other treatments. In regard to relapse rate and treatment acceptability, combined treatment approaches appear to result in faster treatment success and reduce risk of relapse.

Acupuncture

Evidence has emerged supporting the use of acupuncture and electroacupuncture in the treatment of NE. It is hypothesized that acupuncture influences spinal micturition centers and parasympathetic innervation to the urinary tract. Additionally, acupuncture is believed to modulate brain function through the descending serotonergic system (Bower & Diao, 2010). To treat NE, acupuncture interventions generally last 10–15 sessions. Traditionally, studying the effectiveness of acupuncture in the treatment of NE has been challenging due to difficulty standardizing treatment procedures. Electroacupuncture, a pulsating electrical current that is applied to acupuncture needles, is purported to be easier to standardize as stimulation is continuous and the practitioner performance is less likely to vary. Additionally, treatment dosage can be objectively monitored and assessed.

Evidence of efficacy of acupuncture for NE is around 70% (Bower & Diao, 2010; Tüzüner, Keçik, Ozdemir, & Canakçi, 1989). Few studies exist however comparing it to simple behavioral interventions, alarms, or medications or examining the long-term effectiveness. Electroacupuncture over traditional acupuncture is found to improve outcomes and has few reported negative side effects. Treatment of NE with acupuncture is an emerging area of research and may be a viable option for families interested in less traditional interventions.

Conclusion

Alarm interventions are highly effective in treating NE; however, relapse rates are fairly high. Combining alarms with other behavioral interventions such as overlearning, dry-bed training, and positive reinforcement can reduce relapse rates. Medications such as desmopressin and imipramine are effective in treating NE quickly, but effectiveness declines significantly when the medication is discontinued. Therefore, duration of treatment is longer when using alarms, but unlike medications, their effectiveness persists posttreatment. In cases where children appear to be highly resistant to treatment or immediate success is needed, a combination of medication and alarms is recommended. Combining medication and alarm interventions provides quick results due to the medication but also increases the likelihood of long-term treatment success because of the alarm interventions. Thus, interventions with an alarm component are considered best practice, garnering considerable research support, and crucial for successful treatment of NE.

Hypnosis and other cognitive interventions do not have as much research support as medication or behavioral/conditioning interventions (e.g., alarms, simple behavioral techniques) and currently do not appear to be any more effective. However, continued study of cognitive interventions is beneficial for families who are hesitant to try medication and find behavioral interventions time-consuming and aversive. Acupuncture is another alternative option for the treatment of NE and has produced promising effects, but well-controlled research is still needed comparing its effectiveness to other interventions and examining long-term outcomes.

One area of study that appears to be lacking with regard to treatment of NE, and may be worth attention, is if certain clinical features or demographic variables affect treatment success. Identifying patient characteristics that predict treatment outcomes would be beneficial for professionals when discussing treatment options with families to increase success rate and treatment satisfaction. That being said, the state of research with regard to treatment of NE is overall in a good place as there are many empirically supported interventions to treat this common childhood problem.

References

American Psychiatric Association. (2013). *Diagnostic and statistical manual of mental disorders* (5th ed.). Arlington, VA: American Psychiatric Publishing.

Aikawa, T., Kasahara, T., & Uchiyama, M. (1998). The arginine-vasopressin secretion profile of children with primary nocturnal enuresis. *European Urology*, *33*(3), 41–44.

Axelrod, M. I., Tornehl, C., & Fontanini-Axelrod, A. (2014). Enhanced response using a multicomponent urine alarm treatment for nocturnal enuresis. *Journal for Specialists in Pediatric Nursing*, *19*, 172–182.

Azrin, N. H., Sneed, T. J., & Foxx, R. M. (1974). Dry-bed training: Rapid elimination of childhood enuresis. *Behaviour Research and Therapy*, *12*(3), 147–156.

Azrin, N. H., & Thienes, P. M. (1978). Rapid elimination of enuresis by intensive learning without a conditioning apparatus. *Behavior Therapy*, *9*(3), 342–354. https://doi.org/10.1016/S0005-7894(78)80077-X.

Banerjee, S., Srivastav, A., & Palan, B. M. (1993). Hypnosis and self-hypnosis in the management of nocturnal enuresis: A comparative study with imipramine therapy. *American Journal of Clinical Hypnosis*, *36*(2), 113–119.

Bollard, J., & Nettelbeck, T. (1981). A comparison of dry-bed training and standard urine-alarm conditioning treatment of childhood bedwetting. *Behaviour Research and Therapy*, *19*(3), 215–226. https://doi.org/10.1016/0005-7967(81)90005-X.

Bower, W. F., & Diao, M. (2010). Acupuncture as a treatment for nocturnal enuresis. *Autonomic Neuroscience, 157*(1–2), 63–67. https://doi.org/10.1016/j.autneu.2010.07.003.
Bradbury, M., & Meadow, S. (1995). Combined treatment with enuresis alarm and desmopressin for nocturnal enuresis. *Acta Paediatrica, 84*(9), 1014–1018. https://doi.org/10.1111/j.1651-2227.1995.tb13818.x.
de Jonge, G. A. (1973). Epidemiology enuresis: A survey of the literature. In I. Kolvin, R. C. MacKeith, & S. R. Meadow (Eds.), *Bladder control and enuresis - clinics in developmental Medicine* (pp. 39–46). PA, Lippincott: Washington Square.
DiBianco, J. M., Morley, C., & Al-Omar, O. (2014). Nocturnal enuresis: A topic review and institution experience. *Avicenna journal of medicine, 4*(4), 77.
Edwards, S. D., & Spuvy, H. I. J. V. (1985). Hypnotherapy as a treatment for enuresis. *Journal of Child Psychology and Psychiatry, 26*(1), 161–170. https://doi.org/10.1111/j.1469-7610.1985.tb01635.x.
Fergusson, D. M., Hons, H., Horwood, L. J., & Shannon, F. T. (1986). Factors related to the age of attainment of nocturnal bladder control: An 8-year longitudinal study. *Pediatrics, 78*(5), 884–890.
Fielding, D. (1985). Factors associated with drop-out, relapse and failure in the conditioning treatment of nocturnal enuresis. *Behavioural Psychotherapy, 13*(3), 174–185.
Fitzwater, D., & Macknin, M. L. (1992). Risk/benefit ratio in enuresis therapy. *Clinical Pediatrics, 31*(5), 308–310.
Friman, P. C. (2008). Evidence-based therapies for enuresis end encopresis. In R. G. Steele, T. D. Elkin, & M. C. Roberts (Eds.), *Handbook of evidence-based therapies for children and adolescents: Bridging science and practice* (pp. 311–333). New York: Springer.
Fonseca, E. G., Bordallo, A. P., Garcia, P. K., Munhoz, C., & Silva, C. P. (2009). Lower urinary tract symptoms in enuretic and nonenurtic children. *Journal of Urology, 182*(4), 1978–1983.
Forsythe, W. I., & Redmond, A. (1974). Enuresis and spontaneous cure rate. *Archives of Disease in Childhood, 49*, 259–263.
Foxman, B., Valdez, R. B., & Brook, R. H. (1986). Childhood enuresis: Prevalence, perceived impact, and prescribed treatments. *Pediatrics, 77*(4), 482–487.
Glazener, C. M. (2008). Alarm interventions for nocturnal enuresis in children. *Cochrane Database of Systematic Reviews, 1*. Retrieved from http://search.ebscohost.com/login.aspx?direct=true&db=chh&AN=CD002911&site=ehost-live.
Glazener, C. M. A., Evans, J. H. C., & Peto, R. E. (2005). Alarm interventions for nocturnal enuresis in children. *The Cochrane Database of Systematic Reviews, 2*, CD002911.
Glazener, C. M., Evans, J. H., & Peto, R. E. (2004). Treating nocturnal enuresis in children: Review of evidence. *Journal of Wound Ostomy & Continence Nursing, 31*(4), 223–234.
Henrikson, N., & Peterson, S. (2013). Behavior treatment of bedwetting in an adolescent with autism. *Journal of Developmental and Physical Disabilities, 25*, 313–323.
Jarvelin, M. R., Huttunen, N. P., Seppanen, J., Seppanen, U., & Moilanen, I. (1990). Screening of urinary tract abnormalities among day and nightwetting children. *Scandinavian Journal of Urology and Nephrology, 24*(3), 181–189.
Kristensen, G., & Jensen, I. N. (2003). Meta-analyses of results of alarm treatment for nocturnal enuresis: Reporting practice, criteria and frequency of bedwetting. *Scandinavian Journal of Urology and Nephrology, 37*(3), 232–238.
Lovibond, S. H. (1963). The mechanism of conditioning treatment of enuresis. *Behaviour Research and Therapy, 1*, 17–21.
Mellon, M. W., & McGrath, M. L. (2000). Empirically supported treatments in Pediatric Psychology: Nocturnal enuresis. *Journal of Pediatric Psychology, 25*(4), 193–214. https://doi.org/10.1093/jpepsy/25.4.193.
Meltzer, L. J., Johnson, C., Crosette, J., Ramos, M., & Mindell, J. A. (2010). Prevalence of diagnosed sleep disorders in pediatric primary care practices. *Pediatrics, 125*(6), 1410–1418.
Mowrer, O. H., & Mowrer, W. M. (1938). Enuresis—A method for its study and treatment. *American Journal of Orthopsychiatry, 8*(3), 436–459. https://doi.org/10.1111/j.1939-0025.1938.tb06395.x.

Nettelbeck, T., & Langeluddecke, P. (1979). Dry-bed training without an enuresis machine. *Behaviour Research and Therapy*, *17*(4), 403–404.
Neveus, T. (2011). Nocturnal enuresis - theoretic background and practical guidelines. *Pediatric Nephrology*, *26*, 1207–1214.
Olness, K. (1975). The use of self-hypnosis in the treatment of childhood nocturnal enuresis. A report on forty patients. *Clinical Pediatrics*, *14*(3), 273.
Oppel, W. C., Harper, P. A., & Vider, R. V. (1968). The age of attaining bladder control. *Pediatrics*, *42*(4), 614–624.
Page, M. E., & Valentino, R. J. (1994). Locus coeruleus activation by physiological challenges. *Brain Research Bulletin*, *35*, 557–560.
Roche, E. F., Menon, A., Gill, D., & Hoey, H. (2005). Clinical presentation of type 1 diabetes. *Pediatric Diabetes*, *6*, 75–78.
Ronen, T., Wozner, Y., & Rahav, G. (1992). Cognitive intervention in enuresis. *Child & Family Behavior Therapy*, *14*(2), 1–14. https://doi.org/10.1300/J019v14n02_01.
Sukhai, R. N., Mol, J., & Harris, A. S. (1989). Combined therapy of enuresis alarm and desmopressin in the treatment of nocturnal enuresis. *European Journal of Pediatrics*, *148*(5), 465–467.
Taylor, P. D., & Turner, R. K. (1975). A clinical trial of continuous, intermittent and overlearning "bell and pad" treatments for nocturnal enuresis. *Behaviour Research and Therapy*, *13*(4), 281–293.
Tüzüner, F., Keçik, Y., Ozdemir, S., & Canakçi, N. (1989). Electro-acupuncture in the treatment of enuresis nocturna. *Acupuncture & Electro-Therapeutics Research*, *14*(3–4), 211–215.
Warzak, W. J. (1993). Psychosocial implications of nocturnal enuresis. *Clinical Pediatrics*, *32*(1), 38–40.
Watanabe, H., & Azuma, Y. (1989). A proposal for a classification system of enuresis based on overnight simultaneous monitoring of electroencephalography and cystometry. *Sleep*, *12*, 257–264.
Wille, S. (1994). Primary nocturnal enuresis in children. *Background and treatment. Scandinavian Journal of Urology and Nephrology. Supplementum*, *156*, 1–48.
Wille, S. O. R. E. N. (1986). Comparison of desmopressin and enuresis alarm for nocturnal enuresis. *Archives of disease in childhood*, *61*(1), 30–33.
Williams, P. G., Sears, L. L., & Allard, A. (2004). Sleep problems in children with autism. *Journal of Sleep Research*, *13*, 265–268.
Yazbeck, S., Shick, E., & O'Regan, S. (1987). Relevance of constipation to enuresis, urinary tract infection, and reflux. A review. *European Urology*, *13*, 318–321.
Yeung, C. K., Sit, F. K., To, L. K, Chiu, H. N., Sihoe, J. D., & Wong, C. (2002). Reduction in nocturnal functional bladder capacity is a common factor in the pathogenesis of refractory nocturnal enuresis. *British Journal of Urology*, *90*, 302–307.
Yeung, C. K., Sihoe, J. D., Sit, F. K., Bower, W. F., Sreedhar, B., & Lau, J. (2004). Characteristics of primary nocturnal enuresis in adults: An epidemiology study. *British Journal of Urology*, *93*, 341–345.

Medical Issues

GenaLynne C. Mooneyham, Jessica Xiaoxi Ouyang, and Cassie D. Karlsson

Introduction

Toilet training is often as much about the "accidents" as it is the "successes." On the road to continence, episodes of both daytime and nighttime wetting are a part of normal development. Most parents can share stories about the struggles of achieving this coveted milestone. However, there are times in which toilet training troubles fall outside the realm of normal, and recognizing these scenarios is often key to obtaining an appropriate medical workup when indicated. There are times in which medication management (in addition to behavioral interventions) may be warranted.

This chapter examines enuresis and constipation as medical diagnoses, providing an overview of the subtypes of each condition, common medical and psychiatric issues that may be associated with ongoing symptoms, as well as management options. In addition, times in which referral to a specialist would be warranted are discussed.

G.C. Mooneyham, MD, MS
Department of Psychiatry and Department of Pediatrics, Duke University School of Medicine, 2301 Erwin Road, Durham, NC 27710, USA
e-mail: genalynne.mooneyham@duke.edu

J.X. Ouyang, MD
Indiana University School of Medicine, 705 Riley Hospital Dr, Indianapolis, IN 46202, USA
e-mail: xouyang@iupui.edu

C.D. Karlsson, MD (✉)
Department of Psychiatry, Indiana University School of Medicine, 705 Riley Hospital Dr., Suite 4300, Indianapolis, IN 46202, USA
e-mail: ckarlsso@iupui.edu

J.L. Matson (ed.), *Clinical Guide to Toilet Training Children*, Autism and Child Psychopathology Series, DOI 10.1007/978-3-319-62725-0_12

Enuresis

The Diagnostic and Statistical Manual of Mental Disorders, Fifth Edition (DSM 5) defines enuresis as the "repeated voiding of urine into inappropriate places" (American Psychiatric Association, 2013, p. 355). The subtypes outlined allow for a differentiation between nocturnal and diurnal symptoms as well as for a combination of both. The DSM does provide a minimum chronological age requirement for the diagnosis of enuresis as being 5 years, but also emphasizes the importance of the developmental assessment. Children with intellectual disabilities may fulfill the chronological age requirement for the diagnosis of enuresis, but they may not have met the developmental milestones necessary to initiate a toilet training regimen.

The DSM 5 diagnostic criteria outlined for the diagnosis of Enuresis 307.6 includes the following (American Psychiatric Association, 2013, p. 355):

A. Repeated voiding of urine into bed or clothes, whether involuntary or intentional.
B. The behavior is clinically significant as manifested by either a frequency of at least twice a week for at least three consecutive months or the presence of clinically significant distress or impairment in social, academic (occupational), or other important areas of functioning.
C. Chronological age is at least 5 years (or equivalent developmental level).
D. The behavior is *not* attributable to the physiological effects of a substance (e.g., a diuretic, an antipsychotic medication) or another medical condition (e.g., diabetes, spina bifida, a seizure disorder).

Specifiers include: "nocturnal only" for passage of urine during night sleep only, "diurnal only" for passage of urine during wakeful hours, and "nocturnal and diurnal" when a combination of symptoms is present.

Classifications of Enuresis

A variety of terms to describe enuresis are utilized in practice. This can be particularly confusing to both clinicians and families. The International Children's Continence Society (ICCS) proposed a clarification of terms in its 2006 article "Standardization of Terminology of Lower Urinary Tract Function in Children and Adolescents" (Neveus, von Gontard, Hoebeke, et al., 2006).

Primary enuresis is the descriptor utilized when urinary continence has yet to be established. Alternatively, secondary enuresis describes the scenario in which an individual previously attained urinary continence at one point in time, but has since regressed or lost this capacity. For example, if a 7-year-old male presents to the office for urinary incontinence, the clinician needs to focus on understanding whether the child had attained toilet training proficiency but subsequently *lost* this skill set or whether the child had never been fully toilet trained in the first place. Primary enuresis due to a neurodevelopmental disorder is not uncommon, particularly if there is an underlying etiology that is associated with neurogenic bowel or bladder. The differential diagnosis for enuresis may be vast, ranging anywhere from trauma to medication side effects or other discrete disease processes. Whether the enuresis is primary or secondary, collateral information from the family or caregivers, along with a thorough physical exam, are recommended for children with prolonged or treatment refractory enuresis.

The etiologies and treatment recommendations differ between the subtypes of enuresis. Medications are far more likely to be utilized as an adjunct to behavioral strategies when nighttime enuresis is the primary presenting problem. As such, when addressing toileting issues, the first point of clarification must include the timing of wetting episodes. Enuresis, "bed-wetting," and intermittent nocturnal incontinence are considered to be synonymous. These terms refer to any intermittent discrete amounts of urine leakage throughout the night. However, children often have wetting episodes during the daytime as well. In spite of its inclusion in the Diagnostic and Statistical Manual of Mental Disorders, the term "diurnal enuresis" has fallen out of favor with urologists, and in its place are the terms daytime incontinence and nighttime incontinence. Children with both day- and nighttime symptoms have dual diagnoses within the medical framework. According to the European consensus, daytime symptoms should be treated prior to attempting to treat nocturnal enuresis if both are present, since the presence of daytime symptoms indicates a higher likelihood that a structural and/or organic etiology is present (Vande Walle et al., 2012; Neveus et al., 2010).

The second element that needs to be assessed is the frequency of wetting episodes. Are they happening continuously or intermittently? In terms of risk stratification, children with continuous incontinence may have a higher likelihood of being diagnosed with congenital malformations or neurological etiologies for their symptoms.

One example of a neurodevelopmental disorder that is closely associated with incontinence is spina bifida. Spina bifida is a neural tube defect in which the spinal cord fails to develop properly. This is commonly due to a nutritional deficiency of folate during pregnancy. There are many people in the general public who may have an asymptomatic mild form of spina bifida. On physical exam you may simply find a dimple near the base of the spine, a birthmark, or even a patch of hair. This is referred to as "spina bifida occulta" and is often an incidental finding. However, with more severe forms of the neural tube defect, the spinal fluid itself may leak out forming a swelling beneath the skin. This phenomenon is known as a meningocele. The most severe form of spina bifida is known as a myelomeningocele. In this scenario the nerves at the base of the spinal cord may be visible and they are often damaged. Patients who have spina bifida may present with motor weakness in the lower limbs as well as sensory deficits. The nerves which control the bowel and bladder sensations as well as the muscles required for continence are often affected. As a result, children with spina bifida may display urinary and/or stool incontinence.

Case Vignette 1

A 13-year-old male with past medical history of spina bifida occulta presents to the primary care physicians office with his mother. His mother is concerned that the patient has been having nighttime enuresis episodes. The family has already been using a pharmacologic intervention without success. The patient's mother insists that the child has been taking the medication prior to sleep onset each night. The most likely explanation is which of the following:

A. *Noncompliance.*
B. *The presence of spina bifida occulta significantly affects the response to treatment in patients with nocturnal enuresis.*
C. *The diagnosis of spina bifida occulta is incorrect.*
D. *The patient is taking illicit substances.*
E. *The patient has renal cell carcinoma.*

Answer: B.

In this study the records of 160 pediatric patients with nocturnal enuresis were reviewed. Patients were excluded if they had clear organic urological disease or symptoms that were highly suggestive of spinal dysraphism. The groups of children with spina bifida occulta and those without spina bifida occulta were compared in terms of their response to treatment for nocturnal enuresis. Of the 160 children included, spina bifida occulta was detected in 43 (26.9%). Children without spina bifida occulta had higher likelihood of a complete response to treatment. However none of the children with spina bifida occulta who had primary non-monosymptomatic nocturnal enuresis showed a complete response to treatment (Shin, Im, Lee, et al., 2013).

Lower Urinary Tract Symptoms

According to the International Council on Continence Society, lower urinary tract symptoms may include hesitancy, frequency, urgency, straining, and a weakened urinary stream (Neveus, Eggert, Evans, et al., 2010). Patients may also display evidence of dribbling after a void, pain in the genitalia, pain with urination, and the use of maneuvers intended to hold in urine (Vande Walle, Rittig, Bauer, et al., 2012) (Table 1). Daytime incontinence frequently occurs when there are lower urinary tract symptoms. The workup for lower urinary tract symptoms often includes a urinalysis, given that urinary tract infections are a common source of secondary enuresis with abrupt onset or a noticeable change in pattern. Urinary frequency is considered to be increased when the child is experiencing eight or more voiding events per day, whereas urinary frequency is considered to be decreased when they are experiencing three or less voiding events per day. Another important note is when holding maneuvers are observed, they are only clinically relevant when a child has previously had bladder control. Urgency is often the presenting feature of an overactive bladder.

Table 1 Lower urinary tract symptoms

Increased/decreased voiding frequency
Daytime incontinence
Urgency
Hesitancy
Straining
Weak stream
Intermittency of stream
Holding maneuvers
Feeling of incomplete emptying
Post void dribble
Genital/lower tract pain or dysuria

Neveus et al. (2010), Vande Walle et al. (2012)

Daytime Incontinence

According to Graham and Levy (2009), daytime incontinence has a prevalence of 2–3% in 7-year-old boys and 3–4% in same age girls and declines gradually with age. Daytime incontinence can be conceptualized either as a *s*torage problem or an emptying problem (Graham & Levy, 2009). Bladder filling and bladder storage are both mediated by the sympathetic nervous system, while bladder emptying is controlled by the parasympathetic nervous system. With bladder storage difficulties, the patient may have normal neurological function but simply be unable to store urine even at low bladder pressures. Alternatively, they may have abnormal neurological function with urine leakage when the bladder is under high pressure. Other storage issues may be centralized around hypersensitivity to bladder distention or decreased sphincter tone. In terms of emptying problems, some patients may experience "functional" symptoms in which there is no aberrancy from a neurological perspective, yet the patient cannot fully relax the sphincter during efforts to void. Alternatively, the ability to empty the bladder may be caused by anatomical differences or neurological deficits.

Two other types of daytime wetting are vaginal reflux and giggle incontinence (Graham & Levy, 2009). Vaginal reflux is routinely seen in females who are obese and is a phenomena associated with urine pooling within the vagina or the vaginal canal. As a result, urine leakage typically occurs in the window of time shortly after urinating. On clinical interview, patients often report having damp underwear the majority of the day. Vaginal reflux may be diagnosed by completing a Valsalva and finding urine leakage immediately after the patient has emptied their bladder. Positional changes during toilet sitting are often encouraged with children who have vaginal reflux as a way to offset or avoid the pooling of urine in the vaginal canal. One example is the use of rear facing toilet sitting (such that the child is facing the back of the toilet). In theory, this will allow for more effective balancing on the toilet and thereby may allow for more effective full bladder emptying (Maternik, Krzeminska, Zurowska, et al., 2015). Giggle incontinence occurs when a patient loses full bladder control with complete emptying during laughter in spite of normal urodynamic studies. This is a

Table 2 Diagnosis: Giggle Incontinence vs. Vaginal Reflux

Giggle incontinence	Vaginal reflux
• Complete bladder emptying with extreme laughter • Girls 10–20 years old • Normal urodynamics • Mechanism thought to be related to a cataplectic phenomenon that also mediates narcolepsy • Treated with methylphenidate	• Urine dribbling after voiding • Overweight girls and thin girls who have trouble balancing on the toilet • Other risk factor include labial adhesions • Damp underwear most of the time • Diagnosed with Valsalva post void that leads to urine flow • Treated with repositioning when voiding

Maternik et al. (2015), Graham and Levy (2009)

rare diagnosis found most often in females between the ages of 10–20 years. Some theorize that this is related to a cataleptic phenomenon and thus there may be an association between narcolepsy. Methylphenidate has been proposed as a treatment for this pattern of daytime incontinence (Graham & Levy, 2009) (Table 2). Regardless of the etiology of daytime wetting, non-pharmacologic interventions should be incorporated. These interventions will be covered elsewhere in this manual. However, from a primary care perspective, physicians often recommend strategies which target the elements of bladder distention and bladder overflow. Some of these strategies include the use of "double voiding" in which a patient is asked to empty their bladder, wait, and then attempt to urinate again. Another common strategy is to complete scheduled voiding every 2 h. The interplay between constipation and stool burden leading to enuresis will be covered in the next section of this chapter. Strategies to treat constipation are often incorporated into the treatment of daytime incontinence.

Expected Bladder Capacity

A child's expected bladder capacity (EBC) may be calculated by the following equation: EBC = 30 + (age in years × 30) mL (Vande Walle et al., 2012). As an example, a 5-year-old child's expected bladder capacity is 30 + (5 × 30) mL = 180 mL.

Polyuria

Polyuria is an overproduction of urine. In general, the differential diagnosis for polyuria is quite vast and may include anything from a common urinary tract infection, urinary incontinence, kidney stones, diabetes, interstitial nephritis, psychogenic polydipsia, benign prostatic hypertrophy, etc. The symptoms of polyuria (increased urine production) and polydipsia (increased thirst) are classic features of new onset diabetes mellitus. As such, patients who exhibit polyuria and polydipsia should be screened for diabetes. Children with new onset diabetes may present with vague symptoms to include generalized fatigue and malaise. They may also exhibit nausea, vomiting, gastrointestinal distress, and weight loss. If untreated, patients with type 1 diabetes can progress to diabetic ketoacidosis which is a life-threatening condition requiring admission to an intensive care unit. With any new evaluation for incontinence, the clinician must be conscientious to ask about both polyuria and polydipsia. If these symptoms are present, then the patient should be referred to their primary care provider. A typical workup for new onset polyuria with polydipsia will, at a minimum, include a basic metabolic panel (to screen for electrolyte abnormalities and blood glucose) and a urinalysis (to screen for glucose being spilled into the urine). The urinalysis will also provide information about any abnormal concentration of the urine (specific gravity). While this chapter is certainly not meant to explore the diagnosis of diabetes, it is critical for nonmedical clinicians who may interface with families during an incontinence evaluation to be aware of the importance of the symptoms of polyuria and polydipsia.

Nighttime Incontinence

Nocturnal enuresis can be further divided into primary monosymptomatic nocturnal enuresis (PMNE) and non-monosymptomatic nocturnal enuresis.

- *Primary Monosymptomatic Nocturnal Enuresis (PMNE):* These children have never achieved nighttime continence (thus the use of the term "primary"), yet they do not have daytime wetting episodes. Additionally, patients with PMNE do not have a history of bladder dysfunction or concurrent lower urinary tract symptoms. PMNE may occur even if a child has normal bladder storage capacity and normal urine output volumes. A bladder diary may be used clinically to assist with tracking symptoms. When using this strategy within the medical setting (such as an inpatient admission), the volume of the urine output is recorded. By evaluating the expected bladder capacity and tracking the volume of urine output, polyuria can be diagnosed.
- *Non-monosymptomatic Nocturnal Enuresis:* In keeping with the medical model, nighttime wetting is conceptualized as a symptom. When this symptom occurs simultaneously with lower urinary tract symptoms (outlined previously in this chapter), the clinical presentation is best described by the "non-monosymptomatic" nocturnal enuresis category.

According to Bayne and Skog, nocturnal polyuria (NP) can be considered when a child's bladder diary demonstrates urine production exceeding 130% of their expected bladder capacity (2014). This subtype is often suspected if a child is wetting in the first third of the night, has a large first void volume, and has soaked bed linens during enuretic periods. Desmopressin (a synthetic analogue of vasopressin) is particularly useful in this population.

Small bladder capacity should be suspected when the maximum volume of individual voids (Maximum Voided Volume MVV) is less than 50–65% of the expected bladder capacity (Vande Walle et al., 2012). Desmopressin and anticholinergics can be useful adjunctive medications if first-line treatments fail (Bayne & Skog, 2014).

Both nocturnal polyuria and small bladder capacity can be present and detected successfully with the voiding diary tool. When using this strategy within the medical setting (such as an inpatient admission), the volume of the urine output is recorded. By evaluating the expected bladder capacity and tracking the volume of urine output, polyuria can be diagnosed

Comorbidities

Children with constipation and other comorbidities like ADHD may require treatment for these issues prior to addressing enuresis. According to Grahm and Levy, "surveys show that children who have ADHD have a 30% greater chance of enuretic events" (p 166, 2009). This was once thought to be due solely to inattention, but there is a developing movement toward looking at a potential neurochemical effect for this relationship. Likewise, parents of children with nighttime enuresis often report that their child is a deep sleeper. However, the role of sleep arousal problems in enuresis remains controversial. Speculation that being a deep sleeper leads to enuresis has essentially fallen out of favor within the medical community given that nocturnal enuresis events and sleep stages are often independent of each other. Nonetheless, children with sleep-disordered breathing, including obstructive sleep apnea (OSA) and primary snoring, are more likely to have nocturnal enuresis (Jeyakumar, Rahman, Armbrecht, et al., 2012). "Tonsillectomy, adenoidectomy, or both have been shown to cure enuresis to a significant extent in this select group" (Grahm & Levy, p 166, 2009).

Case Vignette 2

A 6-year-old male presents to your pediatric primary care office with his parents. The parents report that the child had been fully continent since the age of 3. The parents endorse a new concern that the child is "regressing" over the past few days, and when asked to clarify the nature of their concerns, they cite the following: (1) The child has started having nocturia and wetting himself overnight leading to high stress in the household due to cleaning up the wet linens. (2) The child has been getting in trouble for waking up in the middle of the night and going to the kitchen without permission. Furthermore, his parents believe that he has been drinking "all of the lemonade and orange juice" in the house which has increased their grocery bill. (3) The child has been "trying to get out of things by asking to go to the bathroom all of the time or saying he has a stomach ache even when he is at school."

What should your care disposition for this family include?

A. *Send the family home with a behavioral diary to track number of requests to go to the bathroom, number of overnight accidents, and number of juice containers consumed over the next 4 weeks.*

B. *Send the family to a urologist to evaluate for bladder size less than anticipated for body size.*
C. *Send the patient to your in-office lab to complete a urinalysis and obtain a basic metabolic panel (electrolytes, kidney function, and glucose).*
D. *Send the patient to the store to purchase a bell and pad system and follow up with your office in 2 weeks if no improvement.*

Answer: C.

The information obtained from the parents is concerning for both polyuria (increased volume and frequency of urination) and polydipsia (increased thirst which may include drinking large amounts of any fluid that is available). Furthermore, they are describing a child who was previously continent and now has secondary nocturnal enuresis. Each of these elements may be seen as a symptom of hyperglycemia. As such, this child needs to be screened for diabetes mellitus. By obtaining a urinalysis, you can assess whether there are ketones and/or spilled glucose in the urine. Likewise, the basic metabolic panel will tell you what the child's current blood glucose value is along with providing information about potential acidosis. This will greatly assist you in risk stratification for the disposition. If your screening labs are indeed concerning for new onset diabetes, then this child is at risk for the development of diabetic ketoacidosis. DKA is a life-threatening condition that will require emergent hospitalization often within an intensive care unit (Lamb, 2014).

Medical Workup of Enuresis

The medical workup of enuresis will include a thorough history, review of systems, physical exam, and any laboratory or imaging studies necessary to clarify the diagnosis.

Patient History In general, the history of the present illness needs to include a thorough overview of the clinical symptoms to include elucidating the age of toilet training, pattern of wetting, volume of wetness, number of wetting episodes per day, primary vs. secondary enuresis, time of day and activity when incontinence occurs, history of UTI, total voids per day, presence of nighttime wetting, prior evaluation and treatments, bowel function, social history for stressors, and family support (Vande Walle et al., 2012).

As previously mentioned, when evaluating children presenting with a chief complaint of enuresis, the first question is whether there has ever been a period of continence. If the answer is yes, then the current presentation of incontinence would be considered a secondary enuresis pattern. However, those without a historical period of continence would qualify as having primary enuresis. Is the incontinence solely occurring during the daytime? Or is the incontinence occurring at night? If the incontinence is occurring during the daytime, is it a storage problem, an emptying problem, or a combination thereof?

The history obtained during an enuresis workup must also include the toilet training profile, the patterns of voiding (i.e., number of accidents per night and/or per week, daytime voiding patterns), and bowel habits. Sleep patterns are helpful to assess, as are drinking habits. The family response cycle can also provide insight into the clinical presentation as a shame and/or guilt complex may be inherently introduced into the enuresis pattern, whether or not this had been the intention. Likewise, when completing an enuresis evaluation, the trauma history and risk assessment for trauma is of great importance. Is there any evidence of maltreatment, neglect, or abuse?

After you have established a clear understanding of the presenting symptoms, the next elements to be addressed include the developmental history, the past medical history, screening for comorbid conditions, and the family history. Does the child have a history of a neurodevelopmental delay? Are there any medical comorbidities? Is there a family history of bed-wetting? Of note, a child has a 44% chance of having enuresis if one parent had enuresis as a child. The risk increases to 77% if both parents had enuresis. Age of resolution in a parent is predictive of the age of the child's resolution (Graham & Levy, 2009). Is there a history of constipation? Reviewing the medication list is also a key element of the patient encounter. The provider should inquire about whether there have been any changes or additions in the medication list.

A thorough review of systems must include whether or not the following are present: polyuria, polydipsia, abnormal urine stream, dysuria, frequency, urgency, pain, burning, constipation, diarrhea, or the need for abdominal pressure in order to have a successful void.

For daytime incontinence, the initial differential diagnosis may include urinary tract infection, constipation, vaginal pooling or reflux, post void dribble, ADHD, poor attunement to body sensations/cues, diabetes mellitus, diabetes insipidus, or daytime frequency syndrome. Other more rare etiologies may include neurogenic bladder, urethral obstruction, ectopic ureter, or a host of other structural defects. For nighttime incontinence the differential diagnosis is relatively unchanged although vaginal reflux and post void dribble are unlikely etiologies.

Case Vignette 3

A 7-year-old female presents to the pediatricians office with her parents. They report increasing frustration with attempts to toilet train over the years. The child's parents describe a lack of response to behavioral modification strategies and are desperate for help. The patient's teacher also sent a note explaining how difficult it has been to keep the child in the mainstream classroom because of toileting issues requiring 1:1 attention. The teacher and the parents both comment that the child "constantly dribbles" in her underwear and doesn't seem to pay attention to cues of having a full bladder or needing to go to the bathroom. Furthermore, when taken to the bathroom for scheduled toilet breaks, the child often sits for long periods and has to strain with increased abdominal pressure to pass urine. What should your treatment recommendations include?

A. *Referral to a urologist to evaluate for neurogenic bladder*
B. *Referral to a local psychologist who specializes in biofeedback*
C. *Referral to a local bookstore with recommendation of a toilet training manual*
D. *Referral to a family therapist to address the increasing frustration verbalized by the parents*
E. *Referral to a behavioral specialist to address school disruption*

Answer: A

The need to use abdominal pressure to initiate voiding stream, constant dribbling, and apparent lack of response to voiding cues are all potential red flags for neurogenic bladder. A referral to a urologist would be indicated for future evaluation (Issenham et al. 1999; Neurogenic Bladder, Johns Hopkins Medicine Health Library).

Testing All children who are experiencing enuresis should have a urinalysis (UA). In fact, apart from a pertinent and thorough history and physical exam, the International Children's Continence Society states that the only mandatory screening test for enuresis is the urinalysis (Neveus et al., 2010). However, the National Institute for Health and Clinical Excellence 2010 guideline on nocturnal enuresis questions whether the UA is actually a cost-effective recommendation. Nonetheless, the UA holds many pieces of information that can help guide next steps. Proteins or blood in the urine as well as glucose, ketones, and urinary tract infections can readily be identified with the UA. The specific gravity can also be a helpful piece of information for diagnoses like diabetes insipidus. If there is any evidence from the UA that would suggest a urinary tract infection, then the specimen should be sent for culture. If the culture is positive, sensitivities for antimicrobial management should be requested.

Despite the above recommendations, it is not uncommon to see other laboratory and radiologic investigations pursued in the medical workup of enuresis. Abdominal x-rays are sometimes obtained to evaluate for stool burden. Further discussion regarding constipation will be addressed in a later section of this chapter. Serum electrolytes may be checked but are not always necessary and would thereby not be considered a mandate or part of the standard of care per se. Examples of situations in which serum electrolytes may be required would include the evaluation of dehydration or when the medical team is concerned about the possibility of diabetic ketoacidosis. In those with a history of urinary tract infections, especially recurrent, clinicians may consider obtaining a renal bladder ultrasound. For some patients, urodynamic studies will be required. The voiding cystourethrogram (VCUG) is a test which uses contrast dye to evaluate the urinary system from both a structural and a functional perspective. X-rays are taken during the voiding process and the dye is visible on imaging throughout the urinary system. The urinary system includes the kidneys, the ureters, the bladder, and the urethra. Anatomical blockages, reflux, posterior urethral valves, strictures, and atypical urinary transit can be detected with this modality. The American Academy of Pediatrics encourages the use of the voiding cystourethrogram as part of the workup for children with recurrent urinary tract infections if the renal ultrasound shows hydronephrosis or scarring (Newman, 2011).

In addition to this, uroflow testing is a modality that assesses the urine stream and should be helpful for evaluating the amount of urine passed, the rate of flow, and the amount of time until the voiding process has been completed (Hoebeke, Bower, Combs, DeJong, & Yang, 2010). During urination the bladder contracts and flattens, whereas during storage it relaxes and expands. Urologists typically favor obtaining uroflow studies in children with daytime incontinence. A Mag 3 scan is a nuclear medicine study that shows the kidney size, shape, and function. Stone studies (CT or ultrasound) may be used to look for kidney stones if there is evidence of pain out of proportion for physical exam or if there is any evidence of obstruction. MRI may be used to assess for tumor burden or other structural anomalies. However, it is also reasonable to consider subspecialty referral to a urologist prior to the initiation of extensive testing so that a more directed approach can be taken.

Case Vignette 4

An 8-year-old female presents to her child psychiatry appointment for ADHD follow-up. Her parents complete the review of systems questionnaire which is concerning for new onset nocturnal enuresis, low-grade fever, and abdominal discomfort within the last 3 days. The child wears cotton underwear, is fully toilet trained, and has had no major life changes or stressors that you can identify. What should your next step be?

A. *Obtain a clean catch specimen for point of care urinalysis and then culture/microscopy.*
B. *Order a full-body CT scan due to concern of an occult malignancy.*
C. *Write a letter to the school special education committee requesting an IEP and psychoeducational testing.*
D. *Order a child protection team consultation due to likely sexual abuse.*
E. *Obtain a suprapubic bladder specimen and send for stat microscopic analysis.*

Answer: A

Urinary tract infections are a common source of new onset nocturnal enuresis. Your pretest probability for a UTI is also increased by the symptoms of abdominal discomfort with a low-grade fever. Females are at a higher risk for UTIs because of the anatomical proximity of the urethra and rectum. Furthermore, elementary-aged females who are learning to become independent in their self-hygiene are at an even greater risk for unintentional cross contamination leading to a UTI. Obtaining a suprapubic aspirate is unnecessary for the first step in evaluation. As such, obtaining a point of care urinalysis and then sending for culture and microscopy is an appropriate intervention at this time (Newman, 2011; Nickavar & Sotoudeh, 2011).

Ancillary Data A frequency-volume chart is recommended as part of the workup to help provide supportive data for further evaluation. At least 2 days of fluid intake and output recording should be completed along with 1 week of data on other bladder-related symptoms and bowel movements (Bayne & Skoog, 2014). A great deal of clinically salient information can be obtained from the toileting diary (see Appendix 1). Ideally, families will be able to document the timing, volume, and the description of voids and stools. This can help to establish maximum volume and thus bladder capacity. Any co-occurring constipation should be identified and treated before managing enuresis (Vande Walle et al., 2012). Highlighting the importance of this tool for diagnosis and treatment is an important message to families, as completing the chart requires consistency and motivation. Reviewing the natural history of enuresis with families is also essential. Overall, there is a slight male predilection with about 10–15% of 7-year-olds affected. They should be aware that nocturnal enuresis has a spontaneous remission rate of 15% a year such that by age 15, 99% of children are dry (Graham & Levy, 2009).

The child's drinking and voiding pattern can be highly informative. Is the child drinking large volumes of fluid in the evening or near bedtime? Is the child able to drink fluids with ease during the school day? Is the child avoiding the bathroom at school? A distressed and tired parent may not always recognize these patterns.

Examining fluid intake can be a valuable piece of the history and evaluation. For many families, there is a fair amount of guesswork involved in establishing how much and when their child should be drinking. What should the fluid intake pattern look like? According to the National Institute for Health and Care Excellence (2010), the recommended fluid intake per day for children is as follows:

- 1–1.4 L for children 4–8 years old
- 1.2–2.1 L for girls 9–13 and 1.4–2.3 L for boys of the same age
- 1.4–2.5 L for girls 14–18 and 2.1–3.2 L for boys of the same age

The rule of thirds for timing of fluid consumption suggests that children with enuresis, especially PMNE, should have two-thirds of their fluid intake before the school day is over and one-third in the early evening with no fluids 1–2 h before bed (Bayne & Skog, 2014). The International Children's Continence Society is more stringent and recommends 200 mL or less in the evening. This may be difficult to adhere to if a child engages in a lot of physical activity or sporting events in the evening or nighttime; adequate hydration should be the primary goal in this case. Finally, inquiring about bathroom anxiety is important, as some children will drink most of their fluids for the day at home in order to avoid using the restroom at school.

Physical Examination The physical exam should focus on the neurological, gastrointestinal, and urogenital systems. On neurological examination, it is important to note the child's overall tone, reflexes, coordination, and sensation (Bayne & Skoog, 2014). The back must be examined for a tuft of hair, sacral dimple, or other markings that would suggest underlying spinal cord issues like spina bifida, spina bifida occulta, or a tethered cord. In terms of the abdominal exam, the physician will note whether the abdomen is distended or whether there are any palpable masses – for example, bladder, kidney, stool burden, or others. The urogenital exam should include inspection of the phallus and meatus of the penis in males to look for meatal stenosis or phimosis. Likewise, the introitus should be inspected in females looking for urethral abnormalities or labial adhesions (Grahm & Levy, 2009).

Table 3 Enuresis: causes for concern

Weight loss
Sacral dimple or tuft of hair on lower spine
Neuro exam abnormalities
Genitourinary exam abnormalities
Weak or intermittent urine stream
Continuous dribbling or incontinence
Straining to void
Treatment refractory enuresis

Zywicke & Rozzelle (2011), Vande Walle et al. (2012)

Organic Etiologies The organic causes of enuresis are numerous and highly variable. Some of the most common causes for enuresis are constipation, UTIs, impactions, urolithiasis, diabetes, physical trauma, and medication side effects. Other more rare causes of enuresis include spinal cord tumors, vascular phenomena including infarction or thrombosis, neurogenic sequelae of surgical procedures, metabolic disorders, genetic conditions, and bladder spasticity. These will usually be refractory to conservative management and will have more severe clinical presentations (Table 3).

Nonorganic Etiologies There are also many nonorganic etiologies of enuresis, as reviewed elsewhere in this book. Some of these may include psychosocial stressors such as trauma, physical abuse, sexual abuse, adjustment disorders, anxiety disorders, ADHD, developmental delays, and intellectual disabilities. Consideration of these factors should be included in a comprehensive medical evaluation.

Medications The most commonly used medications for the treatment of pediatric enuresis are from three categories: antidiuretic hormone analogues, anticholinergic medications, and tricyclic antidepressants. DDAVP or desmopressin is the synthetic formulation of antidiuretic hormone. Desmopressin is known to be an effective and well-tolerated medication for pediatric nocturnal enuresis. The mechanism of action is via increased water permeability within the renal tubules causing an antidiuretic effect which reduces nocturnal urine output. The short-term direct effects of DDAVP are very good. However, when discontinuing DDAVP, the underlying behavioral elements are unaffected, thus leaving high relapse rates upon discontinuation. Anticholinergic agents such as oxybutynin (which theoretically provides antispasmodic and anti-muscarinic effects) and hyoscyamine (which works by reducing the secretion of fluid by blocking the actions of acetylcholine) are options for treatment adjunct when behavioral interventions alone are unsuccessful. However, the side effect profile for anticholinergic agents can quickly lead to toxicity with atropine-like effects and central nervous system depression. Signs of anticholinergic toxicity may include: flushing, fever, tachycardia, dry skin, dry mucous membranes, urinary retention, tremulousness or myoclonic jerks, hypertension, and altered mental status. Any treatment must include risk and benefit assessment with families. Tricyclic antidepressants such as amitriptyline, nortriptyline, and imipramine help with sleep onset and also provide downregulation of the beta-adrenergic system as well as anticholinergic effects. Table 4 serves as a guideline for medication dosing, duration, and potential side effects when using for the management of nighttime enuresis.

Alpha-agonists such as tamsulosin may be used in the adult population but are not FDA approved for on label usage in pediatrics. Other medications have been utilized in the treatment of enuresis, but these are generally reserved for children in the care of subspecialists, and many require further research. Mirabegron is used in idiopathic overactive bladder refractory to other anticholinergic agents. It is a selective beta-3 adrenoceptor agonist that is currently approved in adults, but with limited studies in children at this time. Beta-3 receptors in the bladder have a role in detrusor muscle relaxation, and in theory, stimulation of the receptors will lead to increased bladder capacity and improvement of overactive bladder symptoms. At this time, oxybutynin remains the only anticholinergic agent approved for use in the pediatric population in North America (Blais, Nadeau, Moore, et al., 2016). Solifenacin is another agent with promising new evidence for treating enuresis, but again with limited data in the pediatric population. It is a selective acetylcholine antagonist at muscarinic receptors and it is used in the treatment of overactive bladder. One small study found that a 5 mg dose of solifenacin was associated with 85% response rate (full and partial) in children who previously were nonresponsive to oxybutynin or tolterodine (Maternik et al., 2015). Botulinum toxin has also been studied in treating enuresis. In skeletal muscles, botulinum toxin produces a paralytic effect, but in smooth muscles it produces a relaxation effect. It has been studied in neurogenic detrusor-sphincter dyssynergy or intractable bladder overactivity. Electrical stimulation techniques are also being studied, but these and local botulinum toxin injections are deferred to urology subspecialists (Schurch & Corcos, 2005).

Discontinuing Medications

In a pediatric population, expected duration of treatment must remain at the forefront of our risk-benefit analysis. While potentially efficacious, the medications used to treat enuresis are not without side effects. Further, as mentioned earlier in the chapter, the rate of remission of enuresis as the child ages is high, and it is important to avoid ongoing medication if not warranted. Desmopressin is the synthetic analogue of antidiuretic hormone. It is suggested that, as with other hormone-related therapies, withdrawal syndromes or hormone deficiency can result with abrupt cessation of the medication. A recent meta-analysis published in Pediatrics concluded that successful cessation of this medication involves a structured withdrawal compared to an abrupt one (Chua, Silangcruz, Chang, et al., 2016).

When thinking about tricyclic antidepressant medications, the gradual downward titration in a stepwise fashion is highly recommended so as to avoid any discontinuation side effects. Tricyclic antidepressants have a known risk of serotonin

Table 4 Medication options for enuresis

Drugs	Dose	Duration	Advantages/uses	Caution
Desmopressin (vasopressin analogue)	Oral formulation preferred: 0.2 mg–0.5 mg/day for use in ages 6 and up. Taken 1 h before sleep	Initial duration 2–6 weeks for effect. Can be used for years, but important to have regular short drug holidays. Guidelines suggest withdrawal every 3 months	• FDA approved in children 6+ • Urine production at night decreases, especially useful in nocturnal polyuria without bladder overactivity • Well-tolerated • 70% effect size • Immediate response	• Evening fluid intake should be restricted to 6 ounces to avoid water intoxication and hyponatremia • Relapse upon discontinuation is higher than that for the alarm • Side effect: headache, nausea, vomiting • Avoid self-titration of medication • Caution in HTN and von Willebrand
Anticholinergics (oxybutynin)	For ages 5+, 5 mg PO once daily; dose may be increased weekly in 5 mg increments; Max 20 mg/day	Effect within 1–2 weeks of medication initiation Attempt to withdraw regularly, about every 3 months	• Reduces bladder contraction by suppressing detrusor overactivity, therefore useful with **small bladder capacity or overactive bladder** by history • Useful in 40% in initial treatment failure • Can be used in conjunction with DDAVP for refractory enuresis	• **Not a first-line** therapy for nocturnal enuresis • Side effects related to anticholinergic include constipation (most bothersome) and increased residual volume after voiding. • Start only after establishing regular voiding habits, excluded/treated constipation, excluded post void residual/low voiding frequency by way of voiding diary and bladder scans • Only indicated in whom standard treatment has failed • Caution in: narrow-angle glaucoma, obstructive uropathy

Tricyclic antidepressants (imipramine)	25–50 mg starting dose at bedtime, larger dose given to children >9–12 years	• Evaluate effect after 1 month • Regular drug holidays of at least 2 weeks every 3 month • Drug holidays necessary to avoid tolerance, reduce risk of cardiotoxicity	• FDA approved in age 6+ • 50% response rate in treatment resistance • Affordable	• **Third-line therapy** at tertiary care facilities • **Overdose can be fatal** • If partial response: add desmopressin • Taper to the lowest effective dose • Lock medicine to avoid accidental ingestions • Avoid in history of palpitation, syncope, or family history of sudden cardiac death, unstable arrhythmia • EKG prior to treatment should be considered to rule out long QT • Side effects appear earlier than beneficial effect and include mood changes, nausea, and insomnia. Waiting strategy usually works for moderate side effects • Avoid in narrow-angle glaucoma • Avoid use with SSRI and MAOI • Relapse rate > 90% after stopping

Maternik et al. (2015), Neveus et al. (2010), Lexicomp Online (2017)

syndrome if used concurrently with selective serotonin reuptake inhibitors (SSRIs) or serotonin norepinephrine reuptake inhibitors (SNRIs). Cross titration between agents is often required.

Case Vignette 5
A 12-year-old child with an intellectual disability presents to the emergency room with a member of his group home staff. He wears a diaper product during the day, but staff report that he has not had a wet diaper in greater than 18 h. They are also concerned that he is behaving "differently" and are worried that he is "not feeling well." When asked to clarify, they indicate that the patient has been "staying in bed all day just moaning and not participating in things he usually loves like going bowling or watching TV." They also report that he has been "picking at things in the air when there is nothing there." On your exam the patient is found to have tachycardia and dry mucous membranes. You obtain a bladder scan and find that he has retained urine greater than 700 mL. On cardiac monitors you also notice an intermittent arrhythmia and as a result you obtain a 12-lead ECG. The ECG shows a prolonged PR interval. Which one of his home medications is most likely to cause this clinical presentation?

A. *Nystatin powder applied to the diaper region due to concerns for fungal dermatitis*
B. *Augmentin which was recently started due to concerns for a possible ear infection*
C. *Levocarnitine used to treat a possible mitochondrial disorder*
D. *Imipramine used to treat nocturnal enuresis*
E. *Calcium carbonate used intermittently to treat symptoms of acid reflux*

Answer: D.

The patient most likely has a hypoactive delirium propagated by the anticholinergic effects of imipramine. Imipramine is a tricyclic antidepressant this is also used to treat enuresis, migraines, and chronic pain syndromes. Imipramine toxicity may include urinary retention, constipation, tachycardia, tremor, blurred vision, ECG changes (i.e., *increased PR, QRS, and QT intervals), and delirium. These effects are primarily due to its anticholinergic properties. Individuals with intellectual disabilities are potentially at a higher risk of being treated with pharmacological agents for nocturnal enuresis simply due to the burden associated with frequent linen changes and caregiver burnout as opposed to a true medical mandate for intervention. Furthermore, delirium may go unrecognized for prolonged periods in a nonverbal/nonambulatory patient. Awareness of the risk-benefit analysis with any pharmacological agent used to treat enuresis is of great importance* (Bentley, 2014).

Constipation

Constipation is a common childhood problem, with prevalence ranging from 0.7% to 29.6% worldwide (Mugie, Benninga, and Di Lorenzo, et al., 2011). When constipation is undiagnosed or untreated, it can cause significant delays in reaching normal toileting milestones or potentially lead to more serious or chronic health concerns. Constipation has been shown to have a significant impact on healthcare utilization and costs, with estimated costs three times that of children without constipation (Liem, Harman, Benninga, et al., 2009). For a large number of children with constipation, symptoms emerge as early as the first year of life (Loening-Baucke, 1993), and a recent retrospective chart review found the median age of onset of functional constipation in children was 2.3 years (Malowitz, Green, Karpinski, et al., 2016).

The prevalence and definition of constipation varies per child's age, and knowledge of normal stooling patterns in early childhood is necessary to determine if the presenting bowel pattern is abnormal. The frequency of normal bowel movements decreases as children progress through early childhood, with infants generally stooling 3–4 times per day and toddlers having 2–3 bowel movements daily. An adult bowel frequency and pattern, with one stool daily, is generally achieved by the age of 4, which is the expected age of bowel continence (Steer, Emond, Golding, 2009; Corazziari, Staiano, Miele, et al., 2005, Colombo, Wassom, Rosen, 2015).

Etiology

In many children, constipation is associated with infrequent, hard, and sometimes painful defecation, as well as fecal incontinence (also known as encopresis). It is often a source of significant distress for the child and family. The medical evaluation of constipation assesses whether there is an underlying neurologic, anatomic, or other systemic etiology or whether it can be classified as functional (nonorganic) constipation. Functional constipation comprises 95% of pediatric constipation presentations (Loening-Baucke, 2005). Other etiologies are rare and often present in early infancy with failure to pass meconium or other patterns of irregular stooling from birth. For systemic etiologies, constipation is rarely the sole presenting symptom of the disorder. Table 5 offers the mnemonic VITAMIN CDEF, a popular tool in medical education for organizing a differential diagnosis based on etiology. It is useful here when recalling potential organic etiologies of constipation which are then systematically excluded through history, physical examination, and other laboratory or imaging studies if warranted. The primary focus of this section is the evaluation and management of functional constipation. If in the course of history and physical examination concerns for other etiologies of constipation arise, referral to a pediatric specialist is often indicated. A more thorough discussion of the initial evaluation of constipation is detailed later in this chapter.

Functional Constipation

The North American Society for Pediatric Gastroenterology, Hepatology, and Nutrition (NASPGHAN) and the European Society for Pediatric Gastroenterology, Hepatology and Nutrition (ESPGHAN) recommend the diagnosis of functional

Table 5 Differential diagnosis of constipation in infants and children

*V*ascular: not typically seen
*I*nfectious/inflammatory: Inflammatory bowel disease, botulism
*T*rauma/toxic: sexual abuse, postoperative complications, spinal cord injury, heavy metal poisoning
*A*utoimmune: celiac disease, dietary protein allergy, lupus
*M*etabolic/musculoskeletal: hypokalemia, hypercalcemia, abnormal abdominal muscle tone (prune belly, gastroschisis, Down syndrome)
*I*diopathic/iatrogenic: vitamin D intoxication, medication side effects (anticholinergics, opiates, antidepressants, chemotherapy)
*N*eoplastic: pelvic mass, spinal cord mass, brain tumors, colon cancer, multiple endocrine neoplasia type 2B
*C*ongenital: cystic fibrosis, Hirschsprung disease, anal achalasia, colonic inertia, anatomic malformations, imperforate anus, small left colon syndrome
*D*egenerative: not typically seen
*E*ndocrine/environmental: hypothyroidism, diabetes mellitus, low-fiber diet, decreased fluid intake
*F*unctional: functional constipation, infant dyschezia, nonretentive fecal soiling

Tabbers et al., 2014; Colombo et al., 2015

constipation, as well as other functional gastrointestinal disorders (FGIDs), be founded on the symptom-based Rome criteria (Tabbers, DiLorenzo, Berger, et al., 2014). The Rome Foundation is an independent not-for-profit organization that has played a pivotal role in operationalizing the research and disseminating the knowledge surrounding FGIDs (Drossman, 2016). The Rome IV criteria were released in May 2016, and the criteria for diagnosing functional constipation in infants and children are outlined in Table 6. Components of the functional constipation diagnosis include two or fewer defecations per week, history of excessive stool retention, painful or hard bowel movements, large-diameter stools, and a fecal mass in the rectum. One primary change in Rome IV from the previous version is the differentiation between children who are toilet trained and those who are not. Additional criteria which may be met for toilet-trained children include at least one episode of incontinence per week (after achieving toilet training skills) and large-diameter stools that may obstruct the toilet. The new criteria are now the same for both the infant and toddler age group and children and adolescents (Zeevenhooven, Koppen, Benninga, et al., 2017).

Stool withholding behavior is felt to play a large role in functional constipation. Constipation can lead to large, painful bowel movements, and painful defecation can promote fear about future bowel movements for a child. As a result of stool withholding, the rectum can become distended, and the urge to defecate diminishes. The longer that stool remains in the rectum, the harder it becomes, increasing the pain and difficulty the child will experience when passing it. Continued withholding creates a vicious cycle of painful constipation, and disimpaction is often required in order to restore regular stooling patterns.

Table 6 ROME IV diagnostic criteria for functional constipation in infants and toddlers

Must include 1 month of at least 2 of the following in infants up to 4 years of age:
Two or fewer defecations per week
History of excessive stool retention
History of painful or hard bowel movements
Large fecal mass in rectum
History of large-diameter stools
In toilet-trained children, the following additional criteria may be used:
At least one episode/week of incontinence after the acquisition of toileting skills
History of large-diameter stools that may obstruct the toilet

Adapted from Benninga, Faure, Hyman, St. James Roberts, et al., 2016

Encopresis

Encopresis (fecal incontinence) occurs as the result of constipation in more than 80% of patients (Rasquin, Di Lorenzo, Forbes, et al., 2006). This is the result of soft or liquid stool leaking around a large bolus of hard stool in the rectum, also clinically described as "constipation with overflow." Encopresis is often misunderstood by families. Parents may believe that their child is having diarrhea or has simply not achieved bowel continence, which can delay evaluation and appropriate treatment. Encopresis differs from diarrhea or delayed bowel training in that this particular type of accident is often seen when small amounts of stool are leaked without the child being aware. As mentioned earlier, because bowel continence is expected to occur by the age of 4 years, encopresis is not a normal developmental variation after this age (Colombo et al., 2015).

In a minority of children, encopresis occurs in the absence of constipation and without any evidence of fecal retention (Rasquin et al., 2006). This phenomena is known as nonretentive fecal incontinence (NRFI). Children with NRFI tend to have increased problems with both daytime and nighttime urinary incontinence, possibly suggesting an overall delay in recognizing the physiological stimuli necessary for toilet training (Bongers, Tabbers, Benninga, 2007). The mechanism for fecal incontinence in these cases is poorly understood. In general, NRFI is believed to be multifactorial with gastric motility, genetic predisposition, and the potential for underlying psychological factors playing a role. Treatment has primarily been targeted at slowing gastric motility and behavioral interventions (Stein, Beninga, Felt, 2017).

The Link Between Constipation and Enuresis

It is widely recognized that constipation and enuresis often occur simultaneously. Likewise, chronic constipation may cause or exacerbate abnormal urine voiding patterns, as is discussed earlier in this chapter. When children are constipated, the burden of fecal mass may constrain the bladder and limit capacity. Furthermore, as the bowel wall becomes distended, the sensorineural response to the stimuli of urge to defecate and urge to urinate may become physiologically confusing, particularly at a young age. Previously known as dysfunctional elimination syndrome, the International Children's Continence Society named this condition bladder and bowel dysfunction (BBD) (Austin, Bauer, Bower, et al., 2016). Children presenting to a gastroenterologist for functional constipation and those presenting to a urologist for voiding dysfunction show similar patterns and severity of bladder-bowel dysfunction (Wolfe-Christensen, Manolis, Guy, et al., 2014). The comorbidity of pediatric urinary and gastrointestinal dysfunction is likely due to multiple factors, including a shared origin in fetal development, close anatomical proximity, and connected neural pathways between the pelvic organs (Malykhina, 2007).

Case Vignette 6

A 10-year-old previously continent male who has autism spectrum disorder presents with his father for evaluation of new onset incontinence of urine. The child has niche interests in John Deere tractors and spends the majority of the visit referencing tractors. His father reports that the patient sleeps well and likes to run. However, he has recently been struggling to get his son to eat anything other than chicken nuggets. The child is average height and weight and BMI is 19. His vitals are all within normal limits. What is the most likely explanation for the new onset of incontinence?

A. *The child has been traumatized and wants to go back to wearing pull-ups.*
B. *The child has a nutritional deficiency that is causing a transient neurogenic bladder.*
C. *The child has inserted one of the tires from a toy tractor into his penis causing an obstruction.*
D. *The child is not incontinent and is engaging in intentional maladaptive voiding behaviors.*
E. *The child has a low-fiber diet with niche food preferences and is at risk for constipation.*

Answer: E.

Constipation can lead to a high stool burden and colonic distention. This can result in aberrant voiding patterns and new onset or worsening of urinary incontinence. Aggressive management of constipation is often necessary to restore urinary continence. The importance of screening for constipation must not be overlooked in the medical management of enuresis (Issenman et al., 1999; Tu & Baskin, 2017).

Medical Evaluation

The NASPGHAN and ESPGHAN consensus guidelines (Tabbers et al., 2014) state that the diagnosis of functional constipation should be based predominantly on history and physical examination. Rectal examination to evaluate for possible impaction and rectal tone is recommended only if full Rome criteria for functional constipation are not met or there are other concerning signs and symptoms related to intractable constipation. While plain radiographic films of the abdomen are used in some settings, the guidelines recommend against routine use of radiographic images to diagnose functional constipation. Exceptions to this include situations where fecal impaction is suspected, but physical examination is unreliable or unable to be completed. In addition, the routine use of colonic transit studies and/or rectal ultrasound to diagnose functional constipation is not recommended.

As stated previously, functional (nonorganic) constipation comprises 95% of pediatric constipation cases. Although constipation may have several etiologies, in the vast majority of cases, no underlying neurologic or systemic illness is found. However, in the diagnostic evaluation, it is prudent to be alert to certain symptoms which would prompt further medical workup, especially those that may warrant immediate medication attention. Severe abdominal distention, abnormal growth or developmental delay, bloody stools, perianal fistula, absent anal wink (poor tone), or sacral dimple indicate a need for further neurologic and medical workup. This workup may include additional laboratory tests and diagnostic imaging (Colombo et al., 2015).

As part of the medical history, reviewing the child's current medication list is also important. If the child is breastfed, it becomes relevant to review any medications the mother is taking as well. Medications associated with constipation can include anticholinergics, narcotics, antidepressants, antipsychotics, and antihistamines, among others.

Guide to the Constipation Diagnostic Assessment

A diagnosis of functional constipation requires focus on specific aspects of the history and physical examination in order to exclude other possible diagnoses. The following is a guideline for initial assessment:

- *History of Presenting Illness*: Establish current stooling pattern and timeline of symptoms. Identify any precipitating factors, including diet or major life changes, and attempts at toilet training. Presence of withholding posturing? (standing on tip toes, holding onto furniture, extending and crossing legs, avoiding the squatting position). Presence of enuresis? Fecal incontinence? Abdominal pain or rectal bleeding?

- *Medical History*: Any delay in meconium passing? The differential diagnosis for delayed meconium passage may include anatomical abnormalities, Hirschsprung disease, or cystic fibrosis. The growth chart should be reviewed along with any developmental screenings completed by history.
- *Past Medications/Treatments*: Trials of oral laxatives, enemas, suppositories, herbals, behavioral treatments (including duration), and reason for cessation should be discussed.
- *Social History*: Any disruption of family life, interaction with peers, temperament, sexual abuse history, and depression symptoms should be addressed.
- *Family History*: Hirschsprung disease, food allergies, inflammatory bowel disease, celiac disease, urinary or kidney disorders, thyroid disease, and cystic fibrosis are all examples of conditions which should be discussed.
- *Examination*: Height and weight should be measured. Visual inspection of the skin and anatomical structures of the lumbosacral/gluteal regions should be completed in order to screen for dimples and/or a tuft of hair (which may indicate neural tube defects). Visualization of the anus and surrounding area for fissures/skin tags/inflammation, abdominal exam to palpate possible fecal mass, neurological examination of gait, assessment of lower extremity muscle tone, strength, and reflexes should all be completed in the physical exam.

(Colombo et al., 2015; Tabbers et al., 2014; Rajindrajith & Devanarayana, 2011)

Treatment of Constipation

Constipation management relies on a multifactorial approach, often including behavioral modification, dietary changes, and medication. Education for the patient and family involves setting expectations for the duration of treatment and, if medications are prescribed, highlighting the importance of adherence. Families need to be aware that treating constipation may take many months of medication and behavioral modification and that relapses are not uncommon. In a systematic review, only about 60% of children treated for 6–12 months for functional constipation were symptom-free at the end of treatment (Pijpers, Bongers, Benninga, et al., 2010).

Children must often undergo disimpaction at the onset of treatment in order to achieve normal stooling patterns. Methods of disimpaction include oral clean out, rectal enema/suppository, and sometimes manual disimpaction. The latter is rarely needed and not advised for routine use. General anesthesia or conscious sedation may be necessary if manual disimpaction is indicated in order to decrease the potential for trauma associated with the procedure (Colombo et al., 2015; Tabbers et al., 2014). A number of maintenance strategies exist to help treat functional constipation to include various classes of oral medications as will be discussed below.

Diet

Constipation is often associated with changes in diet, which are quite common in young children as they are exposed to new foods and new environments. During this time, children may also develop niche dietary preferences which contribute to a pattern of chronic constipation.

The relationship of cow's milk and the development of constipation in young children has been debated. Some have proposed that cow's milk protein (CMP) could play a role in constipation through an immune-mediated mechanism, potentially a late manifestation of food allergy. Irastorza, Ibanez, Delgado-Sanzonetti, et al. (2010) showed that in an open-label crossover study of 69 children with Rome III diagnosed constipation, over 50% showed improved symptoms when cow's milk was removed, though no clear mechanism related to allergy was established. Other proposed mechanisms for the association of cow's milk and constipation are that children who consume more dairy products also consume less fiber containing foods like vegetables and fruits. However, this notion was not supported in the 2010 study. Interestingly, this same study showed that in children with developmental delays and comorbid constipation, 78% were responders to a cow's milk-free diet. As this population frequently presents with high rates of constipation, more research is needed to understand underlying mechanisms and potential association with CMP. Data on cow's milk protein allergy and constipation is conflicting, and at this time, routine CMP allergy testing is not recommended as part of the general workup for functional constipation (Tabbers et al., 2014).

The role of diet modification in treating functional constipation has been studied. Fiber, fluid therapy, and pre-/probiotics have not shown clear efficacy in treating constipation in children. Evidence does not support fiber supplements for treatment of constipation based on the latest clinical guidelines available for physicians in the 2014 NASPGHAN publication (Tabbers et al., 2014). Maintaining adequate hydration, while not proven to change bowel movement habits alone, remains an important factor for many other physiological functions and therefore is a safe recommendation for families (Colombo et al., 2015).

Behavior Modification

Empathizing with parents during this stressful and frustrating time can help to strengthen the therapeutic alliance and maintain the commitment and motivation to continue treatment. Setting appropriate treatment expectations for families is vital. The role of behavioral modification in the setting of toilet training is discussed extensively elsewhere in this book and will not be repeated here. However, support and recommendations for behavioral modification from medical providers is beneficial for patients and their families. When necessary, the combination of medical treatments and behavioral modification are recommended to ensure the most successful outcomes. Incorporating scheduled time on the toilet at routine intervals after meals can take advantage of the physiological gastrocolic reflex, thereby increasing the chance of a successful stooling pattern. In addition, placing the child in a position where defecation is more feasible, such as with feet supported on a step stool, increases the likelihood of the child having a bowel movement. This success will also reinforce future adherence to the toileting plan. Children are often "very busy" in their playtime and forget to use the restroom or fail to recognize physiologic cues when distracted by their play (a problem which may be further exacerbated in children with attention-deficit/hyperactivity disorder or developmental delays). Scheduled toileting routines can also be helpful in these situations and may help to avoid accidents while also decreasing the tendency for the child to engage in withholding stool (Colombo et al., 2015; Tabbers et al., 2014).

Pharmacotherapy

The medications primarily used in the treatment of constipation can be divided into different classes based on their mechanism: osmotic, stimulant, stool softeners, and rectal laxatives/enema.

Mechanism of action of medication classes:

1. Osmotic agents (lactulose, polyethylene glycol (PEG), magnesium hydroxide/citrate) draw fluid into the lumen of the intestine, promoting peristalsis secondary to colon distention.
2. Stimulants (bisacodyl, senna) stimulate the myenteric plexus and smooth muscle of the colon to promote peristalsis.
3. Stool softeners (mineral oil, docusate) decrease surface tension of the stool and allow increased water absorption to enhance stool softness.
4. Enema/suppositories (bisacodyl, sodium docusate, hypertonic phosphate, sodium phosphate, saline, mineral oil, glycerin) – Hyperosmotic effects of sodium-based preparations draw extra water into the colon which promotes stool evacuation. Stimulating agents increase peristalsis. Mineral oil can soften and lubricate stool, making it easier to pass.

(Colombo et al., 2015; Epocrates, 2017).

Overall, the quality of evidence supporting the use of these medications is low, especially regarding dose ranges and length of treatment. That being said, bowel regimens are often the mainstay of both disimpaction and maintenance therapy in children. Table 7 outlines current medication recommendations per NASPGHAN recommendations and a recent Pediatrics in Review guideline (Tabbers et al., 2014; Colombo et al., 2015).

In general, polyethylene glycol (PEG) is considered a first-line therapy due to its efficacy, low side effect profile, and safety for both disimpaction and maintenance. It allows for easy titration to optimize stool consistency. Prune juice and apple juice

Table 7 Medications for disimpaction and constipation maintenance therapy

Drug	Drug class	Dosing+	Duration (per NASPGHAN)	Pitfalls/side effects
PEG 3350, Miralax	*Osmotic*	D: 1–1.5 gm/kg/day (oral) M: 1 gm/kg/day and adjust to clinical response	D: 3–6 days. M: at least 2 months or when symptoms resolve for 1 month before discontinuing *gradually*	• Bloating and diarrhea • Pitfall: parents discontinue too soon
Magnesium citrate	*Osmotic*	D: 4 mL/kg/day	D: 2 consecutive days	• Abdominal cramping
Magnesium hydroxide (milk of magnesia)	*Osmotic*	M (in ml/kg/dose) <2 y.o.: 0.5 2–5 y.o.: 5–15 ml/day 6–11 y.o.: 15–30 ml/day 12+: 30–60 ml/day		• Avoid in infants and patients with renal insufficiency
Lactulose	*Osmotic*	M: 1–3 ml/kg total for 1–2 times/day	Usually well tolerated long term	• Flatulence, abdominal cramps • Difficult to titrate to stool consistency • Some reports of decreased efficacy with prolonged use
Normal saline	*Rectal enema*	D: 10 ml/kg	D: Once a day for 3–6 days for disimpaction if PEG unavailable	
Sodium phosphate	*Rectal enema*	D: 1.125–4.5 oz. depending on age	D: 3 consecutive days	• Risk of electrolyte disturbances: low phosphate, low potassium, low calcium
Mineral oil	*Softener*	D: enema 2.25–4.5 oz. D: oral 15–30 ml per age in year (up to 240 ml) M: 1–3 ml/kg/day (kids 5–15 ml/day, teens 15–45 ml/day)	D: 3 consecutive days	• Can leak from rectum, not palatable in oral route • Not for oral use in children <1 or with known/at risk of *aspiration* • M forms not for children <18 months

(continued)

Table 7 (continued)

Drug	Drug class	Dosing+	Duration (per NASPGHAN)	Pitfalls/side effects
Docusate	*Softener*	M: 5 mg/kg/day (up to 400 mg/day)	Intermittent	• Minimal side effects • Less efficacy than other agents
Senna	*Stimulant*	M: (in mg/day) 1 month–2 years: 2.2–4.4 2–6 y.o.: 4.4–6.6 6–12 y.o.: 8.8–13.2 12+: 17.6–26.4	Intermittent, rescue therapy	• Abdominal cramping, but is self-limited and reduced by dose reduction
Bisacodyl	*Stimulant*	M: (in mg/day) 3–12 y.o.: 5–10 12+: 5–15	Intermittent, rescue therapy	• Can cause abdominal cramping, so reserved as rescue medicine

Adapted from Tabbers et al., 2014; Colombo et al., 2015
D disimpaction, *M* maintenance therapy

contain sorbitol, which is also an osmotic and can be used as an adjunctive treatment (Tabbers et al., 2014; Colombo et al., 2015).

The goal of treatment should be to achieve one soft formed stool per day. Adhering to medication, close communication, and follow-up with the prescribing physician (regarding efficacy and side effects) are important aspects of treatment. Achieving a stable stool pattern before lowering medications is strongly advised.

In 2014, the Department of Health and Human Services posted a Request for Applications (RFA) for the Use of Polyethylene Glycol in the Pediatric Population. It indicated that the FDA had found trace amounts of ethylene glycol and diethylene glycol in some samples of polyethylene glycol (PEG), used in the treatment of constipation. These findings raised some concerns regarding the safety of PEG for chronic use in children. There have been reports to the FDA of neurological and psychiatric symptoms in children taking PEG. Thus far, no long-term follow-up studies have linked acute or chronic polyethylene glycol with these adverse events (DHHS, 2014). The latest Cochrane study pooling 25 studies and 2310 children on various medications to treat chronic constipation was published in August 2016 (Gordon, MacDonald, Parker, et al., 2016). It found that the minor side effects reported with polyethylene glycol were lower than that with other agents. However, long-term safety and optimal dosing studies for polyethylene glycol warrant ongoing research.

As with all medications used to treat constipation, ensuring that the lowest effective doses are utilized is routinely recommended. Likewise, medications should be combined with diet and behavioral modifications in order to minimize risk and improve outcomes. While the majority of medications used to treat chronic constipation in children are not FDA approved for this use, it is important to recognize that chronic constipation is a serious health issue. If untreated, it can have significant physical and behavioral consequences. As with any treatment, it is important to weigh the benefits and risks when discussing options with patients and families in order to facilitate shared decision making.

Families who have been given a prescriptive bowel regimen often discontinue or decrease the medications based on effect (i.e., the balance between soft formed stools vs. diarrheal stools vs. hard formed stools that are difficult to pass). At times, families or providers may discontinue a stool softener or stimulant-based laxative product due to the propensity for diarrhea. It is helpful to emphasize that passing liquid stool around a solid or semisolid stool mass routinely occurs. This may lead families to believe that their child has diarrhea when in fact they are still quite constipated. Routine follow-up in the provider's office, accompanied by follow-up history and physical examination, is important in order to determine if the child has reached a normal stooling pattern before considering discontinuation of treatment. The 2014 NASPGHAN guidelines suggest that maintenance treatment should continue for at least 2 months, with all symptoms of constipation being resolved for 1 month, before slow discontinuation of the medication is attempted (Tabbers et al., 2014).

The constipation recovery rate is significantly higher when treatment is initiated before the age of 2 (Loening-Baucke, 1993), emphasizing the importance of early intervention to prevent persistent and chronic constipation in older children. Follow-up studies have shown that symptoms of functional constipation persist into adulthood for one-fourth to one-third of affected children (Bongers, van Wijk, Reitsma, et al., 2010; van Ginkel, Reitsma, Buller, et al., 2003). Thus, referral to a pediatric gastroenterologist should not be delayed if preliminary treatment for constipation is inadequate, regardless of compliance.

Conclusion

Constipation and enuresis are common problems in childhood that may often be undiagnosed and untreated. Failure to recognize medical issues that arise in the setting of toilet training can result in delays in reaching developmental toileting milestones. This delay in diagnosis may lead to chronic issues that are more difficult to treat. Awareness of the signs and symptoms of constipation and abnormal voiding patterns along with a thorough history and physical examination are often sufficient to elucidate the need for a more thorough diagnostic workup. Close follow-up is required to ensure patient progress and to provide ongoing education and guidance for the family. When there is a lack of response to first-line treatments, including behavioral interventions and medications, referral to a pediatric specialist is often warranted. A thoughtful multidisciplinary approach to the evaluation of childhood enuresis and constipation allows for the greatest treatment success.

Appendix 1: Voiding Diary

	Voiding and Stooling Diary Chart Day# ____					
	Void time	Void type*	Volume of void (mL)	Drink time	Fluid in (mL)	Type of fluid
AM						
			Total AM			
PM						
			Total PM			
Sleep						
bedtime						
________						
Rise time ________			Total overnight			
Total						
*Stool? y/n and describe						

References

American Psychiatric Association. (2013). *Diagnostic and Statistical manual of mental disorders* (5th ed.pp. 355–360). American Psychiatric Association: Arlington, VA.

Austin, P. F., Bauer, S. B., Bower, W., et al. (2016). The standardization of terminology of lower urinary tract function in children and adolescents: Update report from the standardization committee of the International Children's Continence Society. *Neurourology and Urodynamics, 35*(4), 471–481.

Bayne, A. P., & Skoog, S. J. (2014). Nocturnal enuresis: An approach to assessment and treatment. *Pediatrics in Review, 35*(8), 327–334.

Benninga, M. A., Faure, C., Hyman, P. E., St. James Roberts, I., et al. (2016). Childhood functional gastrointestinal disorders: Neonate/toddler. *Gastroenterology, 150*, 1443–55.e2.

Bentley, S. (2014). Imipramine level. Emedicine by medscape. Retrieved from http://emedicine.medscape.com/article/2090130-overview

Blais, A. S., Nadeau, G., Moore, K., et al. (2016). Prospective pilot study of Mirabegron in pediatric patients with overactive bladder. *European Urology, 70*, 9–13.

Bongers, M. E., Tabbers, M. M., & Benninga, M. A. (2007). Functional nonretentive fecal incontinence in children. *Journal of Pediatric Gastroenterology and Nutrition, 44*, 5–13.

Bongers, M. E., van Wijk, M. P., Reitsma, J. B., et al. (2010). Long-term prognosis for childhood constipation: Clinical outcomes in adulthood. *Pediatrics, 50*(3), 256–268.

Chua, M. E., Silangcruz, J. M., Chang, S., et al. (2016). Desmopressin withdrawal strategy for pediatric enuresis: A meta-analysis. *Pediatrics, 138*(1), 1–10.

Colombo, J. M., Wassom, M. C., & Rosen, J. M. (2015). Constipation and encopresis in childhood. *Pediatrics in Review, 36*(9), 392–401.

Corazziara, E., Staiano, A., Miele, E., et al. (2005). Italian Society of pediatric gastroenterology, hepatology, and nutrition. Bowel frequency and defecatory patterns in children: a prospective nationwide survey. *Clin Gastroenterol Hepatol, 3*(11), 1101–1106.

Department of Health and Human Services. (2014). The use of polyethylene glycol in the pediatric population. Retrieved from https://grants.nih.gov/grants/guide/rfa-files/RFA-FD-14-002.html

Drossman, D. A. (2016). Functional gastrointestinal disorders: History, pathophysiology, clinical features, and Rome IV. *Gastroenterology, 150*, 1262–1279.

Epocrates. (2017). Epocrates Plus for Apple iOS (Version 17.3). Mobile Application Software. Retrieved from www.epocrates.com

Gordon, M., MacDonald, J.K., Parker, C.E., et al. (2016). Osmotic and stimulant laxatives for the management of childhood constipation. *Cochrane Database of Systematic Reviews*, issue 8. Art. No.: CD009118. doi:10.1002/14651858.CD009118.pub3

Graham, K. M., & Levy, J. B. (2009). Enuresis. *Pediatrics in Review, 30*(5), 165–173.

Hoebeke, P., Bower, W., Combs, A., et al. (2010). Diagnostic evaluation of children with daytime incontinence. *The Journal of Urology, 183*(2), 699–703.

Irastorza, I., Ibanez, B., Delgado-Sanzonetti, L., et al. (2010). Cow's-milk-free diet as a therapeutic option in childhood chronic constipation. *JPGN, 51*(2), 171–176.

Issenman, R. M., Filmer, R. B., & Gorski, P. A. (1999). A review of bowel and bladder control development in children: How gastrointestinal and urological conditions relate to problems in toilet training. *Pediatrics, 103*(3), 1346–1352.

Jeyakumar, A., Rahman, S. I., Armbrecht, E. S., et al. (2012). The association between sleep-disordered breathing and enuresis in children. *Laryngoscope, 128*(3), 1873–1877.

Lamb, W.H. (2014). Pediatric diabetic ketoacidosis. Emedicine by medscape. Retrieved from http://emedicine.medscape.com/article/907111-overview

Lexicomp Online. (2017). Wolters Kluwer Clinical Drug Information. Retrieved from www.lexi.com.

Liem, O., Harman, J., Benninga, M., et al. (2009). Health utilization and cost impact of childhood constipation in the United States. *The Journal of Pediatrics, 154*, 258–262.

Loening-Baucke, V. (1993). Constipation in early childhood: Patient characteristics, treatment, and long-term follow up. *Gut, 34*, 1400–1404.

Loening-Baucke, V. (2005). Prevalence, symptoms and outcome of constipation in infants and toddlers. *The Journal of Pediatrics, 146*, 359–363.

Malowitz, S., Green, M., Karpinski, A., et al. (2016). Age of onset of functional constipation. *Journal of Pediatric Gastroenterology and Nutrition, 62*, 600–602.

Malykhina, A. P. (2007). Neural mechanisms of pelvic organ cross-sensitization. *Neuroscience, 149*(3), 660–672.

Maternik, M., Krzeminska, K., & Zurowska, A. (2015). The management of childhood urinary incontinence. *Pediatric Nephrology, 30*, 41–50.

Mugie, S. M., Benninga, M. A., & Di Lorenzo, C. (2011). Epidemiology of constipation in children and adults: A systematic review. *Best Practice & Research. Clinical Gastroenterology, 25*(1), 3–18.

Neurogenic Bladder. Johns Hopkins Medicine Health Library. Retrieved from http://www.hopkinsmedicine.org/healthlibrary/conditions/adult/kidney_and_urinary_system_disorders/neurogenic_bladder_85.P01487/

Nevéus, T., Eggert, P., Evans, J., et al. (2010). Evaluation of and treatment for monosymptomatic enuresis: A standardization document from the International Children's Continence Society. *The Journal of Urology, 183*, 441–447.

Nevéus, T., von Gontard, A., Hoebeke, P., et al. (2006). The standardization of terminology of lower urinary tract function in children and adolescents: Report from the standardisation committee of the International Children's Continence Society (ICCS). *J Urology, 176*(1), 314–324.

Newman, T. B. (2011). The New American Academy of Pediatrics urinary tract infection guideline. *Pediatrics, 128*(3), 572–575.

Nickavar, A., & Sotoudeh, K. (2011). Treatment and prophylaxis in pediatric urinary tract infection. *Int J Prev Med, 2*(1), 4–9.

NICE clinical guideline 111. (2010). Nocturnal enuresis: The management of bedwetting in children and young people. National Clinical Guideline Centre. Retrieved from www.nice.org.uk/guidance/CG111

Pijpers, M. A. M., Bongers, M. E. J., Benninga, M. A., et al. (2010). Functional constipation in children: A systematic review on prognosis and predictive factors. *Journal of Pediatric Gastroenterology and Nutrition, 50*(3), 256–268.

Rajindrajith, S., & Devanarayana, N. M. (2011). Constipation in children: Novel insight into epidemiology, pathophysiology and management. *J Neurogastroenterol Motil, 17*(1), 35–47.

Rasquin, A., Di Lorenzo, C., Forbes, D., et al. (2006). Childhood functional gastrointestinal disorders: Child/adolescent. *Gastroenterology, 130*, 1527–1537.

Schurch, B., & Corcos, J. (2005). Botulinum toxin injections for paediatric incontinence. *Current Opinion in Urology, 15*(4), 264.

Shin, S. H., Im, Y. J., Lee, M. J., et al. (2013). Spina bifida occulta: Not to be overlooked in children with nocturnal enuresis. *International Journal of Urology, 20*(8), 831–835.

Steer, C. D., Emond, A. M., & Golding, J. (2009). The variation in stool patterns from 1 to 42 months: A population-based observational study. *Archives of Disease in Childhood, 94*(3), 231–233.

Stein, M. T., Beninga, M. A., & Felt, B. T. (2017). An 8-year old boy with treatment-resistant encopresis. *Journal of Developmental and Behavioral Pediatrics, 38*, S19–S22.

Tabbers, M. M., DiLorenzo, C., Berger, M. Y., et al. (2014). Evaluation and treatment of functional constipation in infants and children: Evidence-based recommendations from ESPGHAN and NASPGHAN. *JPGN, 58*(2), 258–274.

Tu, N.D., Baskin, L.S. (2017). Nocturnal enuresis in children: Management. UpToDate. Retrieved from https://www.uptodate.com/contents/nocturnal-enuresis-in-children-management

Van Ginkel, R., Reitsma, J. B., Buller, H. A., et al. (2003). Childhood constipation: Longitudinal follow-up beyond puberty. *Gastroenterology, 125*, 357–363.

Vande Walle, J., Rittig, S., Bauer, S., et al. (2012). American Academy of Pediatrics; European Society for Paediatric Urology; European Society for Paediatric Nephrology; International Children's Continence Society. Practical consensus guidelines for the management of enuresis. *Eur J Pediatr, 171*(6), 971–983.

Wolfe-Christenson, C., Manolis, A., Guy, W. C., et al. (2014). Bladder and bowel dysfunction: Evidence for multidisciplinary care. *The Journal of Urology*, *190*(5), 1864–1868.
Zeevenhooven, J., Koppen, J., & Benninga, M. (2017). The new Rome IV criteria for functional gastrointestinal disorders in infants and toddlers. *Pediatr Gastroenterol Hepatol Nutr*, *20*(1), 1–13.
Zywicke, H., Rozzelle, C. (2011). *Pediatrics in Review, 32*(3), 109.

Special Populations: Toilet Training Children with Disabilities

Michael A. Cocchiola Jr. and Caroline C. Redpath

Defining Developmental Disabilities

Developmental disabilities are a wide-ranging spectrum of long-term conditions that occur secondary to physical and mental skill deficits (CDC, 2013). The term "developmental disabilities" is an expansive term, with many diagnoses that fit under its canopy, some that have a negative influence on intellectual functioning and others that have an impact solely on physical conditions. For the purposes of this chapter, all diagnoses that fit under the umbrella of a "developmental disability" will be considered for the purposes of toilet training and their impact on children with skill deficits that may negatively affect toilet training.

The terms *intellectual disability* and *developmental disability* are often used interchangeably across clinical and academic settings to replace older terms such as physically handicapped or mentally retarded or any of a collection of more archaic terms used to identify people with cognitive, social, or physical challenges. Clinical experts responsible for the nosology of these disorders have progressively moved from a sterile, clinical label onto a diagnostic classification that sheds value on dignity and respect within the term that categorizes specific diagnoses. Nosology is the branch of medical science that deals with categorizing specific symptoms into concrete disorders, for the purposes of identifying disorders and providing treatment practices available in the scientific field. For the purposes of clarity, developmental disabilities and intellectual disabilities are different based on the following:

- *Intellectual disability*: a group of disorders characterized by a limited mental capacity and difficulty with adaptive behaviors such as managing money, schedules and routines, or social interactions. An intellectual disability typically

M.A. Cocchiola Jr. (✉) • C.C. Redpath (✉)
Capitol Region Education Council-River Street Autism Program,
601 River Street, Windsor, CT 06095, USA
e-mail: mcocchiola@crec.org; credpath@crec.org

J.L. Matson (ed.), *Clinical Guide to Toilet Training Children*, Autism and Child Psychopathology Series, DOI 10.1007/978-3-319-62725-0_13

requires an IQ below 70 and originates before the age of 18. It may result from physical causes, such as autism or cerebral palsy, or from nonphysical causes, such as lack of stimulation and adult responsiveness during early stages of development.

- *Developmental disability*: a severe, long-term disability that can affect cognitive ability, physical functioning, or both. These disabilities appear before age 22 and are likely to be lifelong. The term "developmental disability" encompasses intellectual disability but also includes physical disabilities without cognitive impairment. Some developmental disabilities may be solely physical, such as blindness from birth. Others involve both physical and intellectual disabilities stemming from genetic or other causes, such as Down's syndrome and fetal alcohol syndrome disorder.

(Source: https://report.nih.gov/nihfactsheets/ViewFactSheet.aspx?csid=100).

Either one of the above definitions may include a person with an autism spectrum disorder (ASD), cerebral palsy, language and learning disorder, fetal alcohol syndrome disorder (FASD), and other disorders that occur during the developmental period and negatively impact key areas of functioning to a notable degree. Weaknesses in these key functional areas may include a delay in academic progress, especially in the absence of support based on individualized needs. Progress in the domains of social skills, communication skills (expressive, receptive, nonverbal), self-help skills, self-preservation, and self-advocacy may be negatively impacted as well.

Recent research by Boyle, Boulet, Schieve, Cohen, Blumberg, Yeargin-Allsopp, Visser, and Kogan (2011) provides information that 1 in 6, or nearly 17%, of children were diagnosed with a developmental disability in the USA during the period between 1997 and 2008. These numbers are not restricted to the USA; the World Health Organization (WHO, 2011) reports similar numbers worldwide with a range of 16–19% based on comparable classifications of developmental disorders. Boyle et al. (2011) also provide an insightful study in conjunction with the National Institute of Health (NIH) that combined both diagnoses of developmental disability and intellectual disability to complete a sample analysis of children in the USA from 1997 to 2008. Data revealed a decrease in the number of children with hearing impairments though an increase in the number of children with autism and other developmental delays, perhaps based on an increase in awareness of autism spectrum disorders over the past 10–15 years.

To provide a blended, differentially qualified term that maintains a reasonably sensitive definition for the terms "developmental disability" and "intellectual disability," the American Association on Intellectual and Developmental Disabilities (AAIDD) offers a global description that effectively encapsulates the targeted group. AAIDD (2013) stated that regardless of vogue labels and details of the diagnostic process, three essential elements have remained intact over the past 50 years that identify what now can be considered an intellectual or developmental impairment. They include:

- Compromised intellectual functions or physical functions that delay learning
- Behavioral limitations that negatively impact adapting to environmental changes
- Early age of onset, specifically before the age of 18 for individuals with an intellectual disability and before the age of 22 for individuals with a developmental disability

Dominant diagnoses identified by AAIDD (2013) include specific criterion-referenced labels below. The list is non-exhaustive, though the strands that bind all diagnoses include compromising delays, most commonly in the areas of cognitive development, language development, activities of daily living (ADLs), and social and emotional development. In order to meet any of these criteria, delays need to be well below the normed value of age-related peers (CDC, 2013).

Typical diagnoses that fall under the umbrella of developmental disabilities most frequently include, though are not limited to:

- Autism spectrum disorders (ASDs), in which up to 80% of people with ASD demonstrate deficits with intellectual measures. Specific deficits are in the domains of adaptive social interaction, adaptive communication, and the need for sameness to the point that it impairs adaptive engagement in the school, community, or home setting.
- Down's syndrome, when children and adults have an extra copy of chromosome 21. This chromosomal disorder negatively affects cognitive and physical functioning in the individual when compared to age-related peers.
- Cerebral palsy (CP), when significant delays impair motor and postural ability. These impairments negatively affect basic skill development to include activities of daily living (ADLs) and effective communication and are often related to cognitive delays and other self-help skills.
- Fetal alcohol syndrome disorders (FASD) is a disorder that impacts a diverse set of physical, behavioral, social, emotional, and behavioral achievements based on age-related peers. FASD is 100% reliant on the amount of alcohol consumption of an expecting mother during pregnancy, with an increased risk contingent on the frequency and amount of alcohol consumed during pregnancy (Chudley et al., 2005). Emotional regulation, difficulty with attention, and hypotonic motor skills are all factors that cause a delay in typical development and impact skill growth in the areas of daily living, to include toilet training.

Finally, according to the Centers for Disease Control (2013), some people are born with a health condition that impairs life functions, while other people experience disability secondary to illness, injury, or poor living conditions (e.g., poor nutrition, limited shelter, attachment deficits, reduced exposure to learning). In addition, people with disabilities may also be diagnosed with less frequent diagnoses such as spina bifida, muscular dystrophy, traumatic spinal cord injury, and children with hearing, visual, physical, communication, and nonspecific intellectual deficits. Some people may have a single deficit, while others may be diagnosed with multiple deficits. That is, a person with cerebral palsy may have deficits with adaptive communication, mobility, and intellectual ability. The intricate interaction between a specific diagnosis, the environment the person is raised in, and personal factors means that each child's experience of disability is different (Phillips, 2012).

Individuals with developmental disabilities have notable deficits in major life activities to include language, mobility, cognitive learning, self-help, and independent living. Specific developmental disabilities such as autism, cerebral palsy, hearing impairments, or cognitive impairments, to name a few, may be identified anytime during development and up to 21 years of age. Deficits often last throughout a person's lifetime, though early intervention with effective treatment may reduce or mask the specific deficits noted in a diagnosis (Boyle et al., 2011).

According to Yoo (2010), children with developmental disabilities likely face increased obstacles when toilet training is initiated compared to people without diagnoses that compromise learning. Obstacles may partly be due to the person's deficits in physical development and motor coordination, adaptive communication, effective social interaction, sensory sensitivity, adaptation to changes, or behavioral regulation. A brief overview of these deficits follows below.

Impact of Developmental Disabilities on Learning

Motor Deficits and Delays

Professional medical assessment is generally recommended before moving forward with behavioral interventions to treat a delay in toileting ability. Children with Down's syndrome, for example, may have a host of genitourinary issues that complicate toilet training. Surgical or pharmacological intervention may be recommended before considering behavioral interventions (Handel, 2003).

Children with cerebral palsy have their own unique issues with toilet training as well. They have an increased risk for urinary tract infections, due to spasticity and hypotonia in muscles that control bladder and bowel. Excitement or tension may create unintentional muscle tone changes that interfere with adaptive training. Indeed, medical complications in children with cerebral palsy draw out the average age of bladder and bowel training to 3.9 and 3.8 years of age, respectively (Osturk, Oktem, & Kisioglu, 2006).

In conjunction with motor concerns, visual and auditory factors should also be taken into account before moving forward with a more intensive behavior intervention. Recommendations include support and input from specialized experts, to include physical therapists to suggest adaptive positioning, an audiologist to recommend adaptive equipment for hearing, or vision specialist to provide tactile materials. Although 98% of typically developing peers are toilet trained by age 3 years (Cocchiola, Martino, Dwyer, & Demezzo, 2012), the simple notion that toileting is not intact by age 3 does not necessarily mean that behavior interventions are the most prudent, especially as a stand-alone intervention. Best practice is to gain the insight of experts in the core deficit area and move forward with intervention based on their recommendations.

Cognitive Deficits and Delays

The complexities of processing information through receptive language, applying its relevance and permanence to a life skill, and then maintaining that skill are often immeasurable. Typically developing children are able to take in interactions in their environment, interpret an abundance of observations, and apply a germane skill secondary to observational learning or operant conditioning. Indeed, it is remarkable when we consider how much learning occurs in the natural environment with little to no formal teaching.

In contrast, learning with skill deficits in any areas required for learning (vision, hearing, working memory, modeling, etc.) often requires direct instruction with learning objectives altered from a complex task into smaller chunks of information. This method of direct instruction may require repeated trials and highly relevant reinforcers for learning to be permanently imprinted. Dalrymple and Ruble (1992) provide some evidence that children with cognitive deficits develop toileting skills on average of 1.6 years after age-related peers with no cognitive delays. In addition, nearly 50% of the children included in their study needed supplementary support to enhance learning the skill of toilet training, to include visual schedules and other nonverbal support systems.

Social Deficits and Delays

Typically developing 1-year-old infants display behaviors that indicate a cognitive awareness of other people whose attention and interaction serve as meaningful and socially reinforcing. The desire to interact and social responses to their actions are highly reinforcing and serve as a driving force to support simple imitation and social engagement (Carpenter, Nagell, & Tomasello, 1998). Learning happens most effectively due to developing social awareness of attention that elicits behaviors. In contrast, children with disabilities may have difficulty understanding social interaction or simply be disinterested due to cognitive deficits inherent to their disorder. In essence, typically developing children are more likely to be highly motivated by social contingencies, while the desire to make meaningful social connection with a caretaker may be an absent skill in children with disabilities (Stadtler, Gorski, & Brazelton, 1999), thus negatively impacting learning momentum.

Communication Deficits and Delays

Communication deficits also play a role in a child's ability to understand verbal and nonverbal directions, as well as respond to and interact with the language in the environment. Deficits in receptive and expressive language have a global impact on learning, therefore negatively influence a child's capacity to toilet train at the expected age.

The point is that in the absence of effective receptive language skills, the learner starts at a deficit, not clearly understanding the expectations or sequence of expected behaviors. In addition, deficits in the domain of adaptive requests (mands) impair effective requests to use the toilet effectively.

Issues with Perseveration and Sameness

Changes or novel learning processes may increase a level of noncompliance to nearly any skill acquisition process. The presence of an underlying diagnosis present in children with disabilities can frustrate the child, as well as the caregiver attempting to teach a skill including toilet training (Baily, Hatton, Mesibov, Ament, & Skinner, 2000). Simple activities such as going into a novel bathroom, removing a diaper, or sitting in a relaxed state in the bathroom may be barriers to learning when it is a novel experience. The issue of perseveration and the desire for sameness may trump any immediate reinforcers secondary to a chaining of negative behaviors, making toilet training an aversive procedure as a starting point for the child.

Behavioral Regulation

Behavioral regulation can be described as the spontaneous or intentional modification of a person's emotional status as a means to promote adaptive or goal-directed behavior (Mazefsky et al., 2013). People with disabilities have an increased likelihood of deficits that interfere with regulated emotions under times of distress. They may instead react with behaviors that provide immediate escape from less preferred, short-term expectations at a cost of long-term learning, such as activities of daily living. Behaviors such as tantrums or aggression may occur as a reaction to changes or less preferred expectations with notable deficits in the ability to modify their emotional state.

A Review of Obstacles

In summary, compromised development in the areas of (a) neuro-physical control and coordination, (b) cognitive ability, (c) fluency in expressive and receptive communication, (d) adaptive and meaningful social interaction, (e) the desire for sameness, and (f) the ability to regulate emotions are important to take into account when considering skill acquisition and retention. The saliency of social reinforcement, an understanding of verbal and nonverbal language, rigidity in routines, and the simple trait of wanting to please an adult or peer are often viewed as the bridges of behavioral cusps. A behavioral cusp is the mastery of a new skill that provides an opportunity for the learner to access novel and powerful contingencies, new settings, and a new series of behaviors that compete with older, less effective behaviors (Smith, McDougall, & Edelen-Smith, 2006). For example, learning to walk is a behavioral cusp that increases a child's ability to explore his or her world beyond the simple and rudimentary act of crawling. Toilet training is considered a behavioral cusp as well, increasing a child's independence, adaptive communication, body awareness, and opportunities for socialization.

Unfortunately, children not toilet trained by age 8 were found not likely to attain continence (Singh, Masey, & Morton, 2006) and, more importantly, had decreased opportunities to learn across an expansive range of adaptive, prosocial behaviors. In addition, research also suggests that failures in toilet training may be due to incomplete training and inadvertent reinforcement of incontinence by caregivers who give the individual a great deal of attention in response to soiling (Cicero & Pfadt, 2002; Cooper, Heron, & Heward, 2007).

Parent Perspective on Toilet Training Children with Disabilities

Toilet training for children with developmental disabilities continues to be one of the most frequently researched self-help skills (Konarski & Diorio, 1985). Even for individuals without developmental disabilities, toilet training can be a difficult developmental milestone. The venture frequently demands time, energy, and patience on the part of the caregiver and youngster alike. Regardless, nearly all children without developmental disabilities are successfully toilet trained by age 3. In contrast, individuals with developmental disabilities face greater obstacles with toilet training than typically developing peers, based on impairments described above.

Research over the past several decades supports the notion that toilet training children with developmental disabilities often requires (a) enhanced support and training from interventionists, (b) an increased amount of learning time to develop the skill of toilet training when compared to typically developing peers, (c) an increased amount of direct instruction, and (d) persistence on the part of the caregiver. Multiple barriers may exist that delay toilet training at the same age as typically developing peers. Adding to this complex development issue, research supports the notion that a delay in toilet training beyond 3 years of age results in an increased difficulty with training (Singh, Masey, & Morton, 2006). Enhanced support to teach this skill needs to come into place soon after age 3 to move the process forward and provide dignity and independence to the individual.

Research by Joinson et al. (2013) supports findings that teaching adaptive toilet training may become more difficult as the individual ages. Delays in instructional teaching and support increase the amount of time an individual will depend upon caregivers for toileting needs. Learning patterns reinforced over a prolonged period, such as urinating in a diaper, need to be unlearned. Children not successfully toilet trained by 8 years old were found to be increasingly unlikely to attain toilet training at all (Singh et al., 2006).

Yoo (2012) and her colleagues from the New York State Office for People with Developmental Disabilities (NYS-OPWDD) provide a detailed report and step-by-step training guidelines for interventions on what they call "Targeting the Big 3." The Big 3 refers to three specific barriers that prevent people with disabilities from integrating with age-related peers and integrating with the inclusive population at large. The Big 3 includes (a) toilet training, (b) meal time behavior, and (c) challenging behaviors. Yoo and colleagues define toileting as a crucial target skill necessary to provide optimal integration, first in school and then in the community at large.

Yoo (2010) provides a relevant list of concerns that help bring the issue and concerns of toilet training to the forefront of the clinician's attention.

- A child with autism spectrum disorders and other developmental disabilities faces greater obstacles with toilet training than children without these relevant issues.
- The child's relative weaknesses with communication, social interaction, or level of comfort with changes may be barriers to learning toileting skills without direct support.
- Research suggests that failures in toilet training may be related to ineffective training or unintentional reinforcement by interventionists who provide an abundance of attention or reward for accidents.
- Longer delays in toilet training frequently lead to an increased duration to achieve continence.
- Interventionists (e.g., parents, teacher, consultants) may experience a degree of stress associated with attending to the incontinent individual's toileting needs, which increase as the child ages.
- A lack of bladder and bowel control is one of the most frequently cited reasons for abuse to children, secondary only to episodes of severe emotional dysregulation.
- Societal expectation is that all people have an effective degree of continence.
- Effective interventions to treat incontinence should be a focus soon after a child is identified as delayed in this area, typically by 3 years old.

Research does support the notion that a child should demonstrate prerequisite skills (e.g., an interest in the bathroom, a desire to sit on the toilet, facial expressions, and body movements that illustrate discomfort with a full bladder) before considering toilet training initiation. Although this may be fruitful with a typically developing child, a child who presents with neuro-atypicality may have significant deficits in nonverbal expression, a decreased interest in the actions of others secondary to a deficit in theory of mind, and the issue of remaining cognitively locked on sameness. A proportion of children diagnosed with autism or developmental disabilities may demonstrate no prerequisite skills and therefore move into a prolonged period of no toilet training well beyond the expected norm of 3 years. Current research supports the notion that early and intense intervention to address toileting skills is essential for skill acquisition (see Cicero & Pfadt, 2002; Cocchiola et al., 2012; Baker & Brightman, 1997) and requires focused and prolonged intervention in order to become toilet trained.

The inability to remain continent may expose individuals with disabilities to social isolation at best, or worst, overt ostracization, making it difficult to integrate into the community at large. Some activities such as maintaining a job or recreating in a public pool may not be available to a person with disabilities who is incontinent (Smith & Chaneb, 2016). To be sure, continence and appropriate toileting are important self-help skills that enhance self-esteem, increase effective hygiene, and increase opportunities for inclusion in schools, peer relations, employment, recreation, and success in community-based settings (Brown & Peace, 2011; Luxem & Christophersen, 1994; Sells-Love, Rinaldi, & McLaughlin, 2002).

Most caregivers will experience a great deal of stress associated with attending to the incontinent individual's toileting needs. Stress may increase as the individual gets older. Failure to gain bladder and bowel control is one of the most frequently cited reasons for intentional abuse or injury to children, second only to crying (Pivato, 2009; Silva & Schalock, 2012). Vermandel et al. (2008) cites negative outcomes for late or no toilet training for children to include (a) social isolation and disapproval, (b) restricted access to inclusion in school and gainful employment as an adult, (c) cost of incontinence supplies, (d) physical complications such as skin irritation and infection, (e) lack of privacy and independence, and (f) monetary and social stressors on parents, caregivers, and teachers.

Interestingly, the process and intervention options for toilet training children with disabilities are similar to toilet training typically developing peers caveat; the hurdles faced with typically developing peers are often higher for a child with developmental disabilities. Additional support, training, more expansive periods, and extraordinary diligence with precision teaching are required from the caregivers. It typically requires increased patience, an increased period to reach full independence, more direct support, and more specific guidelines to reach success (Greenspan, Wieder, & Simons, 1998; Stadtler et al., 1999; Cocchiola et al., 2012). To better quantify hurdles along a timeline, children with disabilities require an average duration of 1.6 years from the onset of programming to full toileting independence, while typically developing peers require an average of 3–6 months for full independence (Dalrymple & Ruble, 1992).

Unfortunately, despite parents and caregivers rating toilet training as one of their child's most important accomplishments in their first 3 years (Rinaldi & Mirenda, 2012), toilet training frequently becomes a secondary or tertiary goal when pronounced delays in language, socialization, or learning readiness are present. Educational planning teams develop learning objectives in the child's school and often direct their focus on long-term academic planning at a cost to simpler skills such as toilet training, an adaptive behavioral cusp, that brings a person into contact with new contingencies that have far-reaching consequences (Rogers, 2010; Rosales-Ruiz & Baer, 1997). Rogers (2010) states that it may be counterproductive to delay toilet training too long beyond 3 years old even if some academic or language progress is noted. Indeed, the lack of toilet training and other fundamental early learning skills may allow time for a child to develop maladaptive behaviors, which then become barriers to toilet training, as well as other adaptive, functional skills.

A Historic Development of Toilet Training

For millennia, toilet training children has been an expectation of parenting and of the child, passed on through intergenerational convention, generally effective across cultures with bladder and bowel control intact across nearly all children by 2–3 years old. Authoritative yet simple guidelines consisted of basic rules and procedures passed on as a new generation emerged, with relative success across over 90% of the population. Children with what would be defined as developmental deficits according to current standards were not included in this group.

Past practices included toilet training as early as several weeks after birth and trip training intact in some instances as early as 6 months. More commonly in recent history, parents would simply wait for the child to demonstrate an interest in the skill. Factors that motivated parents to early or later toilet training included family and social influences, the expense or time commitment to prolonged diaper use, or parent concern regarding toileting as a relevant skill.

In the 1940s, Dr. Benjamin Spock, an American pediatrician, provided a novel series of parenting guidelines, which included what he deemed "best practice" for teaching toileting skills to children. Spock's seminal writing of *Baby and Child Care* (Spock, 1946) helped to launch ongoing guidance to parents regarding adaptive and authoritative support for child and adolescent growth, as well as scientific research for measurable outcomes based on intervention practices. Spock's position relied on a developmental approach, to include signs of "toilet readiness," gentle teaching based on the child's learning readiness, and reinforcement (e.g., social praise, access to preferred items) for adaptive toileting.

In the 1960s, Dr. T. Berry Brazelton refined this approach to include signs of physical as well as social and emotional readiness with a foundation on a desire for independence and a desire to please others. The addition of emotional readiness and social salience proved helpful from a developmental approach for typically maturing children. The underlying supposition shared by both clinicians was based on a framework that developmental readiness varied naturally across children and that each child would be ready for eventual learning once multiple skills were intact to include physical readiness, social awareness, and a desire for independence. A noted weakness that the "Child Ready" approach missed was the issue of outliers, such as children with developmental disabilities. In the presence of a developmental disability, developmental readiness may be significantly delayed or indeed absent. The longer the delay beyond a certain age, the more unlikely toilet training would be.

In the late 1960s and early 1970s, a paradigm shift occurred in the research and intervention models for toilet training. Although most children were readily toilet trained within the range of age-related peers, a small proportion of the population remained untrained, presumably due to deficits in developmental readiness or missed opportunities to teach the skill. Van Wagenen and colleagues (1969), as well as Azrin and Foxx (1971) completed additional research to address toilet training in a population that demonstrated difficulty with learning following the typical developmental model. This research was highly influential, as it provided clinically reliable methods to toilet train people with severe developmental disabilities, the remaining 2–3% of the population typically not toilet trained by age 3 years. Direct and intensive intervention, typically provided by trained clinicians, was necessary, though children and even adults who presented as not trainable became toilet trained.

Since the early 1970s as well as today, articles and books about toilet training are abundant with advice from pediatricians, psychologists, urologists, behavior analysts, and a multitude of other people willing to share their advice. Indeed, toilet training remains one of the most researched and explored topics among parents and caregivers with children who have developmental disabilities in the 1970s and 1980s, with an increase trend across all parents over the past several decades (Matson, 1990). Parents as well as clinicians working in applied settings are seeking recommendations about toilet training, with methods that follow the procedural guidelines outlined below.

The "Child Ready" Model

This toilet training process supports the notion that a child needs to demonstrate emotional and physical readiness before a parent or caregiver initiates toilet training. Criteria include development of and awareness for bladder control, a positive relationship with an interventionist, intact receptive language to understand simpler instruction, and an appeal to control body functions in an adaptive manner (Christopherson, 1991). Research demonstrates a broad span in age for typically developing children, with a range of 18–30 months as a starting point for toilet training readiness. Children who start later in the age continuum frequently have briefer training periods, while those of earlier ages require a longer learning process.

The "Child Ready" concept posited by Spock and Brazelton provided a useful guide to parents. It offered a more relaxed parenting style that supported learning based on developmental readiness and self-directed learning supported by the parents. This method diverged from parent-imposed expectations on a rigid timeline, typically based on social pressures. Advice for parents existed before these publications, though consistent methods advised by skilled professionals were sparse at best and rarely available for an expansive population.

Spock's book sold nearly 50 million copies from 1946 to 1998 in 39 different languages and was often viewed as a reliable resource for parents. The most novel feature of Spock's toilet training is that it regarded toilet training as a developmental milestone, accomplished at different ages based on the child's interest in the skill. Additionally, focused points for parents were (a) that toileting should be addressed when the child demonstrates an interest, (b) that the experience should be positive in nature, and (c) that the use of punishment and other aversive procedures are generally unnecessary and perhaps counterproductive to adaptive toilet training.

Although this method provided a high-yield outcome with minimal training, children with developmental disabilities often remained untrained well beyond the average age of 3. Indeed, conditions that impaired learning often left them developmentally below the cusp of learning throughout the "Child Ready" window, with a delay in important early intervention. A notable percent of children with developmental disabilities continued to remain incontinent well after most all (98%) of age-related peers.

The Use of Rapid Toilet Training

The "Child Ready" model may likely have impaired "trainer ready" interventions for a small proportion of children who developed at an atypical rate and fit the current diagnosis of a developmental delay or disability. Continuing to wait for this child to be ready may be fruitless after a certain age, most frequently at 3 years old. Effective implementation of a more intensive instructional program to teach toileting seemed warranted and indeed efficacious to address this population.

Van Wagenen et al. (1969) provided additional scientific weight to the process of toilet training, moving it from a developmental "Child Ready" model with defined prerequisite skills but minimal procedural guidelines to a more empirically based experimental design. More importantly, this study supported the notion that toilet training for a small minority of people is a true issue beyond the developmental process of typically developing children. Participants in the study of Van Wagenen et al. (1969) included 9 males, ranging in age from 20 years old to 62 years old, with a mean age of 43 years old, all of whom lived in an institution for people with today's definition of developmental disability. None were toilet trained. The duration of long-term institutionalization due to developmental disabilities ranged from 6 years to 45 years with a mean duration of 21 years.

The outcome of the Van Wagenen et al. (1969) intervention demonstrated that within 12 days of the first experimental group, patients were able to remain dry and maintain dryness over an 8-h period, following a 2.5-h daily tripping schedule (e.g., cueing to bathroom every 2.5 h). The overwhelming outcome of this study points to the fact that people with developmental disabilities may be far beyond the reaches of "Child Ready." However, they are capable of toilet training regardless with interventions based on behavioral strategies that teach a skill beyond the premise of developmental readiness before imposing instruction. The outcome revealed that even with a lack of readiness proposed by developmental specialists, intensive intervention with a clear sequence of prompting and responses to incorrect and correct behaviors (consequence-based responses) demonstrated merit across the divides of development, even with subjects who demonstrated delayed development.

Following the Van Wagenen study, Azrin and Foxx (1971) published what is now considered a seminal article in rapid toilet training, titled *A Rapid Method of Toilet Training the Institutionalized Retarded.* This method recognized that people with disabilities were much less likely to respond to the "Child Ready" method, supported by Spock and colleagues, and instead required a much more intensive intervention based on the principles of operant learning. This included (a) eliciting the behavior of urination through the delivery of a discriminating stimulus (Sd), (b) increasing opportunities to urinate through increased fluid intake, (c) delivering reinforcers that motivate adaptive urination, and (d) overcorrection procedures for episodes of wetting. Outcomes proved highly effective for toilet training individuals with compromising developmental delays over brief periods, sometimes in as little as a 24-h period, and more frequently over a weekend period with intense clinical support intact for long-term learning of toilet training skills.

This rapid toilet training procedure became a principal method to toilet train children with disabilities who lagged behind age-related peers in this skill. In addition, it became an option for parents who preferred a "rapid toilet training" sequence rather than a prolonged process or the need to wait for a child to be ready. In the end, parents had effective alternatives to use if they had children typically developing in most other domains who were resistant to toilet training well after a reasonably expected age of mastery.

The concept of rapid toilet training did have its benefits, though some issues permeated over the years. First, the title of Azrin and Foxx's book, *Toilet Training in Less Than a Day* (1973), provided parents with the notion that toilet training could be attained in a brief period, at best a day and perhaps at worst several days. This concept could be misleading to some parents. The issue of weak procedural integrity absent in trained clinical staff (e.g., implementing interventions effectively, in a timely manner, etc.) sometimes extended or perhaps stagnated progress. Parent's expectations of toilet training over a day or a weekend were based on an optimal response from the child and outliers even with typically developing children existed. Also, rapid regression of progress occurs in some cases if all aspects of the program were not implemented effectively or if the child demonstrated some resistance.

Trained clinicians were much more effective to ensure procedural integrity, though infrequently accessible. Availability in the home setting over a full weekend and sometimes for even longer durations continues to be scarce. This procedure often dealt with well-intentioned starts and ineffective outcomes due to the expectation of a rapid and effective outcome. Toilet accidents after a few days seemed to be a common reason to discontinue a program that required intense and ongoing training. Also, the use of punishment for accidents, a component used in the rapid toilet training sequence, was viewed as an unnecessary aversive to teach toilet training (Cicero & Pfadt, 2002).

The field of applied behavior analysis (ABA) and the education community at large moved away from the notion that rapid behavioral changes were required. This was based partly on the notion that a less than rapid training period could be deemed as acceptable, as well as a move away from imposing aversive procedures to attain an unnecessarily rapid outcome. In many cases, the scientific community agreed that aversives were usually unnecessary in clinical practice and only used as a last resort when other methods prove as ineffective and a rapid outcome was necessary.

Operant Conditioning Without a Timeline

Operant conditioning is a learning process following an A-B-C contingency. For the purposes of toilet training, our focus will be on the use of positive reinforcement to strengthen toileting skills. Clinicians and program implementers provide the learner with a specific prompt that elicits urination in the toilet. The occurrence of this behavior directly following the prompt leads to an immediate "payoff" or access to a preferred item or activity.

For example, if the instructor prompts the learner "time for potty" when seated on the toilet and the learner produces urine, then delivery of an edible or another high-preference item immediately follows urination and increases the likelihood of urination in the future under the same A-B-C contingency. The difference with this model versus that provided by Azrin and Foxx (1971) is that a brief timeline to toilet train (e.g., a day, a week) is not necessary to consider the program effective. Indeed, learners gain strength in the skill at an individual rate of learning.

In the early 1980s and forward, clinicians doing research in toilet training began to follow a more tempered approach to interventions on track with ongoing evidence of blending successful interventions identified over several decades of investigation. Recent and current research shifted the concept from "rapid toilet training" to less focus on the rapidity of training and instead on the durability of a life skill readily implemented in nonclinical settings (Cicero & Pfadt, 2002; Kroeger & Sorensen-Burnworth, 2009; LeBlanc, Carr, Crossett, Bennett, & Detweiler, 2005; Stadtler et al., 1999, Cocchiola et al., 2012). Brazelton (1962) proposed that the concept of toilet training for people with developmental disabilities should be altered from a timeline of less than a day to a timeline of less than 100 days. This simple yet important change in the timeline lays the foundation for a paradigm shift. Major changes to teach toilet training included increased patience, simple correction procedures, and acceptance of slow yet measurable progress, with less direct clinical support. Also, with the onset of preschool intervention for developmentally delayed children through IDEA-2004, a migration from home-based programming to school-based programming occurred.

The amount of research regarding toilet training at large and more specifically with children with a developmental disability has been expansive over the past 45 years. The question at the onset of identifying toileting as a challenging learning hurdle is often "what intervention is best to use to toilet train my child?" Klassen et al. (2006) provide a well-written meta-analysis of rapid toilet training outcomes, compared to "Child Ready" practices. Interestingly, Klassen et al. (2006) concluded the following when considering a toilet training program for children.

- The outcomes appear similar for each intervention method across healthy, typically developing children. Clinicians and caregivers can prescribe to any one of the intervention models, generally with a positive outcome to attain adaptive toileting skills.
- Negative social or emotional outcomes appear to be non-salient regardless of intervention method. To clarify, past theories that claimed that rapid toilet training had a negative emotional impact on typically developing children present with no supporting evidence given recent research.
- Nearly all children with developmental disabilities can attain adaptive toileting as a skill repertoire, to a point where at least partial success can be attained. Partial success may mean that prompt reliance is required or that isolated episodes of accidents occur based on the child's developmental profile.
- The range of functionality among children with developmental disabilities varies widely, often in conjunction with physical and behavioral deficits. With this in mind, a toilet training program may need to be more flexible to meet success.
- Toilet training children with developmental disabilities is enhanced considerably when incorporating a multidisciplinary team (e.g., OT, PT, BCBA services working collaboratively), with empirical data-driven decisions in place.
- If a child with a developmental disability has not been toilet trained beyond the far-reaching average of typically developing peers (e.g., 3 years old), toilet training should start soon thereafter, with timelines expanded based on the availability of resources and the child's developmental level.

Research and intervention over the past several decades present promising methods which vary as defined earlier in the chapter; the use of a "package intervention" that utilizes some procedures from the "rapid toilet training" model, others from the "developmental readiness" model, and still others from the "operant conditioning without a timeline" model may be practical and effective. The individual needs of the student appear more salient than selection of a particular program.

IDEA (2004) and Its Impact

Over the past decade, there has been a paradigm shift in special education, moving to a much more global perspective on learning. Reading, writing, math, and other academic skills remain salient, though other life skills pushed aside in the past have taken on increased relevance. A focus is on a more expansive educational progress, with adaptive social behaviors, activities of daily living, self-preservation skills, vocational skills, and communication skills as "front and center" to learning in conjunction with academic and cognitive goals. A germane objective provided by IDEA 2004 is that each child receives adequate skills and training that address multiple functions in life so that they can learn at their optimal level when they are prepared to leave school and enter adulthood (IDEA 2004). School districts are required to teach skills that are beyond the scope of straightforward academic goals; a focus on and accountability for functional life skills is a requirement as well. Education of children who require specialized services needs to address broad issues of learning including adaptive skills that support inclusion (Bryson, Rogers, & Fambonne, 2003). IDEA 2004 provides a clear and succinct definition of "disability" as it relates to education as follows:

"IDEA 'child with a disability' means a child evaluated in accordance with rule 3301-51-06 of the Administrative Code as having a cognitive disability, a hearing impairment, a speech or language impairment, a visual impairment, a serious emotional disturbance, an orthopedic impairment, autism, traumatic brain injury, another health impairment, a specific learning disability, deaf-blindness, or multiple disabilities and who, by reason thereof, needs special education and related services. [The] child must be between the ages of 3–21" (IDEA 2004).

IDEA 2004 definition of a disability is quite clear and provides clear expectations of the task required of all local education agencies (LEAs) under federal law. An LEA is typically a local school district that operates public primary and secondary education, following the mandates of free and appropriate public education (FAPE), guaranteeing education to children with disabilities.

Current federal laws in place mandate LEAs to teach skills that are beyond the scope of straightforward academic goals; a focus on and accountability for functional life skills is required as well. Education of children who require specialized services needs to address broad issues of learning including adaptive skills that support inclusion (Bryson, Rogers, & Fambonne, 2003).

This seemingly subtle change in wording provides a vast change in the responsibility of school districts. It shifts learning from focused academics (e.g., reading, writing, math) to a broad spectrum of learning, to include basic academics but to integrate other basic learning such as fine motor activities, gross motor, adaptive communication, social regulation, and activities of daily living (ADLs) such as toileting (see IDEA 2004, Sec. 602(34)(A)). The point of this clause is to a focus on adaptive living skills and vocational training, with the school's responsibility to develop the prerequisite skills needed to provide optimal opportunity outcomes.

Teaching nonacademic skills to students in school may have been viewed as outside of educators' field of practice a decade ago, though IDEA (2004) clearly defines expectations of a child's school. The positive impact on children with disabilities can be quite convincing. Schools are created to be learning centers with an expansive series of domains, to include learning readiness, academics, social adaptability, time management, self-advocacy, behavioral regulation, and ADLs. Educators and related service providers have specialized training across the spectrum of learning, with curriculum and research that support learning across people. The purpose for education at large is to provide expansive learning across multiple domains so that individuals are ready for independent work and living. The concept of teaching even basic functional skills to students with identified deficits helps to attain this end goal at the end of the educational process: increased adaptive independence.

With the parameters established in IDEA 2004, school districts are not only required to provide instruction with ADLs but also need to use the least restrictive methods to provide learning. That is readily interpreted as researched-based interventions with proven efficacy in learning a skill, absent unneeded aversive procedures.

Current Innovations and Future Practices

The enactment of IDEA 2004 and research over the past 45–50 years supports the notion for direct instruction following empirically validated methods to toilet train children who demonstrate difficulty in learning this skill. An increased urgency of intervention is warranted following a student's third birthday, especially when he or she is diagnosed with a development disability. Effective methods for consideration in this population include rapid toilet training and operant learning without a timeline; the Child Ready process following developmental readiness for toileting may be considered, though after 3 years old, should be removed as an option due to risks of negatively impacting behavioral cusps and setting the stage for negative behavioral patterns.

Over the past decade, "sites of primary intervention" have shifted from the home setting to the school setting. Schools may be the best place to provide treatment for toilet training, and indeed most skill deficits are identified in a child's repertoire when they start preschool. The availability of specialized instruction and "best practice settings" is intact based on IDEA Part B, providing specialized services based on presenting deficits to children at the age of 3 years old and can continue up through a child's 21st year (see IDEA 2004). The foundation of IDEA Part B is to provide early identification to children age 3 through 22 who present with deficits under any of several domains. Examples can include cognitive, academic, social/behavioral, communication, fine motor or gross motor movement, activities of daily living, or any other life skill that is notably below that of age-related peers. Once a team of experts identifies weaknesses, the child receives specific, targeted interventions to address learning in these areas from specialized service providers in their field. Experts may include a speech and language pathologist (SLP) for communication deficits, a special education teacher for academic/cognitive deficits, an occupational therapist (OT) for fine motor issues, or a board certified behavior analyst (BCBA) for behavioral issues. All experts work in unison as interdisciplinary team, to address each issue as a learning module. Toilet training often falls into this collection of identified learning issues.

The amount of specialized service available in schools for early intervention and for continued support through IDEA 2004 Parts 2 and 3 supports the notion that effective intervention can most effectively be taught in schools and then generalized across settings once skill development becomes adequately intact. Specialized services that were sparse in home and community settings are now readily available, with up to 6 or more hours per day, with increased opportunity to address each unique learning need presented by a child, including toilet training.

Indeed, instruction in schools under IDEA 2004 requires that (a) defined objectives, (b) with measurable outcomes, be implemented, (c) in the absence of aversive procedures and (d) in the least restrictive environment. Interventions for school systems exist (see Yoo 2012; Cocchiola et al., 2012; Dalrymple, & Ruble, 1992; Stadtler et al., 1999) providing the most recent procedural guidelines in general that follow along the standards of IDEA 2004, as well as procedural safeguards to include the following:

- Rule out medical as a first step.
- Gain parent consent to initiate a toilet training program.
- Set realistic goals to determine progress over time.
- Use non-aversive procedures to teach toileting as a requisite skill.
- Implement trainer requirements for program integrity.
- Provide ongoing data collection and analysis.
- Move from isolated learning to generalization across people, times, and places.

If adaptive toileting skills are absent when a child starts school and the child is determined to qualify for special education, it is the responsibility of the LEA to address this as a skill for formal instruction. An LEA typically means a student's local school district or a public agency responsible for implementation of education in preschool through high school (pre-K through 12). Goals and objectives are put in place through a formal Individual Education Plan (IEP), to include all domains identified as deficits and activities of daily living such as toileting. The expectation is each learning objective is addressed through formal and valid intervention (e.g., curriculum, research studies, etc.), with data-driven decision making.

Conclusions

Volumes of research support the notion that toilet training is generally an attainable skill for nearly 97–98% of the population by 3 years old. This portion of the population represents children who are typically developing when compared to age-related peers. Intervention options to gain independence are expansive, though generally developmental readiness in the areas of physical, cognitive, and social skills is a key factor to meet success. The initiation of toilet training at an earlier age typically leads to an increase in duration with training, and girls usually become independent with toileting skills at a marginally earlier age.

On the other side of the spectrum lies 3% of the population who may require more time intensive programming to achieve toileting independence, perhaps with precision teaching embedded into process to enhance learning. Support across a multidisciplinary team often yields better results, with a rule-out of medical intervention as a starting point and a formal program to follow based on the child's constellation of skill deficits. When supplemental support is provided effectively, toilet training for the 3% who start as outliers typically is accomplished, though often requires expanded time and dedication to meet the goal.

Some parents may address toilet training their child who has a developmental disability with reasonable success. If skill acquisition does not occur and the child is ready to begin school, the LEA is responsible to implement a toilet training program, though this responsibility is based on the determination of the Planning and Placement Team (PPT) when creating the child's IEP. IDEA (2004) requires that the least restrictive, scientifically based methods of instruction are used across all goals and objectives; therefore the use of aversives is not tolerable. Reasonable, and less aversive options must be attempted with subtherapeutic success first. Schools moving forward into the next generation of learners will continue to hold the responsibility and privilege to move a child for vocational and lifelong success, perhaps starting with behavioral cusps as simple and important as toilet training.

More research is warranted to support the notion of toilet training in the school setting with an enhanced interdisciplinary team intact and trained staff as program implementer versus home-based programming. Specific programs should be used to measure best practice outcomes.

Appendices

Toileting Tracking Sheet

Student's Initials: __________

Codes:
I= incomplete (no urine produced during the interval)
C= correct voiding in toilet
A= accident in pants

Month & Year:______-______

SD: "Time for bathroom"

Date→	1	2	3	4	5	6	7	8	9	10	11	12	13	14	15	16	17	18	19	20	21	22	23	24	25	26	27	28	29	30	31
Time ↓																															
9:00 a																															
9:30 a																															
10:00 a																															
10:30 a																															
11:00 a																															
11:30 a																															
12:00 p																															
12:30 p																															
1:00 p																															
1:30 p																															
2:00 p																															
2:30 p																															
3:00 p																															
Daily % Correct *(C/A+C)*																															

Bathroom Teaching Strategy

Name: **John Doe**	Program: **Bathroom Training Teaching Strategy**
Date Initiated: 01-08-09	Most recent revision:

Objective: Given staff support, John will sit on the toilet and urinate appropriately with 100% accuracy for five consecutive days by 08-31-09. Run this program every day John is at school.	
Materials needed: Task analytic worksheet An established bathroom A monthly data collection sheet Timer set at 3 min 1:1 instruction Edible reinforcers available for correct use of bathroom *(currently M&Ms)* Change of clothes in case of an accident	
Set-up Directions ➔	1. Each day upon arrival at school, John will enter the bathroom to ensure his "pull-up" is off. 2. Every day, John will be cued to the bathroom on the half hr (e.g., 9:00, 9:30, 10:00, etc). 3. Once in the bathroom and seated on the toilet, he will remain seated for 3 min.

SD: "Time for Bathroom"

Task analysis
1. Go to bathroom
2. Lights on
3. Close door
4. Pants down
5. Sit on toilet *(staff to set timer for 3 min)*
6. Stay on toilet *(if cue needed)*
(Upon sound of timer or upon urination) 7. All done
8. Pants up
9. Wash hands
10. Lights off

Staff Instructions

1. If John urinates on the toilet, deliver heavy verbal praise immediately (e.g., within 0.5 s) coupled with *"M&Ms"* as the edible reinforcer.
2. Use the edible reinforcers only for appropriate use of the bathroom

If a wetting accident occurs, simply assist John into the bathroom and help him to put dry clothes on. Interaction during this procedure should remain neutral and matter of fact.

References

AAIDD. (2013). http://aaidd.org/intellectual-disability/definition#.V7STQ455w7A. Retrieved August 7, 2016.

Azrin, N. H., & Foxx, R. M. (1971). A rapid method of toilet training the institutionalized retarded. *Journal of Applied Behavior Analysis*, *4*(2), 89–99.

Bailey, D. B., Hatton, D. D., Mesibov, G., Ament, N., & Skinner, M. (2000). Early development, temperament, and functional impairment in autism and fragile X syndrome. *Journal of Autism and Developmental Disorders*, *30*(1), 49–57.

Baker, B. L., & Brightman, A. J. (1997). *Steps to independence; teaching everyday skills to children with special needs*. Baltimore: Paul H. Brookes.

Brazelton, T. B. (1962). A child oriented approach to toilet training. *Pediatrics*, *29*, 121–128.

Brown, F. J., & Peace, N. (2011). Teaching a child with challenging behaviors to use the toilet: A clinical case study. *British Journal of Learning Disabilities*, *39*(4), 321–326.

Boyle, C. A., Boulet, S., Schieve, L.A., Cohen, R. A., Blumberg, S. J., Yeargin-Allsopp, M., Usser, S., Visser, S., & Kogan, M. D. (2011, June). Trends in the prevalence of developmental disabilities in US children, 1997–2008. *Pediatrics, 127*(6), 1034–1042.

Bryson, S. E., Rogers, S. J., & Fombonne, E. (2003). Autism spectrum disorders: Early detection, intervention, education, and psychopharmacological management. *Canadian Journal of Psychiatry*, *48*, 506–515.

Carpenter, M., Nagell, K., & Tomasello, M. (1998). Social cognition, joint attention, and communicative competence from 9 to 15 months of age. *Monographs of the Society for Research in Child Development*, *4*, 1–174.

Center for Disease Control and Prevention. (2013). Developmental disabilities. Retrieved September 16, 2016.

Chudley, A. E., Conry, J., Cook, J., Loock, J., Rosales, T., & LeBlank, N. (2005). Fetal alcohol spectrum disorder: Canadian guidelines for diagnosis. *CMAJ*, *172*(5 Suppl), S1–S21.

Cocchiola, M. A., Martino, G. M., Dwyer, L. J., & Demezzo, K. (2012). Toilet training childre n with autism and developmental delays: An effective program for school settings. *Behavior Analysis in Practice*, *5*(2), 60–64.

Christophersen, E. R. (1991). Toileting problems in children. *Pediatric Annals*, *20*(5), 240–244.

Cicero, F. R., & Pfadt, A. (2002). Investigation of a reinforcement-based toilet training procedure for children with autism. *Research in Developmental Disabilities*, *23*(5), 319–331.

Cooper, J. O., Heron, T. E., & Heward, W. L. (2007). *Applied behavior analysis* (2nd ed.). Upper Saddle River, N.J: Pearson Prentice Hall.

Dalrymple, N. J., & Ruble, L. A. (1992). Toilet training and behaviors of people with autism; parent views. *Journal of Autism and Developmental Disorders*, *2*(22), 265–275.

Foxx, R. M., & Azrin, H. H. (1973). *Toilet Training the Retarded*. In *Behavior Therapy* (vol. Volume 5, Issue 2, March 1974, pp. 280–282). Champaign, IL: Research Press.

Greenspan, S. I., Wieder, S., & Simons, R. (1998). *The child with special needs: Encouraging intellectual and emotional growth*. Reading, MA, US: Addison-Wesley/Addison Wesley Longman.

Handel, L. B. (2003). Males with down's syndrome and neurogenic bladder. *The Journal of Urology*, *169*, 646–649.

Joinson, C., Heron, J., vonContard, A., Butler, U., Golding, A., & Emond, J. (2013). Early childhood risk factors associated with daytime wetting and soiling in school-age children. *Journal of Pediatric Psychology*, *33*(7), 739–750.

Klassen, T. P., Kiddoo, D., Lang, M. E., Friesen, C., Russell, K., Spooner, C., & Vandermeer, B. (2006). The effectiveness of different methods of toilet training for bowel and bladder. *US Department of Health and Human Services, Evidence Report/ Technology Assessment, 147;* December 2006.

Konarski, E. A., & Diorio, M. S. (1985). A quantitative review of self-help research with the severely and profoundly retarded. *Applied Research in Mental Retardation*, *6*, 229–245.

Kroeger, K. A., & Sorensen-Burnworth, R. (2009). Toilet training individuals with autism and other developmental disabilities: A critical review. *Research in Autism Spectrum Disorders, 6*(3), 607–618.

LeBlanc, L. A., Carr, J. E., Crossett, S. E., Bennett, C. M., & Detweiler, D. D. (2005). Intensive outpatient behavioral treatment of primary urinary incontinence of children with autism. *Focus on Autism and Other Developmental Disabilities, 20*(2), 98–105.

Luxem, M., & Christophersen, E. (1994). Behavioral toilet training in early childhood: Research, practice and implications. *Journal of Developmental and Behavioral Pediatrics, 15*(5), 370–378.

Matson, J. L. (1990). *Handbook of behavioral modification with the mentally retarded*. New York: Plenum Press.

Mazefsky, C. A., Herrington, J., Siegel, M., Scarpa, A., Maddox, B., Scahill, L., & White, S. W. (2013). The role of emotional regulation in autism spectrum disorder RH: Emotional regulation in ASD. *Journal of the American Academy of Child & Adolescent Psychiatry, 52*(7), 679–688.

NIH. https://report.nih.gov/nihfactsheets/ViewFactSheet.aspx?csid=100; updated 05–2013. Accessed September 15, 2016.

Osturk, M., Oktem, F., & Kisioglu, N. D. (2006). Bowel and bladder control in children with cerebral palsy: Case control study. *Croation Medical Journal, 47*(2), 264–270.

Phillips, D. (2012). Early childhood development and disability: A discussion paper. World Health Organization. https://www.Google.Com/search?Q=diagnoses+that+compromise+developmental +disabilities&ie=utf-8&oe=utf-8, access September 12, 2016).

Pivato, E. (2009). Breaching the last frontier: Dignity and the toileting issue for persons with multiple and severe disabilities. *Developmental Disabilities Bulletin., 37*(1), 153–164.

Rinaldi, K., & Mirenda, P. (2012). Effectiveness of a modified rapid toilet training workshop for parents of children with developmental disabilities. *Research in Developmental Disabilities, 33*(3), 933–943.

Rogers, J. (2010). One step at a time: How to toilet train children with developmental disabilities. *Nursing Times, 106*(47), 19–20.

Rosales-Ruiz, J., & Baer, D. (1997). Behavioral cusps: A developmental and programatic concept for behavior analysis. *Journal of Applied Behavior Analysis, 30*, 533–544.

Sells-Love, D., Rinaldi, L. M., & McLaughlin, T. F. (2002). Toilet training an adolescent in the classroom: A case study. *Journal of Developmental and Learning Disabilities, June 2002, 14*(2), 111–118.

Silva, L. M. T., & Schalock, M. (2012). Autism parent stress index; initial psychometric evidence. *Journal of Autism and Developmental Disorders, 42*(4), 566–574.

Singh, B., Masey, H., & Morton, R. (2006). Levels of continence in children with cerebral palsy. *Pediatric Nursing, 18*(4), 23–26.

Smith, G., McDougall, D., & Edelen-Smith, P. (2006). Behavioral cusps: A person-centered concept for establishing pivotal individual, family, and community behaviors and repertoires. *Focus on Autism and Other Developmental Disorders., 21*(4), 223–229.

Smith, J. S., & Chaneb, B. (2016). *Toilet Training. A Handbook of Evidence-Based Practices in Intellectual and Developmental Disabilities* (pp. 943–955). Boston: Springer International Publishing.

Spock, B. (1946). *The common sense book of baby and child care:* New York: Duell., Sloan and Pearce.

Stadtler, A. C., Gorski, P. A., & Brazelton, T. B. (1999). Toilet training methods, clinical interventions and recommendations. *American Academy of Pediatrics, June, 103*, 1359–1368.

U.S. Department of Education. (2004). Building the legacy: IDEA 2004. Retrieved August 7, 2016, from http://idea.ed.gov/archive

Van Wagenen, R. K., Meyerson, L., Kerr, N. J., & Mahoney, K. (1969). Field trials of a new procedure for toilet training. *Journal of Experimental Child Psychology, 1*(8), 147–159.

Vermandel, A., VanKampen, M., Van Gorp, C., & Wyndaele, J. J. (2008). How to toilet train healthy children? A review of literature. *Neurological Urodynamics, 27*, 162–166.

Yoo, H. (2010, December 16th). https://www.opwdd.ny.gov/sites/default/files/documents/Toilet_Training_Trainer Manual.pdf. Retrieved August 10th, 2016.
Yoo, H. (2012). https://www.opwdd.ny.gov/opwdd_community_connections/autism_platform/behavior management/targeting_the_big_3. Retrieved August 7th, 2016.
WHO. (2011). http://www.who.int/disabilities/world_report/2011/report.pdf. Retrieved October 3, 2016.

Overview and State of the Field

Johnny L. Matson

Toilet training is a universal issue for children and one of the most important first steps toward independence. As a result, it constitutes a major achievement for 2–3-year-old children with respect to daytime continence. Nighttime continence typically occurs months or years later since it is a more difficult skill set to master. Boys have more difficulty in achieving this milestone. Additionally, persons with special needs such as intellectual disabilities and autism spectrum disorders are particularly susceptible to difficulties in training. Treatment typically occurs later, is more intense, and takes longer. Also, these difficulties involve delays in training and the need to modify training experiences. Adaptations typically include smaller treatment steps with more therapist and educator input.

Modern toilet training methods date back to the 1930s. As such, this was one of the first childhood problems with successful psychological remedy. The most effective procedures developed since this time has been based on operant and classical conditioning. (The former are now often referred to as applied behavior analysis.) The foundation established early on was followed with studies in the 1970s and 1980s, enhancing the efficiency of the best methods. Also, the number of special population effectively treated increased as well.

Despite all the positive developments noted above, various issues have not been addressed sufficiently. For example, how well prepared professionals can be when confronted with these difficulties? Also, compliance with treatment regimens is often an issue. Difficulties in this area can lead to temper tantrums, aggression, anxiety, and/or low self-esteem. When persistent, these issues need to be addressed by educators and health professionals. This means layers of additional interventions specific to these problems but is also interrelated to the toileting process.

Issues involving challenging behaviors such as tantrums and aggression are more pronounced in special populations such as persons with autism spectrum disorder

J.L. Matson, PhD (✉)
Department of Psychology, Louisiana State University, Baton Rouge, LA 70803, USA
e-mail: johnmatson@aol.com

J.L. Matson (ed.), *Clinical Guide to Toilet Training Children*, Autism and Child Psychopathology Series, DOI 10.1007/978-3-319-62725-0_14

(ASD) (Fodstad, Rojahn & Matson, 2012). The new ASD criteria in DSM-5 may mean even more severe symptoms for the overall group receiving the diagnosis. Additionally, more severe comorbidities such as noncompliance and challenging behaviors may result in even more pronounced side effects for toileting persons with ASD relative to the general population of children (Matson, Kozlowski, Hattier, Horovitz & Sipes, 2012). The move to identify children with special needs at very young ages is also now common practice and has implications for toilet training moving forward (Matson, Boisjoli, Hess & Wilkins, 2010). Methods focused on toilet training should be incorporated in these early intervention programs.

Problems for daytime would be more specific to sitting on a stool by young children. The attempts at daytime toileting would be hard for younger children compared to kids who are being trained at bedtime. Temper tantrums and aggression, while not exclusive to daytime toileting, would be more likely during daytime applications. Nighttime toileting would involve older children where anxiety and low self-esteem would be more problematic than when daytime toileting is ongoing.

Physiological issues can also be present. For children where voiding in the toilet is problematic, urinary infections and constipation may be present. These issues need to be addressed by the child's pediatrician and medical procedures and/or drugs may be required. However, it would be best to coordinate these efforts with psychological treatments specific to the toileting process. At present, this approach is used to some extent, but more and better coordination is still needed.

Compliance is a problem in some instances with children, but it is a much greater problem for parents. Often, in clinical practice, parents report having used a given evidence-based treatment with little or no effect. However, upon discussion of the implementation of the methods it quickly becomes apparent that haphazard and/or sporadic attempts were made. Also, parents often assume change will occur more rapidly than is realistic. These problems are often compounded by professionals who promise results that are unattainable and cause parents to lose faith in proven intervention methods. Additionally, misinformation on toilet training is rampant in the news and on the Internet; these are major sources of parent information.

The good news regarding toilet training is that effective intervention is commonplace at this point in time. A combination of applied behavior analysis and classical conditioning has proven empirical support. These methods date back decades. Having said that, the available technology could benefit from further improvement and updating. The general attention to the topic has trailed off substantially in recent years. This trend is unfortunate for a number of reasons. These topics have been elaborated earlier on in this volume.

The interactions of psychological interventions with life style choices are also worthy of additional study. Parents have for many years used restricted liquid intake close to bedtime as a relevant and often effective intervention. However, this method is often applied haphazardly. It would be useful to develop a technology based on age, gender, physical, and developmental handicaps. Flow charts detailing the amount of liquid intake during the day, the appropriate liquid intake and when to begin restricting intake at night could prove very helpful to parents and professionals, particularly pediatricians. These medical professionals are most frequently the first stop for parents in need of toileting assistance. Also, based on the factors noted above, intake may vary from child to child. Guidelines to assist parents, given their child's specific needs, would be very informative. Also, day- and nighttime toileting are not binary processes. More needs to be known about how restricted intake interacts with other treatments such as applied behavior analysis and classical conditioning. This set of issues is further compounded by how maturation affects this set of combined technologies. Thus, while maturation has been emphasized in the toileting process for many decades, little exists on the specifics of how maturation affects multifactorial liquid intake variables (Brazelton, 1962).

Constipation is the toileting problem most commonly associated with diet. Issues such as a high fiber diet are often recommended along with or before medical interventions such as diuretics are used. Most of the focus is on medical approaches such as the methods just mentioned. This focus is warranted. However, a much greater emphasis on psychological methods is needed as well. The focus should be on both research and clinical application. Voiding of fecal material can be classically conditioned, largely by establishing a consistent toileting schedule. The best time to plan for toileting is 20–40 min post breakfast, lunch, and/or dinner. Voiding should then be followed by praise and tangible reinforcers. Psychological approaches produce a more normalized set of toileting skills. Similarly, the focus shifts to prevention. Regular, regulated toileting results in the decrease or elimination of constipation.

A concern in toileting is the use of medications with children. For constipation, the use of suppositories may be unavoidable. As just noted, greater use of preventative methods, especially psychological procedures, can help in this matter, however. The much larger issue is the continued, widespread use of medications for nighttime bed-wetting. Given the more effective psychological methods which have been available for decades, the former practice is difficult to justify. At this point, the greatest focus moving forward should be on the education of front-line medical staff such as pediatricians and nurses. These professionals could treat, but at a minimum; hence, they should know what procedures work best for bed-wetting and where they can refer the family for treatment.

Parents may not wish to use psychological treatments, or for logistical reasons they cannot carry out these methods. In these instances, the health professional should be able to explain that medication often only works while the drug is being administered. The family should also be given information on the short- and long-term side effects of these drugs for the young child. This information can rebalance what methods the parents will choose.

Little new development has surfaced in the area of treatment for toileting in many years. The major reason for this may be that a number of highly effective treatments already exist as previously noted. An area where considerable strides could be made involves incorporating the vast developments in technology. It is hoped, moving forward, that developments in this area would be considered. Some improvement in effectiveness is likely. However, the greatest gains would most likely be in its ease of application. For example, decreasing labor for intensive treatments and developing more rapid application of contingencies after voiding success and failure are needed. Finally, a much more accurate and comprehensive data collection is needed. In another domain, learning how best to disseminate information to first contact professionals is an area in urgent need of study.

Pediatricians, pediatric nurses, and child clinical psychologists should be among those who have content built into their curriculums how to advise caregivers in the toilet training process. As noted throughout the book, there are several issues with different methodologies that must be considered. These topics include initial toilet training, daytime wetting accidents, fecal accidents, incontinence, and nocturnal enuresis. Each of these issues, while being part of the broader concept of toilet training, are separate issues with separate solutions. Practitioners should also have this training imbedded in internships and resident program. Research is needed on the best ways to conduct this training. Also, board certification and licensure exams should, but rarely do, address this topic.

This book provides a reference work for professionals who frequently are required to deal with childhood toileting problems. As such, the *Clinicians Guide to Toilet Training Children* is by far the most comprehensive review of the toilet training literature to date. This volume is a major contribution on toilet training books produced. Previous books have been almost exclusively aimed at parents via a "how to do it" approach. Several common characteristics in these books are notable. First, they focus almost exclusively on daytime toilet training. Second, the general assumption is that the methods are geared to typically developing children between 2 and 3 years of age. Third, the level of specificity and concrete examples varies markedly from one book to the next. Fourth, the degree to which these books are evidence based varies considerably. To our knowledge, little has been done on evaluating these "how to do it" books in terms of their value in assisting parents with the toilet training process. It seems reasonable to conclude that many, if not all, of these books have value. It would also seem reasonable to assume that their value would vary and that chronicity and severity of the toileting issues, comorbid challenging behaviors, parent motivation and knowledge, and related factors would also be associated with the effectiveness of bibliotherapy for toileting issues. Certainly, "how to do it" books on this topic far outnumber parenting books on most other developmental skills. How therapists use and assist parents using these books also needs further study.

From this writer's perspective, effective toilet training is one of the more successful areas of treatment with respect to essential childhood developmental milestones. This factor is based on the important research developments that have occurred over the years. Also, some topics tend to be fashionable at given points in history. Toilet training is as essential as it has ever been. However, the topic does not receive adequate research attention presently. Areas where additional research is needed have been briefly addressed. Clearly, many new advances are possible. At this point, it is largely a matter of will and focus on the problem that is needed.

Updates in the area of research are needed due to changing services models and an increasing focus on early preschool education. Also, values about culture and childhood education change over time. These topics also are in urgent need of attention in the research literature. In terms of persons involved in the toilet training process, moving forward early childhood educators will inevitably need to become experts in this service delivery area. Thus, while great strides have been made in toilet training children, time marches on and adjustments in strategies are needed. This book then has been an effort to provide a comprehensive accounting of where we have been, where we currently are, and where we need to go.

References

Brazelton, T. B. (1962). A child-oriented approach to toilet training. *Pediatrics, 29*, 121–128.

Fodstad, J. L., Rojahn, J., & Matson, J. L. (2012). The emergence of challenging behaviors in at-risk toddlers with and without autism spectrum disorder: A cross-sectional study. *Journal of Developmental and Physical Disabilities, 24*, 217–234.

Matson, J. L., Boisjoli, J. A., Hess, J. A., & Wilkins, J. (2010). Factor structure and diagnostic fidelity of the baby and infant screen for children with aUtIsm traits: Part 1 (BISQUIT part 1). *Developmental Neurorehabilitation, 13*, 72–79.

Matson, J. L., Kozlowski, A. M., Hattier, M. A., Horovitz, M., & Sipes, M. (2012). DSM-IV vs DSM-5 diagnostic criteria for toddlers with autism. *Developmental Neurorehabilitation, 15*, 185–190.

Index

J.L. Matson (ed.), *Clinical Guide to Toilet Training Children*, Autism and Child Psychopathology Series, DOI 10.1007/978-3-319-62725-0

9783319627243